HUMAN REPRODUCTIVE SYSTEM – ANATOMY, ROLES AND DISORDERS

UTERINE FIBROIDS

EPIDEMIOLOGY, SYMPTOMS AND MANAGEMENT

Human Reproductive System – Anatomy, Roles and Disorders,

Additional books and e-books in this series can be found on Nova's website under the Series tab.

Women's Issues

Additional books and e-books in this series can be found on Nova's website under the Series tab.

HUMAN REPRODUCTIVE SYSTEM – ANATOMY, ROLES AND DISORDERS

UTERINE FIBROIDS

EPIDEMIOLOGY, SYMPTOMS AND MANAGEMENT

SIMONE FERRERO
AND
FABIO BARRA
EDITORS

nova
Medicine & Health

Library of Congress Cataloging-in-Publication Data

ISBN: 978-1-53615-046-9

Published by Nova Science Publishers, Inc. † New York

CONTENTS

PREFACE

Myomas (or fibroids) are the most frequent benign tumors of the female pelvis: generally, 30-40% of their diagnosis are in women older than 40 years, reaching a peak among 45-49 years of age. Because of the high estimated prevalence and costs associated with treatments, the direct and indirect costs of these benign tumors are substantial for both the health care system and the individual patient.

The epidemiology of myomas is currently an interesting investigational topic: several factors have consistently been found to be inversely associated with myomas (such as parity, age at menarche and at first childbirth). On the other hand, until now only conflicting data have emerged for the use of oral contraceptives, smoking history, and metabolic diseases.

In more than 50% of cases, these common tumors are asymptomatic; otherwise, around 30% of women affected may experience multitude of clinical presentations. Importantly, their effect on clinical signs and symptoms and on fertility is largely determined by their location.

Because of the high prevalence in pre-menopausal age, myomas represent a common occurrence in women seeking pregnancy. As submucous myomas has been associated with 5-10% of infertility cases, their most appropriate detection and subsequent management is critical.

Histologically, myomas are benign tumors consisting of smooth-muscle cells and a high amount of extracellular matrix. At macroscopic examination, they appears well-demarcated, solid, whitish, with elastic consistency, often multiple. However, they may show a variety of unusual morphology that the pathologist should accurately consider. Interestingly, the growing knowledge on myomas molecular features may radically change in the near future their management by performing more individualized therapies.

Nowadays, ultrasonography is the first-line imaging modality for detection and evaluation of uterine myomas, as it is easy, accessible, harmless and inexpensive. Overall, it likely allows the differentiation of these benign uterine tumors from other common gynecological conditions such as adenomyosis or endometrial polyps.

Currently, on the basis of their extension in the uterine wall thickness, it is commonly accepted to subdivide myomas into three known main type (subserous, intramural and submucous); this classification tends to have also a not negligible correlation with clinical presentation. Anyway, in the last years, new classifications have been developed in order to better characterize the specific localization and characteristics of these tumors and to better predict technical difficulty and complexity when performing their operative management.

Overall, multidisciplinary approaches are available for treating uterine myomas; the choice of the best modality for the treatment depends on several factors such as age, childbearing aspirations, extent and severity of symptoms, size, number and location of myomas, proximity to menopause.

Medical therapy for myomas tends to be employed for controlling patients' menorrhagia that can be importantly responsible for iron-deficiency anemia. The use of pre-surgical medical treatment has demonstrated not only to reduce the intraoperative blood loss, but also to decrease the volume of uterine fibroids, potentially facilitating minimally invasive surgery. For this purpose, in last two decades gonadotropin-releasing hormone agonist (GnRH-a) have been widely adopted in the clinical practice. Additionally, recent randomized controlled trials succeeded in showing advantages also for the administration of selective progesterone receptor modulator (SPRMs), which thus represent a new clinical opportunity.

In the past years, several minimally invasive treatment options have been introduced and studied; they may not only preserve the uterus and – possibly – fertility, but also decrease morbidity and recovery time in comparison with traditional hysterectomy. Among surgical options, myomectomy represent a valid option, in particular when subsequent childbearing is a consideration. With refinement in endoscopic techniques, the laparoscopic route has gained popularity being characterized by better esthetic outcome, less postoperative pain, and shorter hospital stay in comparison with traditional open surgical methods.

At the same time, radiologic therapies, such as uterine artery embolization and magnetic resonance-guided focused ultrasound have been recently explored, and currently represent emerging non-invasive options for treating these patients.

Thanks to the advances of endoscopy and the introduction of new performant operative resectoscopes, hysteroscopic myomectomy continues to be the standard minimally invasive surgery for the removal of sub mucous myomas. This procedure is supposed to be a safe and effective method to treat associated menstrual disorders and infertility, with success rates reported from 70% to 90%. Interestingly, in the last twenty years, the Versapoint Bipolar Electrosurgical System has been successfully introduced for the hysteroscopic therapy of small submucosal myomas (in general, with largest diameter < 2 cm): in fact, it offers several advantages over conventional hysteroscopic surgery allowing to avoid the risks of anesthesia and the inconvenience of the operating room.

Finally, in the early 2000s, the Food and Drug Administration (FDA) licensed robotic-assisted laparoscopic surgery for the therapy of gynecological diseases. As the consequence, surgeons have started to employ robotic technology also for performing myomectomy. Anyway, to date, there is a lack of knowledge about surgical or fertility outcomes after robotic-assisted myomectomy due to lack of large randomized controlled studies. In the meantime, different types of robotic surgery has been brilliantly improved, such as the robotic single-site surgery and the newly introduced reduced-port robotic surgery. All these innovative procedures surely require further validation about safety, feasibility and effectiveness before being routinely adopted in the clinical practice.

The aim of this book is to introduce latest evidences about epidemiology, pathogenesis, diagnosis and therapy of uterine myomas. We take this opportunity to thank all the authors who, selflessly, worked hard and contributed their knowledge to this book. Our special thanks to the publisher, Nova Publisher for entrusting use with this project.

Fabio Barra, MD
Giulio Evangelisti, MD
Simone Ferrero, MD, PhD

Academic Unit of Obstetrics and Gynecology
University of Genoa
Genoa, Italy

In: Uterine Fibroids
Editors: Simone Ferrero and Fabio Barra
ISBN: 978-1-53615-046-9

Chapter 1

EPIDEMIOLOGY AND RISK FACTORS OF UTERINE MYOMAS

Gloria D'Alessandro[1,2], MD, Fabio Barra[1,2], MD and Simone Ferrero[1,2,*], MD, PhD

[1]Obstetrics and Gynecology, Department of Neurosciences, Rehabilitation, Ophthalmology, Genetics, Maternal and Child Health (DiNOGMI), University of Genoa, Italy

[2]Academic Unit of Obstetrics and Gynecology, IRCCS Ospedale San Martino, Genoa, Italy

ABSTRACT

Leiomyomas are histologically benign tumors and their diagnosis is common during fertile age. They represent the most frequent indication for hysterectomy in the U.S. and Australia, although alternative therapies, such as myomectomy and uterine artery embolization, have been increasing over the years. Their impact on reproductive outcome is relevant, considering that they may affect fertility and even lead to obstetric adverse events during pregnancy. Several theories to explain the spread of the tumors concern genetic factors, specific biochemical pathways and different risk factors. Disorders of endocrine factors, abnormal wound healing and genetic mutations in cell growth regulation may constitute the early causative events in the genesis of myomas. Sex hormones may probably play a crucial role in this process, since fibroids tend to occur during reproductive age. In particular, incidence of myomas increases by age; the majority of these benign tumors are diagnosed among women older than 40 years and they tend to decline after menopause. Several studies show different lifetime risk among different races. In particular, myomas are more frequent among blacks compared to whites and this distribution may explain why their prevalence is higher in U.S. compared to Europe. With

* Corresponding Author's E-mail: simoneferrero@me.com.

regard to this topic, several theories have been proposed, such as an eventual racial difference in the metabolism of estrogens, in the expression of receptors for steroid hormones and in the molecular expression of micro-RNAs. Different risk factors about fibroid onset have recognized, including endogenous and exogenous hormone exposition, different lifestyles, infections, uterine injuries, genetic factors, specific demographic characteristics, hypertension and environmental factor.

Keywords: uterine myomas, epidemiology, risk factor, endogenous hormones, hypertension, environment factors

1. Introduction

Uterine myomas have been known since ancient times. The Greek physician Hippocrates was the first to mention them as "uterine stones" whereas, in the 2nd century A.D, Galen as "scleromas". Moreover, the curator from the Egyptology Department in the English Museum in London reported that some mummies had pelvic calcified masses suggestive of myomas, which have been identified thanks to a radiological exam [1].

In a more recent past (1793), the Scottish physician Matthew Baillie, described these masses, which were named "fibroids" by Rokitansky and Klob in XIX century and subsequently "myomas", since the German Pathologist Virchow demonstrated the origin from the uterine smooth muscle [3].

The surgeon Ephraim McDowell performed the first laparotomy for myomas in 1809 in Virginia; interestingly, the patient operated was the cousin of President Abraham Lincoln [2].

Leiomyomas, currently called "fibroids" or "myomas", according to the 4th edition of World Health Organization (WHO) Classification of Tumors, are histologically benign tumors consisting of smooth-muscle cells and a high amount of extracellular matrix (ECM). These lesions differ from normal myometrium as they show a disorder in the myometrial architecture and an abnormal extracellular ECM deposition. They are surrounded by a pseudocapsule of connective tissue, which fixes the nodule to the myometrium. A typical myoma has 50% more amount of collagen, arranged in a nonparallel way, compared to normal myometrium. The type I collagen is the most represented [4], even if some studies found the presence of type III collagen. When cut, the myoma appears pinkish white with a firm consistency. The vessels origin from the capsule, sending radial branches into the mass. For this reason, the central area, less vascularized, may undergo to a degeneration event; thus, calcifications firstly develop in the peripheral portion along the vessels.

Several theories have been proposed to explain the widespread of myomas. They are based on genetic factors, biochemical pathways and different risk factors. With regard to genetic factors, some studies have revealed that the uterine myoma risk may be inherited, indeed the risk raises 2.5 times among first-degree relatives.

Great levels of myofibroblast cells and specific metalloproteinases (MMPs), MMP2 and MMP11 have been found in uterine myomas, contributing to produce collagen and to remodel the ECM, causing a relevant amount of fibrosis [5]. Some investigators suggest this process to be a mistaken attempt to repair an uterine damage; moreover, this theory is corroborated by the finding of similar genetic characteristics in myomas and keloids [6].

Although the majority of myomas are asymptomatic, they may cause relevant symptoms, affecting patient's quality of life. The most common experienced symptoms are abnormal bleeding, anemia, pelvic pain, dyspareunia, fertility problems and urinary disorders, such as an increased urinary frequency or incontinence [7]. Size, location and number of fibroids influence the symptom onset and its severity: for example, the greater the tumor size, the higher is the risk of self-reported heavy bleeding, as proved by an ultrasound-screening study enrolling 1,349 women [8]. When the symptoms are relevant, medical or surgical approaches are indicated. Endometriosis, adenomyosis and other gynecologic illnesses may concomitant to myomas; in these cases, it results difficult to determine which symptoms are associated with.

The most common diagnostic methods to investigate uterine myomas are abdominal [9] or transvaginal [10, 11] ultrasound. These exams are minimally-invasive and usually had a good sensitivity. Anyway, whenever the uterus is enlarged, affected by multiple fibroids or presenting a fibroid smaller than 0.5 cm [12], the ultrasonographic exam tend to show less diagnostic accuracy; thus, other investigations are needed. Magnetic resonance imaging (MRI) may help to clarify some controversial reports at ultrasound [11], even if the gold standard for the definitive disease confirm is the histological diagnosis. Moreover, the surgical approach is more precise to define size, location, and number of myomas; anyway, it usually represents a second step of treatment, which follows the failure of medical therapy.

The discovery of new strategies for primary and secondary prevention of myomas may become possible after the future identification of the exact etiology of these tumors; anyway, a specific knowledge of risk factors is important to break down the costs of public healthcare and improve women health. Importantly, further researches are needed to understand how risk factors impact fibroid growth; it could be interesting to stratify, based on ultrasonographic and molecular features, the onset of different tumors subtypes after particular exposures.

A relation between myomas and coronary heart disease has been reported, suggesting a common etiologic mechanism. Moreover, some immunological and infectious roles have been related to these tumors, as noticed by the widespread of myomas among HIV-positive patients [13].

Some risk factors are not modifiable, such as age at menarche, premenopausal age, childbearing history and reproductive factors, African ancestry and heritage, whereas others are modifiable, such as obesity, hypertension, lifestyle (diet, caffeine and alcohol consumption, smoking, physical activity and stress), and other environmental factors.

Together with the studies regarding the risk factors for the development of myomas, other researchers aim specifically to find which myoma features are more commonly associated to worsening of symptoms or which molecular characteristics are implicated in their recurrence after myomectomy. For example, Tsuda et al. [12] showed that a high vascularity of the tumors, the fibroid size at initial diagnosis, the position of tumoras well as the age of patient were predictors of an increased tumor growth.

2. Epidemiology of Myomas

A large amount of myomas go undiagnosed and their prevalence results underestimated if it is focused mostly on symptomatic women.

In more recent times, ultrasonographic screening on the general population has allowed a more accurate estimation [18]. Three epidemiologic studies based on ultrasonographic screening from United States (U.S.) [10, 19, 20] and two others from Europe [21, 22] have reported an evaluation of the age-specific prevalence or cumulative incidence of myomas. The only one to give an epidemiological evaluation among young women was performed by Laughlin et al. [10], who showed a higher prevalence of myomas sixed more than 5mm of diameter in the first trimester pregnant women. The pregnant analyzed population, naturally, is not representative of the general population, since fibroids may interfere with fertility; however, the investigators provided evidence about the earlier diagnosis of myomas in black women compared to whites. Moreover, they showed that the cumulative incidence by age 50 was about 70% for white women and more than 80% for blacks. These data are illustrative of an accurate evaluation of lifetime risk among different races. Pregnant Hispanic women from the southern U.S. showed a prevalence of 10%, more similar to whites, and, in another study [23], a high prevalence (67%) was reported among Finnish twins aged 40-47 year old, more similar again to white population. Different epidemiological findings were reported by Borgfeldt et al. [22] among a random sample of asymptomatic Swedish women aged 25-40 years, which showed a prevalence of 5.4% (95% CI 3.0–7.8%), much lower compared to what is described in literature [24, 25].

According to relevant trials, myoma disease represent the most common diagnosis among patients 15-54 years of age, admitted for gynecologic problems in U.S. [26], and the most common indication for hysterectomy in the U.S. and Australia is myoma tumor; particularly the hysterectomies due to myoma range from 40% to 60% [27].

Large prospective cohort studies [28–30] report a rate of approximately 2.0 per 1,000 person-years for hysterectomy-confirmed cases. In the U.S., nearly 30% of all the hysterectomies for fibroids are performed among women 18-44 years of age [31] and the annual healthcare costs amount to approximately $9.4 billion [32].

However, between 1997 and 2005, the hysterectomies for myoma declined from 31.4% to 26.9% [31], in parallel to the increase of other alternative therapies, such as myomectomy and uterine artery embolization [33].

Regarding the incidence of uterine fibroids among pregnant women, even if it could not be considered data regarding the general population considering that myomas may interfere with fertility, various studies [34, 35] move towards an overestimation for two main reasons.

First of all, asymptomatic women with fibroids would not have been seen by a gynecologist if they had not been pregnant, secondly the endocrine impact of the pregnancy over the myoma growth may reinforce the overestimation [10].

Several studies show a relationship between the presence of myoma during pregnancy and obstetric adverse outcome. Common reported complication are malpresentations, with an increase of caesarian section rate, and postpartum hemorrhage due to the risk of uterine atony [36, 37]. Other reports have investigated the association of fibroid disease with placenta previa, placental abruption, preterm delivery and late intrauterine fetal death (IUFD) [36, 38].

During the postpartum period, 36% of myomas should regress [34], regardless their size, pregnancy duration, mode of delivery, choice to breastfeed and delay of menses but black women, compared to whites, present a more limited regression.

However, the protective effect of postpartum period is not longstanding, given that it has been reported a lower myoma risk among women who had delivered 1-3 years before, compared to women who had given birth 16 years before [35].

Fibroids may affect fertility in 3.4%-31.9% of women [39, 40] and they are associated with a decreased rate of live birth and an increased rate of spontaneous abortion, especially submucosal or intramural ones, whereas it has been demonstrated that women with subserosal fibroids have the same pregnancy outcomes of infertile controls with no myomas [41].

It has been also evaluated the effect of myomectomy over infertile women with the result that the surgical procedure does not significantly increase fertility outcomes in cases of intramural myomas; nevertheless, women with submucosal fibroids may benefit from the treatment.

A systematic review [42] corroborated that intramural fibroids which do not warp the cavity are associated to adverse pregnancy outcomes in women undergoing IVF treatment (with 15% lower rate of clinical pregnancy per IVF cycle and 21% lower rate of live birth compared with no fibroids). However, it has not been demonstrated that their removal restore fertility to the levels expected in women without myomas, so the routine myomectomy does not appear justified among these patients.

2.1. Demographic Patterns: Age and Race

Age and race are two important factors related to the risk of myoma development. Regarding the first one, it has been shown that fibroids incidence increases steadily by age [18]. These tumors do not occur before puberty, 20-25% of the diagnosis emerges during fertile age and 30-40% of myomas are diagnosed among women older than 40 years, reaching a peak among 45-49 years of age[24, 40]. However, their incidence tends to decline after menopause [26, 29, 44] (Table 1). The clinical impact is more relevant during perimenopause period, during which symptomatic women require a treatment, and it decreases in postmenopause [45].

Table 1. Estimated number and rate per 10,000 persons-year of patient hospitalizations for uterine myomas by age group among women from USA aged 15–54 years in 1998-2005 [26]

Age	Number	Rate (standard error)
15-24	4,831	0.3 (0.01)
25-29	31,623	4.1 (0.1)
30-34	125,360	15.3 (0.3)
35-39	315,975	35.9 (0.6)
40-44	546,786	59.9 (0.8)
45-49	532,405	62.7 (0.8)
50-54	238,493	31.8 (0.5)
Total	1,795,473	27.5 (0.4)

Myomas are the most frequent in black women and the rarest in women of the Asian race [43]. Several studies report 2-3 times higher prevalence of fibroids among blacks compared to whites [19, 29], after adjustment for age and other risk factors, and lower prevalence in Europe compared to U.S., probably due to racial differences. The specific prevalence of myomas, stratified between different races, has been determined by Laughlin et al. [10] who found: 18% in black women, 8% in white women, 10% in Hispanic women and 13% in "others" group, consisting largely of Asian women.

The high rate of fibroids among black women is found at nearly all ages [29, 46]. The nodules are usually diagnosed at an earlier age than whites, about ten years before [10]. Black women often have multiple and larger tumors and they are affected by a greater symptomatology compared with other ethnic groups [47]. Moreover, their nodules have a quicker rate of growth [48] and tend less frequently to regress after pregnancy compared to myomas in white women [49]. An ultrasonographic screening study among asymptomatic women aged 18 to 30 years old revealed a prevalence of 26% in blacks and 7% in whites, considering adjustment for potential risk factors [29].

The age-specific cumulative incidence, a more accurate measure of lifetime risk, is about 3 times greater in blacks, it steadily increases for 10 years beginning at about age 25 for black women and about age 35 for white and, by age 50, it is about 70% for white women and more than 80% for blacks [19].

In parallel, healthcare costs for hospitalization are higher for blacks; they amount to about 5.3 per 1,000 person-years for black women and to 2.4 per 1,000 person-years for whites [46].

The exact reasons for racial differences in fibroids prevalence are mostly unknown, even if all these data support a genetic basis. Several theories have been proposed, such as a racial difference in the metabolism of estrogens, in the expression of receptors for steroid hormones and an aberrant expression of micro-RNAs (miRNAs)in black women [48, 50]. miRNAs belong to the class of small non-coding RNAs and they have a role in the regulation of cell proliferation, differentiation and apoptosis. Other analyzed causes, which may further clarify the ethnic impact on myoma frequency, include heritage, lifestyle, dietary habits and stress.

3. Etiology

Several pathways are involved in the promoting event of leiomyoma development. The beginning events arise from disorders of endocrine factors, abnormal wound healing and genetic mutations in cell growth regulation [51].

In particular, specific somatic genetic or epigenetic mutations lead to chromosomal abnormalities, which increase sensitivity to growth factors or hormones [24, 52]. Moreover, the different myoma prevalence among races suggests a genetic pathogenesis.

Regarding endocrine factors, sex hormones play a crucial role in the process, considering that fibroids occur during reproductive age [51]. Some studies provide evidence that circulating sex steroid hormones level is the same between women affected by fibroids and women without them [43]; however, patients with myomas show an higher concentration of estrogens nearby the tumor, in part due to a great tissue expression of aromatase, an enzyme with the function of converting testosterone and androstenedione into estrogen [53]. Other authors describe a major expression of steroid hormones receptors and growth factor receptors in fibroid tissue compared to normal myometrium [54, 55]. Progesterone plays a key role in the process [56] and it is considered essential for the maintenance and growth of the nodule [5]. It exerts the action through several pathways, performing both a proliferative and anti-apoptotic activity, through the production of ECM via down-regulation of a tumor suppressor [57, 58] and through a promotion of the anti-apoptotic proto-oncogene bcl-2 action [59], respectively. Ishikawa et al. [60] have suggested a close relationship between estrogen and progesterone and, particularly, that estrogens increase the expression of the progesterone receptors in fibroid cells.

As a consequence of these discoveries, progestins, progestin-releasing intrauterine systems and danazol have been proposed as medical therapy, but their specific effects on fibroids and bulk symptoms were limited and they gave side effects that lead to discontinuation [61–63]. Aromatase inhibitors, progesterone receptor agonists and antagonists, selective estrogen receptor modulators and GnRH agonists represent other therapeutic options, proposed to treat fibroid discomfort and reduce size effect symptoms [60–64].

GnRH agonists have been approved for preoperative setting due to their action of correcting anemia, decreasing blood loss and reducing myoma size [67].

However, they have climacteric side effects, such as vasomotor symptoms, decreased bone density and an initial estrogen flare effect that may exacerbate symptoms before provoking a constant hypoestrogenic state.

In parallel, progesterone receptor modulators (SPRMs), which have mixed agonist and antagonist activity, have shown success for the treatment of women with uterine fibroids [68]. SPRMs were first discovered in 1980, and mifepristone, a powerful progesterone antagonist, was the pioneer drug.

Ulipristal acetate is another compound belonging to the class with great results among symptomatic patients, showing a shrinking effect and a good control of symptomatology [67–70]. It presents a similar effectiveness of GnRH agonists but it is better tolerated because it does not result in menopausal side effects [69].

Lastly, disordered wound healing may have a promoting action in myoma development, following growth factors exposition. Indeed, a myometrial damage leads to an increase of growth factors expression to repair the injury.

They have the common action of incrementing cellular proliferation and of decreasing the apoptosis process [70]. Vascular endothelial growth factor-A (VEGF), fibroblast growth factor, insulin-like growth factor-1 (IGF-1) and transforming growth factor-beta (TGF-β) represent part of involved growth factors.

Most of these have an expression influenced by sex hormones [43] and their concentration is higher in myoma tissue compared to normal myometrium. They play different roles in angiogenesis process and stimulation of ECM through several signaling pathways [24, 71, 72].

4. Risk Factors

Despite further studies are needed to know more about risk factors impacting fibroids onset, the most studied risk factors include endogenous and exogenous hormone exposition, different lifestyles, infections, uterine injuries, genetic factors, specific demographic characteristics, hypertension and environmental factors. A part of them are modifiable but some others are not.

4.1. Markers of Endogenous Hormone Levels

4.1.1. Menarche, Menstrual Patterns, and Menopause

Mitotic activity in the myometrium is greater during luteal phase of the menstrual cycle [73]; therefore, a long exposition to menses may increase myoma risk. Women who present early onset of menses at menarche and a late onset of menopause have a longer exposure to ovulatory cycles. Thus, it is to be expected that this category of women presents a higher occurrence of fibroids.

Many epidemiological studies report a relationship with earlier age at menarche [28, 35, 43, 57, 74]. Anyway, it is difficult, in available literature, to find studies proving a higher risk in case of late menopause [18].

The association between uterine myomas and different menstrual patterns is not clear and the only evidence proving that irregular menstrual cycles and longer menstrual cycle length are associated with decreased myomas onset is reported by the Nurses' Health Study II (NHS II) by Terry et al. [35].

The National Institute of Environmental Health Sciences Fibroid Growth Study (NIEHS - FGS) showed a different myoma growth rate among white women and blacks during premenopausal age. In according to its findings, whites present a lower myomas growth than black women [75]: The study measured a growth rate per 6 months in both races after 45 years of age and it reported a 2% rate for white women and a 15% rate for black women.

The risk of myomas decreases after menopause [28, 76]; this data has been confirmed by several pathologic studies on hysterectomy specimens that have shown uterus with less and smaller nodules among postmenopausal patients in comparison to premenopausal women [77].

4.1.2. Reproductive Factors

Several studies [35, 47, 74, 78, 79] report an inverse association between myoma incidence and parity; indeed, women with a history of more term pregnancies have a lower myoma risk, whereas spontaneous abortions or incomplete pregnancies are not associated to this risk [78, 79].

Parous women present a 20-50% lower risk compared to nulliparous women; in particular, some researchers report that the higher the number of children, the lower is myoma rate. Moreover, the longer the time since the last birth, the higher is the risk of uterine myomas [74, 79].

Multiparous women present a lower myoma occurrence also compared to infertile women. This data may be in part explained by the fact that infertile patients are more likely to have submucous myomas, especially young infertile women [74, 79]. The reason why childbearing seems to have a protective effect, may be explained through both hormonal and non-hormonal mechanisms.

An altered endocrine profile may follow a first or a second pregnancy in late reproductive age: in fact, many trials show a low prevalence of myoma among women of older age at first term birth [35, 47, 80]. In fact, pregnancy induces a decrease of estrogen receptors in myometrial tissue [73].

Moreover, Terry et al. [35] indicated an inverse association between fibroids risk and exclusive breastfeeding, probably due to the suppression of sex hormones during lactation. On the contrary, other authors [47] did not find the same relationship between breastfeeding and risk of developing these tumors; in fact, breastfeeding period may be too short to increase myomas risk.

Regarding non-hormonal hypothesis, a study [6] tried to demonstrate in favor to childbearing, a decrease of collagen and smooth muscle cells in uterine tissue during uterine involution that occurs in postpartum period. Another proposed explanation may be allocated to the ischemic state during delivery and the uterine remodeling [81].

Laughlin et al. [82] recruited 171 women with a single nodule in early-pregnancy and they screened the population in early pregnancy and postpartum period by performing ultrasound and MRI. They found that 36% of the fibroids were eliminated by the time of the ultrasonographic screening, which had been done 3-6 months postpartum; moreover, the persisting nodules decreased in size. They explained the phenomenon through an ischemic process occurring during the observation period. Two previous studies [83, 84] reported an abnormal and reduced vasculature in myoma tissue. Furthermore, delivery implies clots forming but, nearby the fibroid, there is a decrease in fibrinolytic activity, which may contribute to the ischemia [85]. The results of the prospective pregnancy study of Laughlin et al. [82] are consistent with these findings. In fact, MRI screening performed in postpartum period revealed a lack of enhancement after contrast among some of the few persisting fibroids, indicating the probable presence of central ischemia.

4.1.3. Anthropometric Characteristics

Literature shows contrast data about the association between obesity and myoma development [43, 86]. Several studies report no correlation, while other authors found a linear correlation [87, 88] and others a non-linear association (with an increase of the risk among overweight women and a reduction among obese patients) [89, 90].

This non-linear association may be related to the anovulation and the following decreased progesterone level, frequently detected among obese women [91].

An Italian study by Chiaffarino et al. [92] did not find any association between body mass index (BMI, kg/m^2) and fibroids onset, whereas He et al. [93] performed a case-control study providing evidence that Asian obese women presented a major myoma incidence during premenopausal age compared to the controls (they did not observe the same significant association between BMI and fibroids in postmenopausal period). In parallel, a Finnish twin cohort study [23] showed results consistent with this association.

At least, The National Institute of Environmental Health Sciences Uterine Fibroid Study (UFS) [94] reported a positive association only among black patients.

Many further researches did not associate the risk of having myomas in teenagers and young adulthood with high BMI, whereas confirmed an association among women who gained weight during adulthood [88–90].

A prospective cohort study [28], with the aim of describing reproductive and lifestyle correlation with surgically confirmed fibroids, measured an increment of risk for surgical treatment in women who gained weight: the risk was 16% higher among who had an increment of 10-20 kg and 23% higher among who had an increment of more than 20 kg, compared to patients who gained <10 kg; on the contrary, women who had a constant weight or lost weight presented a 13% lower risk of having myomas.

The reason clarifying the association between obesity and myoma incidence might be expected by the great levels of circulating estrogens among obese women. It may be due to the aromatization of androgens in estrogens by peripheral fatty tissues; however, the association cannot be explained by last assumption because the most circulating estrogens in premenopausal women comes from the ovaries [95]. Nevertheless, the lower hepatic production of sex hormone binding globulin (SHBG) may increment in sex hormones bioavailability among obese women [96].

4.1.4. Diabetes and Polycystic Ovary Syndrome (PCOS)

Many epidemiological studies reported a correlation between obesity and diabetes mellitus in the development of fibroids [18, 43, 86, 96]. The insulin resistance, together with the high IGF-I and androgen levels, represents the common factor for probably explaining the high incidence of myomas in these patients.

In vitro studies [97, 98] reported that IGF-1 promotes proliferation of fibroid cells in culture, corroborating the correlation between IGF-1 and fibroid growth. Moreover, the Black Women's Health Study (BWHS) [99] assumed that high dietary glycemic index (GI) and glycemic load (GL) may contribute to increase myomas risk, due to high IGF-1 levels or estrogen bioavailability. BWHS did not find a significant association between GI and myomas risk, but it observed a small positive association among young women of less than 35 years of age (IRR for highest versus lowest quintile: 1.18; 95% CI 1.02–1.37). The investigators of UFS [100] did not confirm any relationship between IGF-1 and myoma growth. On the contrary, they found diabetes as protective factor in the development of fibroids among black women. An explanation of this last result may be researched in a systemic vascular dysfunction in women with hyperinsulinemia and diabetes, which seem to have a less vascularized myometrium, such preventing an eventual tumor development [84].

On the other hand, women with PCOS presenta 65% increased risk of myoma [43, 86] compared to women without PCOS, despite the correlation with hyperinsulinemia [86]. Several hypotheses may clarify this phenomenon: the most important of these is the increased levels of luteinizing hormone (LH) among affected women [101]. Indeed, high levels of LH are related to larger nodules and LH hypothesis is also corroborated by the finding that the effect of PCOS is greater among lean than among obese women. In favor to this supposition, it is important to under light that LH receptor is also shared with human chorionic gonadotropin, the hormone that promote uterine growth during early pregnancy.

4.2. Use of Exogenous Hormones

4.2.1. Oral Contraceptives

Epidemiological data about the relationship between oral contraceptives (OCs) and fibroids are inconsistent [102]. Until now, controversial results have been published by several studies and no clear conclusions have yet emerged.

The BWHS [47] reported no association with any type of progestin or estrogen-based formulation. This study observed just a 40% lower risk in current users of injectable progestin-only compared to non-users, explainable with the down-regulation of estrogen receptors in these benign tumors, which may be likely induced by progestin; moreover, the impact of intrauterine device (IUD) with levonorgestrel is not yet understood [102, 103].

Inconsistent data are available regarding current versus former use of OCs and the duration of their assumption [47, 74, 87, 104]. Some authors [47, 74] showed an 20–29% increased risk among women who started taking OCs before 17 years of age.

Early assumption of OCs is related to precocious beginning of sexual activity and, consequently, to an increased risk of sexually transmitted infections [105]. Therefore, the possible explanation may be ascribed to the infectious etiology. Anyway, another confounding factor is the major incidental diagnosis of fibroids among women who receive OCs prescription for other gynecological conditions, such as endometriosis or dysmenorrhea.

4.2.2. Postmenopausal Hormone Use

Women in postmenopausal age who receive a hormone replacement therapy, such as estrogens only or combined estroprogestins, seem to present a positive association with myoma risk [18]. Consistent findings derive from prospective and case-control studies [53, 66, 78, 106] evaluating the presence of fibroids after surgery. They corroborated an increased occurrence of myoma growth among women who took hormone replacement therapy compared to those who did not take it, reporting 6 times increased risk among the first group of patients.

4.2.3. Depot Medroxyprogesterone Acetate

Several researches [47, 107] have observed an inverse correlation between myomas risk and the use of depot medroxyprogesterone acetate (DMPA). A study [107] carried out among Thai population showed a great inverse association and reported a correlation with the duration of assumption.

The longer the duration of DMPA consumption, the lower may be this risk, because of the more sustained estrogen suppression [108]. In particular, there may be a 90% lower risk among women who took the compound for more than 5 years.

The reason of the inverse correlation may be the limited estradiol concentrations, caused by DMPA, comparable to those observed in postmenopausal age.

4.2.4. Diethylstilbestrol (DES)

A prenatal exposure to diethylstilbestrol (DES) is difficult to assess and the available literature show conflicting results. DES exposure may provide long-term changes in estrogen-related gene expression.

Some authors [109] did not confirm this association, whereas others reported a 21% increased risk among women who self-reported exposure to DES in the first trimester of pregnancy [110]. Other studies [111, 112] are consistent with the last observation, even if these kinds of studies may present recall bias. Additionally, several trials have been performed also in laboratory rodents [113, 114], supporting a correlation with this exposure.

4.3. Lifestyle

It has been demonstrated that lifestyle factors, such as diet, caffeine, alcohol consumption, smoking, physical activity and stress, may have a potential effect on the formation of myomas and their growth [93].

4.3.1. Dietary Factors

Most of studies, evaluating the impact of diet on the risk of fibroid onset, have been carried out using a food frequency questionnaire.

Exogenous hormones in food, such as the phytoestrogens, may have a role in myoma development [115]. In particular, the risk seems to increase eating food with a high glycemic index; otherwise, fruit, especially citrus fruits, and vegetables are protective for many authors [92, 93, 116]. Two studies have assumed that a plant-based diet promote a decreasing risk of myomas due to a lower bioavailability of endogenous hormones [117, 118]. Concerning other kind of food, an Italian case-control study of surgically confirmed cases in Italy by Chiaffarino et al. [92] showed a positive relationship with myoma risk among patients who consumed a great amount of red meat and ham, whereas it did not find any association with dairy consumption. The BWHS [119] provided evidence, for the first time, of an inverse association with calcium, phosphorus and calcium-to-phosphorus ratio (a marker of bioavailable calcium), so with dairy products. It reported similar results for both low-fat and high-fat milk consumption. In particular, the risk was 30% lower among women consuming ≥4 serving/day of total dairy versus women consuming <1 serving/day (95% CI 0.58–0.86; P-trend <0.001).

The BWHS performed a subsequent epidemiological study [120] and it observed a statistically significant linkage with different subtypes of fat, showing an inverse association for saturated fat and a positive one for monounsaturated and polyunsaturated fatty acids. The study also reported a small positive relationship with myoma occurrence among African American women who eat food rich in long-chain omega-3 fatty acids (which are polyunsaturated fatty acids: predominantly *eicosapentaenoic acid, docosapentaenoic acid and docosahexaenoic acid*), such as marine fatty acids (MFA). However, the study did not show a consistent association between the overall risk of myomaandthe total intake of fat or with different fat subtypes.

The Uterine Leiomyomata Epidemiology Project (TULEP) [121] investigated the impact of soy intake measuring urinary isoflavones and lignans and it reported no association with myoma risk, despite it is expected that soy would have an inverse relationship with myomas considering two factors: soy has an antiestrogenic role among women with high endogenous estrogens levels and, secondly, myoma frequency is lower among Asian women, population who typically consume many soy food products. Other authors [122] corroborated the same lack of association, evaluating the soy intake impact, also among population who make a great use of soy, such as Asian women.

Green tea has a potential for myoma treatment due to his protective effect on fibroids development. Animal studies [123] on myoma cells showed an inhibition of cell proliferation and an apoptosis activity with green tea and a cultured study [124] on human myoma cells demonstrated again that gallactocatehingallate (EGCG), an extract of green tea, caused the inhibition of cell proliferation. However, further studies are needed.

Among micronutrients, vitamins have a role in myoma risk, as reported by several investigators. Vitamin D seems to be protective for myoma development. Laboratory and animal studies report that 1,25-dihydroxyvitamin D3 has an inhibition activity and led myoma cells to apoptosis [125]. A further evidence comes from the fact that women with hypovitaminosis D present a higher risk of fibroids [126].

Vitamins C, E, B6, B9 and B12have been not associated to myoma risk in several studies whereas the role of vitamin A is more debated. Martin et al. [127] showed that vitamin A intake had a positive impact on fibroids. On the opposite, others [116] demonstrated an inverse correlation between food plenty of vitamin A and the risk of having fibroid among black women. However, the authors concluded the study with the assumption that the likely protective effect could have caused also by other ingredients present in the food, rather than by vitamin A.

Lastly, carotenoids, that exert a pro-vitamin A activity, has not been related to myomas risk by Terry et al. [128] and by Wise et al. [116].

4.3.2. Alcohol and Caffeine

Caffeine and alcohol have been associated to relevant change of endogenous hormone levels [129].

Literature indicates that alcohol is able to increase estradiol and estrone levels [130] and many investigators appoint it as a risk factor to myomas onset [92, 122, 129], especially among beer drinkers compared to wine ones. Not surprisingly, Chiaffarino et al. [92] did not found any association between alcohol intake and myomas incidence among Italian women, due to the great prevalence of wine consumption rather than beer in their study.

Caffeine has not been associated to myoma risk by different investigators [92], even if BWHS [129] reported an association in young (<35 years) women who drank 3 or more cups for day (500mg or more of caffeine for day).

Furthermore, some authors [131, 132] reported that coffee and caffeine were related to an enhance in sex steroid hormones production, in particular with estradiol increase during early follicular phase.

4.3.3. Cigarette Smoking

The relation between tobacco and myomas is controversial. It has been suggested a protective role, as tobacco may shift the production of estradiol into less potent form [133] and inhibit the action of aromatase enzyme [134]. This hypothesis have found confirm in several studies showing an inverse association between myomas risk and smoking [28, 135, 136].

On the contrary, it has been also suggested that tobacco may have an estrogen-related impact, supporting myoma cells proliferation [137]. However, a more recent report [129]seems to probably exclude this association.

4.3.4. Physical Activity

Contrasting data emerge also regarding physical activity. In a survey study [138] relative to the history of fibroids performed among former college athletes and non-athletes, the results were in support of a protective effect of exercise: non-athletes reported more frequently to have a history of myomas. The California Teachers Study (CTS) [28] did not found any association between lifetime high activity (over 3 hours a week) and the requirement of surgical therapy for myomas. Nevertheless, the UFS [94] showed again an inverse association with a dose-response relation, measuring a 40% lower risk among women who performed 7 or more hours of exercise per week versus those trained less than 2 hours per week. The observations by UFS may be related to the low luteal phase estrogens among women performing a greater physical activity [118].

4.3.5. Stress

A cross-sectional study [139] showed a relation between risk of fibroids and the number of stressful life events. Boynton-Jarrett R, et al. [140] observed that women who had experienced early-life abuse were more exposed to myomas occurrence. Moreover, the risk was lower if woman reported an emotionally supportive relationship in childhood.

Stress may have a role in the increment of adrenal progesterone [141], even if it may also down-regulate gonadotropin synthesis. However, cultural studies on granulosa cells [141, 142] found an up-regulation of secretion of ovarian steroids and other promoting factors, such as growth factors, cytokines, and matrix metalloproteinases, after stress hormones exposure.

4.4. Infection and Uterine Injury

Inflammation and infection have been postulated to have a role in the development of fibroids as early as 1930s [143, 144], following an increment in ECM production and a decrement of apoptosis phenomenon [106]. Faerstein et al. [145] assessed the relationship between the myomas risk and potential uterine infectious or noninfectious irritants, performing a case-controlled retrospective study. They estimated a dose-response association with pelvic inflammatory disease (PID), with 1.8-fold increased adjusted risk among women with a history of PID (keeping out who had had a diagnosis of myoma before the diagnosis of PID). The risk resulted even higher (OR 3.7; 95% CI 0.9–15.9] if women had had 3 or more PID episodes, compared to who did not reported any episode. Chlamydia infection, a common cause of PID, was associated to the fibroid occurrence too, with a 3.2 increased risk; whereas infectious agents which affect mostly the external genitalia, such as genital herpes or warts, were not related in their observational study. On the contrary, a cross-sectional ultrasonographic study [146] reported an inverse association with the bacteria chlamydia and no relationship with other reproductive tract infections. Faerstein et al. [145] evaluated also the association with the use of IUD and the application of talc in the genital area, reporting a little increase of the risk among former or current users of talc but not consistent associations with the status or the duration of IUD use. The authors finally suggested that endometrial inflammation may induce a myometrial response, playing a role in myoma development.

Women with an abnormal Pap test showed a decreased risk in two different studies [81, 147], one of which [147] reported a 39% lower risk among young African-American women who needed a cervical procedure. These findings suggest a protective effect of HPV infection.

A Brazil case-controlled study by Murta et al. [148] proposed the Chagas disease as associated to myoma development, reporting a higher myoma diagnosis among multiparous white women, affected by this infection and subsequently subjected to a surgical procedure for myoma or other gynecological conditions.

Lastly, uterine injury is considered a risk factor, having similar mechanisms of keloids and hypertrophic scars [149]. The remodeling of ECM and collagen during healing process is deeply involved in this common process. Uterine injury and myomas were correlated in a study on African-American women [150]. On the other hand, Harmon et al. [151] did not find any correlation between screened myomas at ultrasound and self-reported keloids and hypertrophic scars among African American population. Otherwise, Sun et al. [152] studied keloid incidence in Asian people, demonstrating a 2-fold myoma incidence in case of keloids.

4.5. Genetics and Epigenetics Factors

"Myoma families" have widely been described in literature [45, 153] and they refer to a familial predisposition to myoma development. The genetic predisposition is proven by familial aggregation studies [154, 155], twin studies [23, 156], and genetic linkage studies among families affected by syndromes associated to fibroids [157, 158].

To corroborate the "myoma families" hypothesis, Uimari et al. [153] reported cases of familial fibroids women, in Finland, where in young women, detected for the disease, undergone to surgery at an earlier age. Two previous twin studies were consistent with the genetic relevance [23, 156], one of which [156] described a twice concordance rate for hysterectomy among monozygotic twins compared to dizygotic twins. Further researches [154, 159] showed an increase of myoma incidence among women who had first-degree affected relatives. Moreover, given that there is a high recurrence of tumors after myomectomy, the presence of inherited genes or a genetic predisposition is even more assumed.

Several genetic linkage analyses were performed to investigate familial forms and they led to identify hereditary leiomyomatosis and renal cell carcinoma (HLRCC) as the most clinically significant syndrome [160]. It is caused by an autosomal dominant mutation of the fumarate hydratase (FH) gene, which results in a loss of tumor suppression [161].

A national prospective cohort study [162] evaluated risk alleles for myomas between African and European American women. Specific loci on chromosomes 2, 4, and 10 were identified as associated to European ancestry, suggesting that multiple loci may have a role for ethnic disparity in tumors and that several genetic alternatives influence a higher incidence of uterine nodules in African Americans.

Cytogenetic analysis [163] identified different chromosomal changes in 40-50% of myoma cases. By these findings, it is reasonable to assume that each tumor develops independently [43] and that specific regions of the genome have a role in the pathogenesis.

In particular, somatic mutations, such as the gene encoding the mediator complex subunit 12 (MED12) and the gene encoding the high-mobility group AT-hook 2 (HMGA2), are associated to the disease [5].

MED12 is considered the most mutated gene in women affected by fibroids, ranging from 50 to 85% [164]. It concerns a heterozygous somatic mutation affecting the mediator complex subunit 12, encoded by a gene located on the X chromosome. Heinonen et al. [164] found the mutation inversely associated to myoma size.

HMGA2 overexpression has also been associated with tumor formation. It comes from a rearrangement involving 12q15, which is responsible to the most common translocation (t [12; 14] (q14-q15; q23-q24)) founded in myoma tissue, with about 20% of incidence [165]. The overexpression of HMGA2 is provoked by the break point located over a gene promoter. The translocation, together with another mutation onchromosome 7q22 (del [7] (q22)), is associated to larger tumors and it is founded more frequently in subserosal and intramural myoma.

The first ever genome-wide association study (GWAS) of myoma was carried out among Japanese population [166]. It found three loci on chromosomes (10q24.33, 22q13.1 and 11p15.5), associated to the tumor. A further subgroup analysis was performed to investigate a possible linkage between each single nucleotide polymorphism (SNP) and clinically symptomatic myomas. The results showed a high relationship with myoma development regardless of presence or absence of hypermenorrhea or dysmenorrhea. The BioVU and Right From the Start cohorts [167] corroborated the findings of the first GWAS, observing SNPs among European Americans. Eggert et al. [168], genotyping further SNPs, identified new connected regions in 10p11, 3p21, 2q37, 5p13, 11p15, 12q14, and 17q25 and they conducted a meta-analysis among two independent cohorts of European women, carrying out a subsequent GWASs. In particular, they reported a SNP on chromosome 17 involving fatty acid synthase (FASN) gene, which they indicated as the initial myoma risk allele. The last but not least mapping analysis within BWHS [162], worthwhile to mention, showed a suggestive linkage with 2q37, 4p16.1, and 10q26.

Varghese et al. [169] identified G protein-coupled receptor 10 (GPR10), whose ligand is prolactin releasing peptide (PrRP), as the most upregulated GPR in fibroid tissue.

The linkage between GPR10 and PrRP stimulates the phosphoinositol-3-kinaseeprotein kinase B/Akt mammalian target of rapamycin (PI3K/AKT/mTOR) pathway, which is involved in proliferation and in increasing survival of myomas cells. Moreover, the authors described a factor having an inhibiting action over the pathway, the RE1-silencing transcription factor/neuron-restrictive silencing factor (REST). Therefore, the loss of this transcriptional repressor results in a GPR10 overexpression and it may impact on fibroid growth.

Concerning epigenetic phenomenon, DNA methylation and demethylation of cytosine residues in CpG islands represent common mechanisms that may interfere with genes expression, especially if they occur closely to the promoter of specific genes. DNA methyltransferases (DNMTs) catalyze the DNA methylation [170] and these enzymes present an irregular expression in fibroid cells compared to myometrial cells [171].

Hypomethylation and demethylation, rather than hypermethylation, have been associated to activation of genes transcription [172], resulting in cell proliferation and synthesis of proteins involved in ECM genesis and, by implication, in promoting the transformation of normal myometrial tissue to myoma.

Among DNMTs, DNMT3A and DNMT3B could have a specific role in fibroid growth because their expression has been found decreased in myoma cells, resulting a hypomethylation of targeted genes [171].

Another studied epigenetic modulation concerns small miRNAs, irregularly expressed in myoma tissue. They are single-stranded RNAs, implicated in regulation of gene expression by inhibition of translation, degradation of specific mRNA or by binding to their promoter regions [173].

They may act on oncogenes or tumor suppressors, having a role in cell transformation [174], and they may be employed in different pathways regarding cell proliferation, inflammation, angiogenesis, cell adhesion, cell matrix formation, transcriptional reprogramming processes and tissue turnover. In particular, they play a role on specific signaling pathways involving mitogen-activated protein kinase (MAPK), wingless integration site (WNT), Janus kinase (JAK), signal transducer and activator of transcription (STAT) and TGF-b [175].

4.6. Other Potential Risk Factors

4.6.1. Demographic Characteristics

It has been shown as married women, with more years of education and a "professional" occupation more frequently undergo detection of myomas [176].

This finding may be related to the major access to medical care of this population category.

4.6.2. Hypertension

Uterine myomas and high blood pressure have been associated since the 1930s to risk of developing fibroids [27]. Many cross-sectional epidemiologic reports [177, 178] confirmed this positive association; many other researchers showed similar results [179, 180]. NHS II [181] described a greater relation especially between women needing surgery and the BWHS [182] found the same association among hysterectomy cases but not among women who undergone to other kind of surgery or received only an ultrasonographic diagnosis of fibroids. The results by Boynton-Jarrett et al. [181], who performed a prospective study about hypertension and risk of uterine LMs, showed again a correlation between myoma risk and the duration of hypertension, probably due to cytokine release or injury to the myometrium.

4.6.3. Environmental Factors

Environmental factors may influence myoma development by multiple mechanisms, such as an endocrine upheaval. Irradiation exposure is one of the studied environmental mechanisms that may have an impact on tumors. A greater detection of myoma was found among women survived the atomic explosion, with a correlation dose-response [183].

Two epidemiologic studies [184, 185] assessed an increased risk with phthalates exposure, ubiquitous chemical compounds used as plasticizers and largely present in consumer products. Lambertino et al. [186] observed an association with self-reported myoma and the exposure to polychlorinatedbiphenyl (PCB), an organic chlorine compound present at every level of the foodchain, as well as to other groups of estrogenic, antiestrogenic and dioxin-likePCBs. A positive association was also found detecting urinary levels of bisphenol A, which has endocrine-disrupting properties [187].

Blood levels of lead, mercury, and cadmium seem to not have any relationship with myoma development [188], whereas high serum levels of dioxin (measurable following Seveso disaster in 1976), showed a protective effect, probably thanks to antiestrogen activity and inhibition of ECM production through TGF-β pathways [189].

References

[1] Flake GP, Andersen J, Dixon D. Etiology and pathogenesis of uterine leiomyomas: A review. *Environmental Health Perspectives.* 2003;111(8):1037–1054.

[2] Bozini N. BEC. The history of myomectomy at the Medical School of University of São Paulo. *Clinics (Sao Paulo).* 2007; 62(3):209-10.

[3] Borahay MA, Al-Hendy A, Kilic GS, Boehning D. Signaling Pathways in Leiomyoma: Understanding Pathobiology and Implications for Therapy. *Mol Med.* 2015;21:242-56.

[4] Brosens I. *Uterine Leiomyomata: Pathogenesis and Management.* Abingdon, England, Inf Heal Taylor Fr. 2006

[5] Koohestani F, Braundmeier AG, Mahdian A, Seo J, Bi JJ, Nowak RA. Extracellular matrix collagen alters cell proliferation and cell cycle progression of human uterine leiomyoma smooth muscle cells. *PLoS One.* 2013;8(9):e75844.

[6] Bulun SE. Uterine Fibroids. *N Engl J Med.* 2013;369:1344-1355.

[7] Ferrero S, Abbamonte LH, Giordano M, Parisi M, Ragni N, Remorgida V. Uterine myomas, dyspareunia, and sexual function. Vol. 86, *Fertility and Sterility.* 2006;86(5):1504-10.

[8] Schwartz SM, Marshall LM, Baird DD. Epidemiologic contributions to understanding the etiology of uterine leiomyomata. *Environ Health Perspect.* 2000;108 Suppl 5:821-7.

[9] Loutradis D, Antsaklis A, Creatsas G, Hatzakis A, Kanakas N, Gougoulakis A, et al. The validity of gynecological ultrasonography. *Gynecol Obstet Invest.* 1990;29(1):47-50.

[10] Fedele L, Bianchi S, Dorta M, Brioschi D, Zanotti F, Vercellini P. Transvaginal ultrasonography versus hysteroscopy in the diagnosis of uterine submucous myomas. *Obstet Gynecol.* 1991;77(5):745-8.

[11] Dueholm M, Lundorf E, Hansen ES, Ledertoug S, Olesen F. Accuracy of magnetic resonance imaging and transvaginal ultrasonography in the diagnosis, mapping, and measurement of uterine myomas. *Am J Obstet Gynecol.* 2002;186(3):409-15.

[12] Hartmann KE, Laughlin SK, Baird DD, Savitz DA, Herring AH. Prevalence of uterine leiomyomas in the first trimester of pregnancy: An ultrasound-screening study. *Obstet Gynecol.* 2009;113(3): 630–635.

[13] Wise LA, Laughlin-Tommaso SK. Epidemiology of uterine fibroids: From menarche to menopause. *Clin Obstet Gynecol.* 2016;59(1):2-24.

[14] Tsuda H, Kawabata M, Nakamoto O, Yamamoto K. Clinical predictors in the natural history of uterine leiomyoma: preliminary study. *J Ultrasound Med.* 1998;17(1):17-20.

[15] Wise LA, Laughlin-Tommaso SK. Uterine Leiomyomata. In: *Women and Health.* 2013;179(2):186–191.

[16] Baird DD, Dunson DB, Hill MC, Cousins D, Schectman JM. High cumulative incidence of uterine leiomyoma in black and white women: Ultrasound evidence. *Am J Obstet Gynecol.* 2003;188(1):100-7.

[17] JK B, PJ S, Sternfeld B, CE L. Black-white differences in hysterectomy prevalence: the CARDIA study... Coronary Artery Risk Development in Young Adults. *Am J Public Health.* 2009;99(2):300-7.

[18] Eskenazi B, Warner M, Samuels S, Young J, Gerthoux PM, Needham L, et al. Serum dioxin concentrations and risk of uterine leiomyoma in the Seveso Women's Health Study. *Am J Epidemiol.* 2007; 166(1):79-87.

[19] Borgfeldt C, Andolf E. Transvaginal ultrasonographic findings in the uterus and the endometrium: Low prevalence of leiomyoma in a random sample of women age 25-40 years. *Acta Obstet Gynecol Scand.* 2000;79(3):202-7.

[20] Luoto R, Kaprio J, Rutanen EM, Taipale P, Perola M, Koskenvuo M. Heritability and risk factors of uterine fibroids - The Finnish Twin Cohort Study. *Maturitas.* 2000;37(1):15–26.

[21] Andersen J, Barbieri RL. Abnormal Gene Expression in Uterine Leiomyomas. *J Soc Gynecol Investig.* 1995;2: 663–672.

[22] Vollenhoven BJ, Lawrence AS HD. Uterine fibroids: a clinical review. *Br J Obs Gynaecol.* 1990;97(4):285-98.

[23] Whiteman MK, Kuklina E, Jamieson DJ, Hillis SD, Marchbanks PA. Inpatient hospitalization for gynecologic disorders in the United States. *Am J Obstet Gynecol.* 2010;202(6):541.e1-6.

[24] Sparic R, Mirkovic L, Malvasi A, Tinelli A. Epidemiology of uterine myomas: A review. *International Journal of Fertility and Sterility.* 2016; 9(4): 424–435.

[25] Templeman C, Marshall SF, Clarke CA, DeLellis Henderson K, Largent J, Neuhausen S, et al. Risk factors for surgically removed fibroids in a large cohort of teachers. *Fertil Steril.* 2009; 92(4):1436–1446.

[26] Marshall LM, Spiegelman D, Barbieri RL, Goldman MB, Manson JE, Colditz GA, et al. Variation in the incidence of uterine leiomyoma among premenopausal women by age and race. *Obstet Gynecol.* 1997;90(6):967-73.

[27] Wise LA, Palmer JR, Stewart EA, Rosenberg L. Age-specific incidence rates for self-reported uterine leiomyomata in the Black Women's Health Study. *Obstet Gynecol.* 2005;105(3):563-8.

[28] Merrill RM. Hysterectomy surveillance in the United States, 1997 through 2005. *Med Sci Monit.* 2008;14(1):CR24-31.

[29] Cardozo ER, Clark AD, Banks NK, Henne MB, Stegmann BJ, Segars JH. The estimated annual cost of uterine leiomyomata in the United States. In: *American Journal of Obstetrics and Gynecology.* 2012;206(3):211.e1-9.

[30] Viswanathan M, Hartmann K, McKoy N, Stuart G, Rankins N, Thieda P, et al. Management of uterine fibroids: an update of the evidence. *Evid Rep Technol Assess (Full Rep).* 2007;(154):1-122.

[31] Laughlin SK, Hartmann KE, Baird DD. Postpartum factors and natural fibroid regression. *Am J Obstet Gynecol.* 2011;204(6):496.e1-6.

[32] Terry KL, De Vivo I, Hankinson SE, Missmer SA. Reproductive characteristics and risk of uterine leiomyomata. *Fertil Steril.* 2010;94(7):2703-7.

[33] Lai J, Caughey AB, Qidwai GI, Jacoby AF. Neonatal outcomes in women with sonographically identified uterine leiomyomata. *J Matern Neonatal Med.* 2012;25(6):710-3.

[34] Klatsky PC, Tran ND, Caughey AB, Fujimoto VY. Fibroids and reproductive outcomes: a systematic literature review from conception to delivery. *Am J Obs Gynecol.* 2008;198(4):357-66.

[35] Stout MJ, Odibo AO, Graseck AS, MacOnes GA, Crane JP, Cahill AG. Leiomyomas at routine second-trimester ultrasound examination and adverse obstetric outcomes. *Obstet Gynecol.* 2010;116(5):1056-63.

[36] Ezeama C, Ikechebelu J, Obiechina N, Ezeama N. Clinical presentation of uterine fibroids in Nnewi, Nigeria: A 5-year review. Ann Med Health Sci Res. 2012; 2(2): 114–118.

[37] Fonseca-Moutinho JA, Silva Barbosa L, Gonçalves Torres D, Morgado Nunes S. Abnormal uterine bleeding as a presenting symptom is related to multiple uterine leiomyoma: An ultrasound-based study. *Int J Womens Health.* 2013; 5: 689–694.

[38] Pritts EA, Parker WH, Olive DL. Fibroids and infertility: an updated systematic review of the evidence. *Fertil Steril.* 2009;91(4):1215-23.

[39] Sunkara SK, Khairy M, El-Toukhy T, Khalaf Y, Coomarasamy A. The effect of intramural fibroids without uterine cavity involvement on the outcome of IVF treatment: A systematic review and meta-analysis. *Human Reproduction.* 2010;25(2):418-29.

[40] Okolo S. Incidence, aetiology and epidemiology of uterine fibroids. *Best Practice and Research: Clinical Obstetrics and Gynaecology.* 2008;22(4):571-88.

[41] Reed SD, Cushing-Haugen KL, Daling JR, Scholes D, Schwartz SM. Postmenopausal estrogen and progestogen therapy and the risk of uterine leiomyomas. *Menopause.* 2004; 11:214–222 154.

[42] Gupta S, Jose J, Manyonda I. Clinical presentation of fibroids. *Best Practice and Research: Clinical Obstetrics and Gynaecology.* 2008;22(4):615-26.

[43] Velebil P, Wingo PA, Xia Z, Wilcox LS, Peterson HB. Rate of hospitalization for gynecologic disorders among reproductive-age women in the United States. *Obstet Gynecol.* 1995;86(5):764-9.

[44] Wise LA, Palmer JR, Harlow BL, Spiegelman D, Stewart EA, Adams-Campbell LL, et al. Reproductive factors, hormonal contraception, and risk of uterine leiomyomata in African-American women: a prospective study. *Am J Epidemiol.* 2004;159(2): 113-23.

[45] Jacoby VL, Fujimoto VY, Giudice LC, Kuppermann M, Washington AE. Racial and ethnic disparities in benign gynecologic conditions and associated surgeries. *American Journal of Obstetrics and Gynecology.* 2010;202(6):514-21.

[46] Sparić R. Uterine myomas in pregnancy, childbirth and puerperium. *Srp Arh Celok Lek.* 2014;142(1-2):118-24.

[47] Othman EE, Al-Hendy A. Molecular genetics and racial disparities of uterine leiomyomas. *Best Pr Res Clin Obs Gynaecol.* 2008;22(4):589-601.

[48] Asada H, Yamagata Y, Taketani T, Matsuoka A, Tamura H, Hattori N, et al. Potential link between estrogen receptor-α gene hypomethylation and uterine fibroid formation. *Mol Hum Reprod.* 2008;14(9):539–45.

[49] Bulun SE, Imir G, Utsunomiya H, Thung S, Gurates B, Tamura M, et al. Aromatase in endometriosis and uterine leiomyomata. In: *Journal of Steroid Biochemistry and Molecular Biology.* 2005;95(1-5):57-62.

[50] Andersen J. Growth factors and cytokines in uterine leiomyomas. *Semin Reprod Endocrinol.* 1996;14(3): 269-282.

[51] Sadan O, Van Iddekinge B, Van Gelderen CJ, Savage N, Becker PJ, Van Der Walt LA, et al. Oestrogen and progesterone receptor concentrations in leiomyoma and normal myometrium. *Ann Clin Biochem.* 1987; 24 (Pt 3):263-7.

[52] Rein MS. Advances in uterine leiomyoma research: The progesterone hypothesis. *Environ Health Perspect.* 2000;108 Suppl 5:791-3.

[53] Moravek MB, Yin P, Ono M, Coon V JS, Dyson MT, Navarro A, et al. Ovarian steroids, stem cells and uterine leiomyoma: therapeutic implications. *Hum Reprod Update.* 2015;21(1):1-12.

[54] Qiang W, Liu Z, Serna VA, Druschitz SA, Liu Y, Espona-Fiedler M, et al. Down-regulation of miR-29b is essential for pathogenesis of uterine leiomyoma. *Endocrinology.* 2014; 155(3): 663–669.

[55] Matsuo H, Maruo T, Samoto T. Increased expression of Bcl-2 protein in human uterine leiomyoma and its up-regulation by progesterone. *J Clin Endocrinol Metab.* 1997;82(1):293-9.

[56] Ishikawa H, Ishi K, Ann Serna V, Kakazu R, Bulun SE, Kurita T. Progesterone is essential for maintenance and growth of uterine leiomyoma. *Endocrinology.* 2010;151(6):2433-42.

[57] Ke LQ, Yang K, Li J, Li CM. Danazol for uterine fibroids. *Cochrane Database of Systematic Reviews.* 2009;(3):CD007692.

[58] Sangkomkamhang US, Lumbiganon P, Laopaiboon M, Mol BWJ. Progestogens or progestogen-releasing intrauterine systems for uterine fibroids. *Cochrane Database of Systematic Reviews.* 2013;(2):CD008994.

[59] Van Voorhis B. A 41-year-old woman with menorrhagia, anemia, and fibroids: Review of treatment of uterine fibroids. *JAMA - Journal of the American Medical Association.* 2009; 301(1):82-93.

[60] Friedman AJ, Daly M, Juneau-norcross M, Gleason R, Rein MS, Leboff M. Endocrinology: Long-term medical therapy for leiomyomata uteri: A prospective, randomized study of leuprolide acetate depot plus either oestrogen-progestin or progestin "add-back" for 2 years. *Hum Reprod.* 1994; 9:1618–1625

[61] Chen YL, Zheng A, Wan Q. Selective estrogen receptor modulators (SERMs) for endometriosis. *Cochrane Database Syst Rev.* 2014; Issue 6. Art. No.: CD011169.

[62] Parsanezhad ME, Azmoon M, Alborzi S, Rajaeefard A, Zarei A, Kazerooni T, et al. A randomized, controlled clinical trial comparing the effects of aromatase inhibitor (letrozole) and gonadotropin-releasing hormone agonist (triptorelin) on uterine leiomyoma volume and hormonal status. *Fertil Steril.* 2010;93(1):192-8.

[63] Ferrero S, Venturini PL, Remorgida V. Letrozole monotherapy in the treatment of uterine myomas. *Fertility and Sterility.* 2010;93:e31.

[64] Leone Roberti Maggiore U, Scala C, Venturini PL, Ferrero S. Preoperative treatment with letrozole in patients undergoing laparoscopic myomectomy of large uterine

myomas: A prospective non-randomized study. *Eur J Obstet Gynecol Reprod Biol.* 2014;181:157-62.

[65] Sabry M, Al-Hendy A. Medical treatment of uterine leiomyoma. *Reprod Sci.* 2012;19(4):339-53.

[66] Spitz IM. Clinical utility of progesterone receptor modulators and their effect on the endometrium. Vol. 21, *Current Opinion in Obstetrics and Gynecology.* 2009;21(4):318-24.

[67] Ferrero S, Alessandri F, Vellone VG, Venturini PL, Leone Roberti Maggiore U. Three-month treatment with ulipristal acetate prior to laparoscopic myomectomy of large uterine myomas: a retrospective study. *Eur J Obstet Gynecol Reprod Biol.* 2016;205:43-7.

[68] Tafi E, Scala C, Leone Roberti Maggiore U, Bizzarri N, Candiani M, Venturini PL, et al. Drug safety evaluation of ulipristal acetate in the treatment of uterine fibroids. *Expert Opin Drug Saf.* 2015; 14(6):965-77.

[69] Ferrero S, Vellone VG, Barra F. Pharmacokinetic drug evaluation of ulipristal acetate for the treatment of uterine fibroids. *Expert Opinion on Drug Metabolism and Toxicology.* 2018;14(1):107-116.

[70] Ferrero S, Vellone VG, Barra F, Scala C. Ulipristal Acetate before Hysteroscopic and Laparoscopic Surgery for Uterine Myomas: Help or Hindrance? Gynecol Obstet Invest. 2018;1-13.

[71] Donnez J, Hudecek R, Donnez O, Matule D, Arhendt HJ, Zatik J, et al. Efficacy and safety of repeated use of ulipristal acetate in uterine fibroids. *Fertil Steril.* 2015;103(2):519-27.e3.

[72] Malik M, Norian J, McCarthy-Keith D, Britten J, Catherino WH. Why leiomyomas are called fibroids: The central role of extracellular matrix in symptomatic women. *Seminars in Reproductive Medicine.* 2010;28(3):169-79.

[73] Lee BS, Nowak RA. Human leiomyoma smooth muscle cells show increased expression of transforming growth factor-beta 3 (TGF beta 3) and altered responses to the antiproliferative effects of TGF beta. *J Clin Endocrinol Metab.* 2001;86(2):913-20.

[74] Arslan AA, Gold LI, Mittal K, Suen T-C, Belitskaya-Levy I, Tang M-S, et al. Gene expression studies provide clues to the pathogenesis of uterine leiomyoma: new evidence and a systematic review. *Hum Reprod.* 2005; 20, 852–863.

[75] Kawaguchi K, Fujii S, Konishi I, Iwai T, Nanbu Y, Nonogaki H, et al. Immunohistochemical analysis of oestrogen receptors, progesterone receptors and Ki-67 in leiomyoma and myometrium during the menstrual cycle and pregnancy. *Virchows Arch A Pathol Anat Histopathol.* 1991;419(4):309-15.

[76] Marshall LM, Spiegelman D, Goldman MB, Manson JE, Colditz GA, Barbieri RL, et al. A prospective study of reproductive factors and oral contraceptive use in relation to the risk of uterine leiomyomata. *Fertil Steril.* 1998;70(3):432-9.

[77] Peddada SD, Laughlin SK, Miner K, Guyon J-P, Haneke K, Vahdat HL, et al. Growth of uterine leiomyomata among premenopausal black and white women. *Proc Natl Acad Sci.* 2008;105:19887–19892.

[78] Parazzini F. Risk factors for clinically diagnosed uterine fibroids in women around menopause. *Maturitas.* 2006;55(2):174-9.

[79] Cramer SF, Patel A. The frequency of uterine leiomyomas. *Am J Clin Pathol.* 1990; 94(4):435–438.

[80] Chen CR, Buck GM, Courey NG, Perez KM, Wactawski-Wende J. Risk factors for uterine fibroids among women undergoing tubal sterilization. *Am J Epidemiol.* 2001;153(1):20-6.

[81] Parazzini F, Negri E, La Vecchia C, Chatenoud L, Ricci E, Guarnerio P. Reproductive factors and risk of uterine fibroids. *Epidemiology.* 1996; 7: 440 442.

[82] Dorgan JF, Reichman ME, Judd JT, Brown C, Longcope C, Schatzkin A, et al. Relationships of age and Reproductive Characteristics with Plasma Estrogens and Androgens in Premenopausal Women. *Cancer Epidemiol Biomarkers Prev.* 1995; 4(4):381–386.

[83] Laughlin SK, Schroeder JC, Baird DD. New directions in the epidemiology of uterine fibroids. *Seminars in Reproductive Medicine.* 2010;28(3):204-17.

[84] Laughlin SK, Herring AH, Savitz DA, Olshan AF, Fielding JR, Hartmann KE, et al. Pregnancy-related fibroid reduction. *Fertil Steril.* 2010;94(6):2421-3.

[85] Wei J-J, Zhang X-M, Chiriboga L, Yee H, Perle MA, Mittal K. Spatial differences in biologic activity of large uterine leiomyomata. *Fertil Steril.* 2006; 85(1):179-87.

[86] Walocha JA, Litwin JA, Miodoński AJ. Vascular system of intramural leiomyomata revealed by corrosion casting and scanning electron microscopy. *Hum Reprod.* 2003;18(5):1088-93.

[87] Burbank F. Childbirth and myoma treatment by uterine artery occlusion: Do they share a common biology? *Journal of the American Association of Gynecologic Laparoscopists.* 2004;11:138e52.

[88] Wise LA, Palmer JR, Stewart EA, Rosenberg L. Polycystic ovary syndrome and risk of uterine leiomyomata. *Fertil Steril.* 2007; 87(5): 1108–1115.

[89] Ross RK, Pike MC, Vessey MP, Bull D, Yeates D, Casagrande JT. Risk factors for uterine fibroids: reduced risk associated with oral contraceptives. *Br Med J (Clin Res Ed).* 1986;293(6543):359-62.

[90] Marshall LM, Spiegelman D, Manson JE, Goldman MB, Barbieri RL, Stampfer MJ, et al. Risk of uterine leiomyomata among premenopausal women in relation to body size and cigarette smoking. *Epidemiology.* 1998; 9(5):511-7.

[91] Terry KL, De Vivo I, Hankinson SE, Spiegelman D, Wise LA, Missmer SA. Anthropometric characteristics and risk of uterine leiomyoma. *Epidemiology.* 2007;18(6):758-63.

[92] Wise LA, Palmer JR, Spiegelman D, Harlow BL, Stewart EA, Adams-Campbell LL, et al. Influence of body size and body fat distribution on risk of uterine leiomyomata in U.S. black women. *Epidemiology.* 2005;16(3):346-54.

[93] Pasquali R, Gambineri A. Metabolic effects of obesity on reproduction. *Reprod Biomed Online.* 2006;12(5):542-51.

[94] Chiaffarino F, Parazzini F, La Vecchia C, Chatenoud L, Di Cintio E, Marsico S. Diet and uterine myomas. *Obstet Gynecol.* 1999;94(3):395-8.

[95] He Y, Zeng Q, Dong S, Qin L, Li G, Wang P. Associations between uterine fibroids and lifestyles including diet, physical activity and stress: a case-control study in China. *Asia Pac J Clin Nutr.* 2013;22(1):109-17.

[96] Baird DD, Dunson DB, Hill MC, Cousins D, Schectman JM. Association of physical activity with development of uterine leiomyoma. *Am J Epidemiol.* 2007;165(2):157-63.

[97] Azziz R. Reproductive endocrinologic alterations in female asymptomatic obesity. *Fertil Steril. 1*989; 52(5):703–725.

[98] He Y, Zeng Q, Li X, Liu B, Wang P. The Association between Subclinical Atherosclerosis and Uterine Fibroids. PLoS One. 2013; 8(2): e57089.

[99] Strawn EY, Novy MJ, Burry KA, Bethea CL. Insulin-like growth factor I promotes leiomyoma cell growth in vitro. *Am J Obstet Gynecol.* 1995;172(6):1837–1843.

[100] Van Der Ven LTM, Van Buul-Offers SC, Gloudemans T, Bloemen RJ, Roholl PJM, Sussenbach JS, et al. Modulation of insulin-like growth factor (IGF) action by IGF-binding proteins in normal, benign, and malignant smooth muscle tissues. *J Clin Endocrinol Metab.* 1996; 81(10):3629–3635.

[101] Radin RG, Palmer JR, Rosenberg L, Kumanyika SK, Wise LA. Dietary glycemic index and load in relation to risk of uterine leiomyomata in the Black Women's Health Study. *Am J Clin Nutr.* 2010; 91:1281-8.

[102] Baird DD, Travlos G, Wilson R, Dunson DB, Hill MC, DAloisio AA, et al. Uterine leiomyomata in relation to insulin-like growth factor-i, insulin, and diabetes. *Epidemiology.* 2009; 20(4):604-10.

[103] Baird DD, Kesner JS, Dunson DB. Luteinizing hormone in premenopausal women may stimulate uterine leiomyomata development. *J Soc Gynecol Investig.* 2006;13(2):130-5.

[104] Berisavac M, Sparic R AR. Contraception: modern trends and controversies. *Srp Arh Celok Lek.* 2009.

[105] Berisavac M, Sparić R, Argirović R, Hudelist G, Zizić V. Application of a hormonal intrauterine device causing uterine perforation: a case report. *Srp Arh Celok Lek.* 2011;139(11-12):815-8.

[106] Parazzini F, Negri E, La Vecchia C, Fedele L, Rabaiotti M, Luchini L. Oral contraceptive use and risk of uterine fibroids. *Obstet Gynecol.* 1992;79(3):430-3.

[107] Winter L, Goldy AS, Baer C. Prevalence and epidemiologic correlates of chlamydia trachomatis in rural and urban populations. *Sex Transm Dis.* 1990;17(1):30-6.

[108] Cramer SF, Padela AI, Marchetti CE, Newcomb PM, Heller DS. Myometrial Hyperplasia in Pediatric, Adolescent, and Young Adult Uteri. *J Pediatr Adolesc Gynecol.* 2003;16(5):301-6.

[109] Lumbiganon P, Rugpao S, Phandhu-fung S, Laopaiboon M, Vudhikamraksa N, Werawatakul Y. Protective effect of depot-medroxyprogesterone acetate on surgically treated uterine leiomyomas: A multicentre case-control study. *BJOG An Int J Obstet Gynaecol.* 1996;103(9):909-14.

[110] Clark MK, Sowers M, Levy BT, Tenhundfeld P. Magnitude and variability of sequential estradiol and progesterone concentrations in women using depot medroxyprogesterone acetate for contraception. *Fertil Steril.* 2001;75(5):871-7.

[111] Wise LA, Palmer JR, Rowlings K, Kaufman RH, Herbst AL, Noller KL, et al. Risk of benign gynecologic tumors in relation to prenatal diethylstilbestrol exposure. *Obstet Gynecol.* 2005;105(1):167-73.

[112] Mahalingaiah S, Hart JE, Wise LA, Terry KL, Boynton-Jarrett R, Missmer SA. Prenatal diethylstilbestrol exposure and risk of uterine leiomyomata in the nurses' health study II. *Am J Epidemiol.* 2014;179(2):186-91.

[113] D'Aloisio AA, Baird DD, Deroo LA, Sandler DP. Association of intrauterine and early-life exposures with diagnosis of uterine leiomyomata by 35 years of age in the sister study. *Environ Health Perspect.* 2010;118(3):375-81.

[114] Baird DD, Newbold R. Prenatal diethylstilbestrol (DES) exposure is associated with uterine leiomyoma development. Vol. 20, *Reproductive Toxicology.* 2005; 20(1):81-4.

[115] Greathouse KL, Cook JD, Lin K, Davis BJ, Berry TD, Bredfeldt TG, et al. Identification of uterine leiomyoma genes developmentally reprogrammed by neonatal exposure to diethylstilbestrol. *Reprod Sci.* 2008;15(8):765-78.

[116] Newbold R. Cellular and molecular effects of developmental exposure to diethylstilbestrol: Implications for other environmental estrogens. In: *Environmental Health Perspectives.* 1995; 103 Suppl 7:83-7.

[117] Wise LA, Palmer JR, Ruiz-Narvaez E, Reich DE, Rosenberg L. Is the observed association between dairy intake and fibroids in African Americans explained by genetic ancestry? *Am J Epidemiol.* 2013; 178(7):1114-9.

[118] Wise LA, Radin RG, Palmer JR, Kumanyika SK, Boggs DA, Rosenberg L. Intake of fruit, vegetables, and carotenoids in relation to risk of uterine leiomyomata. *Am J Clin Nutr.* 2011; 94(6):1620-31.

[119] Fowke JH, Longcope C, Hebert JR. Macronutrient intake and estrogen metabolism in healthy postmenopausal women. *Breast Cancer Res Treat.* 2001; 65(1):1-10.

[120] Michnovicz JJ, Bradlow HL. Dietary and Pharmacological Control of Estradiol Metabolism in Humans. *Ann N Y Acad Sci.* 1990.

[121] Wise LA, Radin RG, Palmer JR, Kumanyika SK, Rosenberg L. A prospective study of dairy intake and risk of uterine leiomyomata. *Am J Epidemiol.* 2010;171(2):221-32.

[122] Wise LA et al. A prospective study of dietary fat and risk of uterine leiomyomata. *Am J Clin Nutr.* 2014; 99(5): 1105–1116.

[123] Atkinson C, Lampe JW, Scholes D, Chen C, Wähälä K, Schwartz SM. Lignan and isoflavone excretion in relation to uterine fibroids: a case-control study of young to middle-aged women in the United States. *Am J Clin Nutr.* 2006;84(3):587-93.

[124] Nagata C, Nakamura K, Oba S, Hayashi M, Takeda N, Yasuda K. Association of intakes of fat, dietary fibre, soya isoflavones and alcohol with uterine fibroids in Japanese women. *Br J Nutr.* 2009; 101(10):1427-31.

[125] Zhang D, Al-Hendy M, Richard-Davis G, Montgomery-Rice V, Sharan C, Rajaratnam V, et al. Green tea extract inhibits proliferation of uterine leiomyoma cells in vitro and in nude mice. *Am J Obstet Gynecol.* 2010;202(3):289.e1-9.

[126] Zhang D, Al-Hendy M, Richard-Davis G, Montgomery-Rice V, Rajaratnam V, Al-Hendy A. Antiproliferative and proapoptotic effects of epigallocatechin gallate on human leiomyoma cells. *Fertil Steril.* 2010; 94(5): 1887–1893.

[127] Halder SK, Sharan C, Al-Hendy A. 1,25-Dihydroxyvitamin D3 Treatment Shrinks Uterine Leiomyoma Tumors in the Eker Rat Model1. *Biol Reprod.* 2012;86(4):116.

[128] Baird DD, Hill MC, Schectman JM, Hollis BW. Vitamin d and the risk of uterine fibroids. *Epidemiology.* 2013;24(3):447-53.

[129] Martin CL, Huber LRB, Thompson ME, Racine EF. Serum Micronutrient Concentrations and Risk of Uterine Fibroids. *J Women's Heal.* 2011;20(6):915-22.

[130] Terry KL, Missmer SA, Hankinson SE, Willett WC, De Vivo I. Lycopene and other carotenoid intake in relation to risk of uterine leiomyomata. *Am J Obstet Gynecol.* 2008;198(1):37.e1-8.

[131] Wise LA, Palmer JR, Harlow BL, Spiegelman D, Stewart EA, Adams-Campbell LL, et al. Risk of uterine leiomyomata in relation to tobacco, alcohol and caffeine consumption in the Black Women's Health Study. *Hum Reprod.* 2004; 19(8): 1746–1754.

[132] Reichman ME, Judd JT, Longcope C, Schatzkin A, Clevidence BA, Nair PP, et al. Effects of alcohol consumption on plasma and urinary hormone concentrations in premenopausal women. *J Natl Cancer Inst.* 1993;85(9):722-7.

[133] Lucero J, Harlow BL, Barbieri RL, Sluss P, Cramer DW. Early follicular phase hormone levels in relation to patterns of alcohol, tobacco, and coffee use. *Fertil Steril.* 2001;76(4):723-9.

[134] Leonard TK, Watson RR MM. The effects of caffeine on various body systems: a review. *J Am Diet Assoc.* 1987;87(8):1048-53.

[135] Michnovicz JJ, Hershcopf RJ, Naganuma H, Bradlow HL, Fishman J. Increased 2-Hydroxylation of Estradiol as a Possible Mechanism for the Anti-Estrogenic Effect of Cigarette Smoking. *N Engl J Med.* 1986; 315(21):1305-9.

[136] Barbieri RL, McShane PM, Ryan KJ. Constituents of cigarette smoke inhibit human granulosa cell aromatase. *Fertil Steril.* 1986; 46(2):232-6..

[137] Parazzini F, Negri E, La Vecchia C, Rabaiotti M, Luchini L, Villa A, et al. Uterine myomas and smoking. Results from an Italian study. *J Reprod Med.* 1996;41(5):316-20.

[138] Romieu I, Walker AM, Jick S. Determinants of uterine fibroids. *Post Mark Surveill.* 1991; 5: 119–133.

[139] Ohtake F, Takeyama K ichi, Matsumoto T, Kitagawa H, Yamamoto Y, Nohara K, et al. Modulation of oestrogen receptor signalling by association with the activated dioxin receptor. *Nature.* 2003;423(6939):545-50.

[140] Wyshak G, Frisch RE, Albright NL, Albright TE, Schiff I. Lower prevalence of benign diseases of the breast and benign tumours of the reproductive system among former college athletes compared to non-athletes. *Br J Cancer.* 1986; 54(5): 841–845.

[141] Vines AI, Ta M, Esserman DA. The association between self-reported major life events and the presence of uterine fibroids. *Women's Heal Issues.* 2010;20(4):294–8.

[142] Boynton-Jarrett R, Rich-Edwards JW, Jun H, Hibert EN, Wright RJ. Abuse in childhood and risk of uterine leiomyoma: the role of emotional support in biologic resilience. *Epidemiology.* 2011; 22(1):6-14.

[143] Puder JJ, Freda PU, Goland RS, Ferin M, Wardlaw SL. Stimulatory effects of stress on gonadotropin secretion in estrogen-treated women. *J Clin Endocrinol Metab.* 2000; 85(6):2184-8.

[144] Ferin M. Clinical review 105: Stress and the reproductive cycle. *Journal of Clinical Endocrinology and Metabolism.* 1999; 84(6):1768-74.

[145] Witherspoon JT BV. The etiology of uterine fibroids. *Surg Gynecol Obs.* 1934;58:57–61.

[146] Witherspoon JT. A possible cause of uterine fibroids. *Endocrinol* (Baltimore). 1933;17:703–708.

[147] Faerstein E, Szklo M, Rosenshein NB. Risk factors for uterine leiomyoma: A practice-based case-controls study. II. Atherogenic risk factors and potential sources of uterine irritation. *Am J Epidemiol.* 2001;153(1):11-9.

[148] Moore KR, Cole SR, Dittmer DP, Schoenbach VJ, Smith JS, Baird DD. Self-Reported Reproductive Tract Infections and Ultrasound Diagnosed Uterine Fibroids in African-American Women. *J Women's Heal.* 2015; 24(6): 489–495.

[149] Moore KR, Smith JS, Laughlin-Tommaso SK, Baird DD. Cervical neoplasia-related factors and decreased prevalence of uterine fibroids among a cohort of African American women. *Fertil Steril.* 2014; 101(1):10.

[150] Murta EFC, Oliveira GP, De Oliveira Prado F, De Souza MAH, Murta BMT, Adad SJ. Association of uterine leiomyoma and Chagas' disease. *Am J Trop Med Hyg.* 2002;66(3):321-4.

[151] Leppert PC, Catherino WH, Segars JH. A new hypothesis about the origin of uterine fibroids based on gene expression profiling with microarrays. *Am J Obstet Gynecol.* 2006;195(2):415-20.

[152] Carrino DA, Mesiano S, Barker NM, Hurd WW, Caplan AI. Proteoglycans of uterine fibroids and keloid scars: similarity in their proteoglycan composition. *Biochem J.* 2012; 443: 361–368.

[153] Harmon QE, Laughlin SK, Baird DD. Keloids and ultrasound detected fibroids in young African American women. *PLoS One.* 2013; 8(12): e84737.

[154] Sun LM, Wang KH, Lee YCG. Keloid incidence in Asian people and its comorbidity with other fibrosis-related diseases: a nationwide population-based study. *Arch Dermatol Res.* 2014;306(9):803-8.

[155] Uimari O, Suomalainen-König S, Sakkinen N, Santala M, Nieminen P, Ryynanen M. Natural history of familial myomas. *Eur J Obstet Gynecol Reprod Biol.* 2006;125(2):255-8.

[156] Kurbanova MKH, Koroleva AG SA. Genetic-epidemiologic analysis of uterine myoma: assessment of repeated risk. *Genetika.* 1989; 25(10):1896-8.

[157] Vikhlyaeva EM, Khodzhaeva ZS, Fantschenko ND. Familial predisposition to uterine leiomyomas. *Int J Gynecol Obstet.* 1995; 51:127–131.

[158] Treloar SA, Martin NG, Dennerstein L, Raphael B, Heath AC. Pathways to hysterectomy: Insights from longitudinal twin research. *Am J Obstet Gynecol.* 1992; 167(1):82-8.

[159] Launonen V, Vierimaa O, Kiuru M, Isola J, Roth S, Pukkala E, et al. Inherited susceptibility to uterine leiomyomas and renal cell cancer. *Proc Natl Acad Sci.* 2001; 98(6):3387-92.

[160] Garcia Muret MP, Pujol RM, Alomar A, Calaf J, De Moragas JM. Familial leiomyomatosis cutis et uteri (Reed's syndrome). *Arch Dermatol Res.* 1988; 280 Suppl:S29-32.

[161] Van Voorhis BJ, Romitti PA, Jones MP. Family history as a risk factor for development of uterine leiomyomas - Results of a pilot study. *J Reprod Med.* 2002; 47(8):663-9.

[162] Kiuru M, Launonen V, Hietala M, Aittomäki K, Vierimaa O, Salovaara R, et al. Familial cutaneous leiomyomatosis is a two-hit condition associated with renal cell cancer of characteristic histopathology. *Am J Pathol.* 2001; 159(3):825-9.

[163] Alam NA, Rowan AJ, Wortham NC, Pollard PJ, Mitchell M, Tyrer JP, et al. Genetic and functional analyses of FH mutations in multiple cutaneous and uterine leiomyomatosis, hereditary leiomyomatosis and renal cancer, and fumarate hydratase deficiency. *Hum Mol Genet.* 2003; 12(11):1241-52.

[164] Wise LA, Ruiz-Narvaez EA, Palmer JR, Cozier YC, Tandon A, Patterson N, et al. African ancestry and genetic risk for uterine leiomyomata. *Am J Epidemiol.* 2012; 176(12): 1159–1168.

[165] Sandberg AA. Updates on the cytogenetics and molecular genetics of bone and soft tissue tumors: Leiomyoma. *Cancer Genetics and Cytogenetics.* 2005;161(1):1-19.

[166] Heinonen HR, Sarvilinna NS, Sjöberg J, Kämpjärvi K, Pitkänen E, Vahteristo P, et al. MED12 mutation frequency in unselected sporadic uterine leiomyomas. *Fertil Steril.* 2014;102(4):1137-42.

[167] Gross KL, Morton CC. Genetics and the development of fibroids. *Clinical Obstetrics and Gynecology.* 2001;44(2):335-49.

[168] Cha PC, Takahashi A, Hosono N, Low SK, Kamatani N, Kubo M, et al. A genome-wide association study identifies three loci associated with susceptibility to uterine fibroids. *Nat Genet.* 2011;43(5):447-50.

[169] Edwards TL, Hartmann KE, Velez Edwards DR. Variants in BET1L and TNRC6B associate with increasing fibroid volume and fibroid type among European Americans. *Hum Genet.* 2013; 132(12): 10.

[170] Eggert SL, Huyck KL, Somasundaram P, Kavalla R, Stewart EA, Lu AT, et al. Genome-wide linkage and association analyses implicate FASN in predisposition to uterine leiomyomata. *Am J Hum Genet.* 2012;91(4):621-8.

[171] Varghese B V., Koohestani F, McWilliams M, Colvin A, Gunewardena S, Kinsey WH, et al. Loss of the repressor REST in uterine fibroids promotes aberrant G protein-coupled receptor 10 expression and activates mammalian target of rapamycin pathway. *Proc Natl Acad Sci.* 2013;110(6):2187-92.

[172] Jin B, Robertson KD. DNA methyltransferases, DNA damage repair, and cancer. *Advances in Experimental Medicine and Biology.* 2013; 754:3-29.

[173] Li S, Chiang TC, Richard-Davis G, Barrett JC, Mclachlan JA. DNA hypomethylation and imbalanced expression of DNA methyltransferases (DNMT1, 3A, and 3B) in human uterine leiomyoma. *Gynecol Oncol.* 2003; 90(1):123-30.

[174] Schübeler D. Function and information content of DNA methylation. Nature. 2015; 517: 321–326.

[175] Karmon AE, Cardozo ER, Rueda BR, Styer AK. MicroRNAs in the development and pathobiology of uterine leiomyomata: Does evidence support future strategies for clinical intervention? *Human Reproduction Update.* 2014; 20(5):670-87.

[176] Wolańska M, Sobolewski K, Bańkowski E, Jaworski S. Matrix metalloproteinases of human leiomyoma in various stages of tumor growth. *Gynecol Obstet Invest.* 2004; 58(1):14-8.

[177] Zavadil J, Ye H, Liu Z, Wu J, Lee P, Hernando E, et al. Profiling and functional analyses of microRNAs and their target gene products in human uterine leiomyomas. *PLoS One*. 2010; 5(8):e12362.

[178] Parazzini F, La Vecchia C, Negri E, Cecchetti G, Fedele L. Epidemiologic characteristics of women with uterine fibroids: a case-control study. *Obstet Gynecol.* 1988; 72(6):853-7.

[179] Silver MA, Raghuvir R, Fedirko B, Elser D. Systemic hypertension among women with uterine leiomyomata: potential final common pathways of target end-organ remodeling. *J Clin Hypertens* (Greenwich). 2005; 7(11):664-8.

[180] Luoto R, Rutanen EM, Auvinen a. Fibroids and hypertension. A cross-sectional study of women undergoing hysterectomy. *J Reprod Med.* 2001; 46(4):359-64.

[181] Takeda T, Sakata M, Isobe A, Miyake A, Nishimoto F, Ota Y, et al. Relationship between metabolic syndrome and uterine leiomyomas: a case-control study. *Gynecol Obs Invest.* 2008; 66(1):14-7.

[182] Haan YC, Oudman I, De Lange ME, Timmermans A, Ankum WM, Montfrans GAV, et al. Hypertension risk in Dutch women with symptomatic uterine fibroids. Am J Hypertens. 2015; 28(4):487-92.

[183] Boynton-Jarrett R, Rich-Edwards J, Malspeis S, Missmer SA, Wright R. A prospective study of hypertension and risk of uterine leiomyomata. *Am J Epidemiol.* 2005;161(7):628-38.

[184] Radin RG, Rosenberg L, Palmer JR, Cozier YC, Kumanyika SK, Wise LA. Hypertension and risk of uterine leiomyomata in US black women. *Hum Reprod.* 2012; 27(5):1504-9.

[185] Kawamura S, Kasagi F, Kodama K, Fujiwara S, Yamada M, Ohama K, et al. Prevalence of uterine myoma detected by ultrasound examination in the atomic bomb survivors. *Radiat Res.* 1997; 147(6):753-8.

[186] Weuve J, Hauser R, Calafat AM, Missmer SA, Wise LA. Association of exposure to phthalates with endometriosis and uterine leiomyomata: Findings from NHANES, 1999-2004. *Environ Health Perspect.* 2010; 118(6):825-32.

[187] Huang PC, Tsai EM, Li WF, Liao PC, Chung MC, Wang YH, et al. Association between phthalate exposure and glutathione S-transferase M1 polymorphism in adenomyosis, leiomyoma and endometriosis. *Hum Reprod.* 2010;25(4):986–94.

[188] Lambertino A, Turyk M, Anderson H, Freels S, Persky V. Uterine leiomyomata in a cohort of Great Lakes sport fish consumers. *Environ Res.* 2011;111(4):565-72.

[189] Zhou F, Zhang L, Liu A, Shen Y, Yuan J, Yu X, et al. Measurement of phenolic environmental estrogens in human urine samples by HPLC-MS/MS and primary discussion the possible linkage with uterine leiomyoma. *J Chromatogr B Anal Technol Biomed Life Sci.* 2013;938:80-5.

[190] Jackson LW, Zullo MD, Goldberg JM. The association between heavy metals, endometriosis and uterine myomas among premenopausal women: National Health and Nutrition Examination Survey 1999-2002. *Hum Reprod.* 2008;23(3):679-87.

[191] Gomez-Duran A, Carvajal-Gonzalez JM, Mulero-Navarro S, Santiago-Josefat B, Puga A, Fernandez-Salguero PM. Fitting a xenobiotic receptor into cell homeostasis: How the dioxin receptor interacts with TGFβ signaling. *Biochem Pharmacol.* 2009;77(4):700-12.

In: Uterine Fibroids
Editors: Simone Ferrero and Fabio Barra

ISBN: 978-1-53615-046-9

Chapter 2

CLASSIFICATION OF UTERINE MYOMAS AND CLINICAL CORRELATIONS

Giulio Evangelisti, MD, Fabio Barra, MD and Simone Ferrero*, MD, PhD

[1]Obstetrics and Gynecology, Department of Neurosciences, Rehabilitation, Ophthalmology, Genetics, Maternal and Child Health (DiNOGMI), University of Genoa, Italy
[2]Academic Unit of Obstetrics and Gynecology, Ospedale San Martino, Genoa, Italy

ABSTRACT

In last three decades, some classifications have been defined in order to better characterize the characteristics of uterine fibroids. Special attention has been reserved to submucous myomas, which present the lowest prevalence among myoma types but are notably responsible of menorrhagia, dysmenorrhea and other reproductive disorders. By the time, hysteroscopic myomectomy has become the treatment of choice for the management of submucous myomas. To better define the outcomes related to their management, Wamstaker et al. developed a specific grading system based on myoma degree of penetration into the myometrium; this classification was later adopted by the European Society for Gynecological Endoscopy (ESGE) and it is currently the most largely used. In 2005, Lasmar et al. developed a more detailed myoma classification for facilitating the hysteroscopic approach (including size, topography, extension, penetration and position on lateral wall), distinguishing them into 3 groups; this classification shows a more accurate correlation with technical operative difficulty and complexity. Moreover, it demonstrates to be a valid instrument to not only predict complete or partial resection of

* Corresponding Author's Email: simoneferrero@me.com.

myomas, but also operative time, fluid absorption, rate and severity of eventual complications. The International Federation of Gynecology and Obstetrics (FIGO) classification system [1] maintains the original division of submucosal myomas in types 0–2, but extends the staging by adding further five categories (3-7 types). The FIGO staging aimed to create a useful tool for both clinical and research practices, although a recent study revealed some important limitations by using it.

Overall, despite of the multiple proposed classifications, it is not yet possible to determine the best one; in fact, each one presents strengths and limits.

The aim of this chapter is to introduce the several classifications adopted for uterine myomas and their clinical correlations.

Keywords: uterine myomas, myomas staging, ESGE classification, STEP-W classification, FIGO Classification

1. INTRODUCTION

Leiomyomas represent the most common benign tumors of the uterus; they are constituted by a large amount of smooth muscle cells associated with fibrous connective tissue. They show a prevalence of 70-80% in women aged 50 [2]. Particularly, black women have a higher risk of developing uterine myomas [3].

Because of the high prevalence in the reproductive ages, myomas can be expected as a common occurrence in women seeking pregnancy. Overall, given the high number of successful pregnancies, it is evident that the majority of fibroids does not cause relevant adverse effects during pregnancy. However, it is estimated that uterine myomas contribute to infertility in 5-10% of cases [4]. Moreover, when other causes of infertility are ruled out, myomas may be considered the single responsible for 1-2.5% of infertility cases [5, 6].

Myomas are distinguished in subserous, intramural and submucous on the basis of their topography; this simple subdivision correlates with characteristics clinical presentation as well as implies different therapeutic measures [7].

Among these types, the submucous myoma has the lowest prevalence, ranging from 5% to 10% of all myomas [5, 8, 9]. Unlike the other two subtypes, submucous myomas can more often cause uterine abnormal bleeding (AUB), even in case of small mass. They represent also a common cause of dysmenorrhea and they can interfere with reproductive processes, potentially causing recurrent pregnancy loss, premature birth and infertility [10].

Hysteroscopic myomectomy has become the treatment of choice for the management of submucous myomas; it is indicated for women who are planning to become pregnant in order to improve fertility rate, or for those who refuse hysterectomy as definitive treatment for a significant and persistent symptomatology [11–16]. Possible complications of this procedure are uterine perforation, injury to adjacent organs, excessive bleeding and fluid overload [15–17]. In rare cases, during the hysteroscopic procedure, excessive fluid absorption can be responsible for pulmonary edema or even death [16].

In the early '90, several attempts to create a uniquely classification system for myomas have been made in order to better evaluate the post-surgical outcomes and to compare result from clinical studies. First steps were done in '93 by Wamsteker et al. [11] who distinguished three degrees of submucosal myoma extension into uterine wall based on hysteroscopic characteristics; this classification was later adopted by the European Society for Gynecological Endoscopy (ESGE). Subsequent classifications were developed by Lasmar et al. [12] and then by FIGO [1]. Overall, each one has different practical application and predictive value.

This chapter aims to shed light on current classifications on uterine myomas, describing their developmental steps, and, in particular, showing their limits or strengths.

1.1. Topographical Classification and Clinical Correlation

The traditional topographical classification subdivides myomas into three groups in relation to their extension in the thickness of the uterine wall; this simple classification has also a relevant correlation with clinical presentation (Table 1). Overall, most women with uterine myomas are symptom-free [9, 18, 19]; furthermore, when symptoms occur, they are related not only to the location, but also to size, or concomitant degenerative changes [20].

Table 1. List of symptoms and other clinical signs related to the uterine myomas

Abnormal uterine bleeding
Menorrhagia Anemia
Pelvic disorders
Urinary frequency Urinary incontinence Difficulty in urination Hydronephrosis Constipation Tenesmus Rectal pressure
Pelvic pain
Reproductive dysfunction
Infertility
Pregnancy related
Myoma growth Red degeneration and pain Spontaneous miscarriage Obstetric complications (e.g., pre-term, abnormal lie, post-partum hemorrhage)
Malignancy
Rare associations (ascites, polycythemia, familial syndromes)

1.1.1. Subserous Fibroids

These benign tumors grow predominantly outside of the uterus; they are sometimes pedunculated, and they can bulge into the abdominal or into pelvic cavity. Subserous fibroids may be characterized by large size before being responsible of clinical symptoms, which often consist in pelvic or abdominal dysfunction; symptoms can occur by distending and compressing the bladder (urinary frequency, urinary incontinence or voiding dysfunctions tend to occur) or bowel (new-onset constipation or abdominal bloating tends to occur). When a myoma becomes particularly large, it may outgrow blood supply subsequently leading to ischemia and necrosis. This degeneration may be associated with severe acute pain, sometimes necessitating immediate surgical exploration. There is general consensus that sub-serous fibroids do not impair fertility; thus, they should not be removed despite of causing relevant clinical symptoms [21].

1.1.2. Intramural Fibroids

They are the most prevalent myomas. Intramural fibroids develop within the muscular uterine wall with an estimated median volume growth rate of 35.2% per year: in particular, it seems that small myomas (<2 cm) grow significantly faster than the larger ones [22, 23]. Overall, their growth can determine bulge either into the uterine cavity or into the abdominal cavity.

Women affected can sometimes experience heavy menstrual bleeding; this is partly due to the obstructive effect on uterine vasculature provoking endometrial venule ectasia; consequently, the myometrial and endometrial congestions may cause profuse menstrual bleeding [24].

Intramural fibroids can increase the likelihood of infertility and pregnancy loss: in fact, the distortion induced by the intramural mass may interfere with embryo implantation and be responsible for mechanical obstruction of both tubal ostia and intramural tubal segment. In addition, it has been assumed that intramural myomas may cause dysfunctional rhythmic uterine contractions hindering sperm motility through the uterus [25, 26]. At the moment, the role of myomectomy for improving fertility of patients with intramural myoma is still debated [21, 27].

1.1.3. Submucous Fibroids

Submucous fibroids grow inside the uterine cavity. They are associated with heavy and prolonged menses and subsequent increased risk of anemia. In general, submucous myomas are more prevalent in women experiencing AUB than in asymptomatic ones [28]. The bleeding pattern consisting in relevant menorrhagia is often the only clinical manifestation [29]. The excessive bleeding may be additionally due to the presence of endometritis in the tissue overlying these myomas (this is a frequent histological finding). Otherwise, pain is not frequent in patients with submucous myoma; in general, whenever occurs, it tends to be associated with torsion of pedunculated myomas, cervical dilatation, red myomas degeneration (associated with pregnancy) [30].

It is largely known that submucous fibroids can be responsible for infertility and miscarriages [21, 31]. Also a higher association between patients' subfertility and presence of submucous myomas has been noted; moreover, it has been estimated a rate of more than 70% of pregnancy wastage in patients with uterine myomas [32]. Even once pregnancy is established, submucous fibroids can cause a premature labor [33–36]. Studies showed that the removal of submucous fibroids may confer benefit in both conception and live birth rates [37].

2. WAMSTEKER/ESGE CLASSIFICATION (1993)

Until early '90, several studies demonstrated the efficacy of hysteroscopic trans-cervical resection of submucous myomas for controlling persistent AUB. Nevertheless, no study has been performed considering the degree of myoma intramural extension; for this reason, it is difficult to compare the post-operative results of these studies.

The first attempt of standardizing the management of submucous fibroids was made by Wamsteker et al. [11], who in 1993 developed a classification system based on hysteroscopic findings (Table 2). This system was adopted later by the ESGE and it is still the most used today: it considers only the penetration depth of the myoma in myometrial layer. In particular, Wamsteker and colleagues performed a 3-year observational study on patients affected by excessive bleeding undergoing trans-cervical hysteroscopic resections of submucous myomas [11]. All the patients enrolled were classified by distinguishing myomas according to their extension into uterine wall: lesions with no intramural extension were classified as type 0, those with <50% of intramural extension as type 1 and those with ≥50% as type 2 (these stages correspond to the 0, 1, 2 stages, respectively, of the most recent FIGO classification; see below [1]) (Figure 1). The authors determined the intramural myoma depth at hysteroscopy by estimating the angle between the mass and the endometrium at the point in which they collide; in order to reduce the margin of error, they suggested to evaluate this angle at various degrees of uterine distention. At this regard, more recently, Leone et al. [38] established the not-inferior efficacy of sonohysterography in comparison to hysteroscopy for the pre-operative evaluation of submucous myomas. Wamsteker et al. [11] proved that higher is degree, lower is the chance-per- procedure to achieve a complete fibroid resection (92% for type 0, 60% for type I, 50% for type II). In their study, the objective of complete resection was achieved in 96% in case of type 0 myomas, 65% in case of type I myomas and 83.3% in case of type II myomas. Applying this new classification, the authors concluded how trans-cervical resection for type 2 myomas should be not routinely performed, as repeated procedures are necessary to achieve a complete resection (however, in this study, no patient needed more than 3 hysteroscopic resections). Moreover, the complete or incomplete myoma removal had also a beneficial effect on bleeding control. In particular, this target was achieved in 97.8% of patients in the complete resection group and in 60% of those in the incomplete resection group; overall, 94.1% of the patients had control of menstrual bleeding after the treatment.

More recently, Mazzon et al. [39] retrospectively collected data from 1244 women with single myoma undergoing hysteroscopic myomectomy. The authors aim to predict success of a single-step procedure in relation to grade and size of myomas, classified by the Wamsteker/ESGE classification. They concluded that grade and size of myomas can affect the result of the single-step hysteroscopic myomectomy. This was consistent with a similar previous study [40]; in the study by Mazzon et al. all hysteroscopic myomectomies of type 0 myomas were completed in a single-step procedure (100%); the chance of success for a single-step treatment was 88.6% and 82.6% for type 1 and type 2 myomas, respectively. Moreover, type 2 myomas with a diameter >3 cm (equivalent to 14.14 cm^3 of volume) had a higher risk of necessitating multiple procedures [11, 39–41]; an inverse correlation between the age of patients and the need of multiple-step procedures was demonstrated [39].

Other authors evaluated the Wamsteker/ESGE classification for predicting pregnancy outcomes after hysteroscopic myomectomy. Overall, the main evidence is that hysteroscopic myomectomy significantly improved pregnancy rates in case of submucosal myomas [42–44]. Casini et al. [42] reported an increase in pregnancy rate after the treatment of type 0 submucous myomas (from 27 to 43%, $P < 0.05$) and for type 1 and 2 myomas (from 15 to 36%, $P < 0.05$). In another study, Ioannis et al. [45] found that hysteroscopic myomectomy was associated with increased pregnancy rate (57.1% for type 0, 42.8% for type I, 25% for type II myomas); in the latter case, patients receiving expectant management had 50% of fertility rate (however, it was not statistically significative). After hysteroscopic myomectomy, delivery at term was reached by 35.7% of patients with type 0 myomas, 28.5% with type I myomas, and 25% with type II myomas [45]. Similar data resulted from other studies reporting higher pregnancy rates among patients with type 0 and type 1myomas after hysteroscopic myomectomy [45–47].

Table 2. The Wamsteker\ESGE classification system for submucous fibroids [11]

Type	Intramural extension
0	None (pedunculated)
1	< 50% (sessile) < 90-degree angle of myoma surface to uterine wall
2	≥ 50% (sessile) > 90-degree angle of myoma surface to uterine wall

3. THE STEP-W CLASSIFICATION (2005)

The classification developed by Wamsteker et al. [11] focused on the pre-surgical evaluation of myomas aiming to reduce morbidity associated to hysteroscopic myomectomy. However, this classification was judged not accurate for determining the complexity of myomectomy (as it is only based on the penetration of myoma into the uterine wall). Therefore, in 2005 Lasmar et al. [12] designed a new classification system (STEP-W) of submucous myomas, in particular, for better predicting the difficulty of hysteroscopic myomectomy.

The STEP-W classification considers four main parameters (Table 3):

- penetration of the myoma into uterine wall (the authors used the same terminology of the ESGE classification to describe the myoma extension into myometrium).

0 point=no penetration/myoma within the uterine cavity;
1 point = penetration in <50% of the myometrium thickness;
2 points= penetration ≥50% of the myometrium thickness.

- extension of myoma in the uterine wall surface.

0 point = ≤1/3 of the whole uterine wall;
1 point = 1/3-2/3 of the wall;
2 points ≥2/3 of the wall.

- position of the nodule in the uterine cavity by dividing the length of the uterine cavity in three parts.

0 point = lower third;
1 point = middle third;
2 points = upper third.

- lateral wall involvement.

If the myoma is situated in lateral uterine wall, an extra point is added;

- size of the fibroid nodule, intended as maximum diameter by using radiological approach (such as ultrasonography, magnetic resonance, etc.).

0 point = diameter <2 cm;

1 point = 2-5 cm;
2 points = ≥ 5 cm.

In case of multiple submucous myoma, clinician should consider that with the highest score.

After summing each parameter (9 points at maximum can be obtained), three levels of complexity for performing hysteroscopic myomectomy are distinguished (Table 4), and higher is the score, more complex is likely the intervention.

Overall, hysteroscopic myomectomy is considered at low complexity when the score ranges from 0 to 4 (defined also as group I), and at high complexity when the score is 5 or 6 (group II); in this latter case, the pre-operatively use of drugs (such as gonadotropin realizing hormone-analogues [GnRH-a]) or a two-step hysteroscopic myomectomy should be considered [48–53]; alternative techniques should be considered when the score is between 7 and 9 (group III).

Table 3. The STEP-W classification developed by Lasmar et al. [12]

Points	Size (cm)	Topography	Extension of the nodule base	Penetration	Lateral wall involvement
0	<2	Low	< 1/3	0	+1
1	2 to 5	Middle	1/3 to 2/3	< 50%	
2	>5	High	>2/3	>50%	

Table 4. Level of complexity and suggested therapeutic options for each STEP-W group [12]

Complexity and therapeutic options	Group	Score
Low complexity hysteroscopic myomectomy. Consider the recurs to direct operative hysteroscopy.	I	0 to 4
High complexity hysteroscopic myomectomy. Consider the GnRH-a use and/or two-steps hysteroscopic myomectomy.	II	5 to 6
Consider alternatives to the hysteroscopic myomectomy.	III	7 to 9

In order to assess this staging system, Lasmar and collegues performed a 4-year retrospective study considering 62 videos of hysteroscopic myomectomies. The assessment was conducted considering four parameters: achievement of complete resection of the myoma, operating time, fluid deficit, frequency of any complications. The results of the study showed statistically significant differences between the STEP-W I and II groups for total resection ($p < 0.001$), operative time ($p < 0.001$) and fluid deficit ($p = 0.02$). Particularly, in the group I all fibroids (100%) were totally excised; in the group II 58.3% of them were totally excised ($p < 0.001$) (Table 5). However, because of the small sample groups, the rate of complications resulted too low to be analyzed. Adopting the ESGE classification, a statistically significant difference between groups was found only for the operative time.

Table 5. Comparison of outcomes of Wamsteker/ESGE and STEP-W classifications by Lasmar et al. [12]

	ESGE	P value for ESGE	STEP-W	P value for STEP-W
Complete resections (n, %) Type 0/Group I Type I/Group II Type II/Group III	 11/11 (100) 31/32 (96.8) 15/19 (78.9)	 0.07	 50/50 (100) 7/12 (58.3) -	 <0.001*
Operative time (median, range; minutes) Type 0/Group I Type I/Group II Type II/Group III	 5.4 (1.3-13.8) 9.1 (1.1-33.2) 18.1 (1.3-38.4)	 0.002*	 8.2 (1.1-33.0) 23.2 (11.7-38.4) -	 <0.001*
Fluid deficit (mean, ml) Type 0/Group I Type I/Group II Type II/Group III	 56.2 123.2 222.0	 0.17	 89.75 335.0 -	 0.02*

*outcomes statistically significative for the specific classification.

Later in 2011, the Lasmar working group [13] carried out a prospective multicentric trial (on 449 patients), aiming to compare the STEPW and ESGE classifications for predicting the partial or complete hysteroscopic removal of submucous fibroids; a secondary outcome was to test the implementation of the STEP-W classification in different international centres (in China, United States, Brazil and Italy). By using the STEP-W classification, a 100% of complete laparoscopic resections was shown for the group I (score 1 to 4), 77.2% for groups 2 and 3 (score > 4); the complete removal of submucous fibroids dropped to 0% when the score reached 8 points. The results for complete myomas removal were different by adopting the ESGE classification (98.8% for type 0, 93.3% for type 1, 85.2% for type 2 myomas). Some complications occurred in the STEP-W groups: the most severe (1 case of uterine perforation and 1 case of fluid overload) occurred in groups II-III.

In 2012, the same authors [54] performed a new trial including only Brazilian women. The purpose of the study was to evaluate the accuracy of the ESGE and STEP-W classifications to predict complete or partial myomas removal, operative time, rate of post-operative complications and fluid balance during hysteroscopic myomectomy. Group I (STEP-W scores <4) and group II-III (score > 4) were considered. This study evaluated 205 hysteroscopic myomectomies performed by 11 skilled surgeons. Mean operative time was 22.7 min for the group I and 47.6 min for groups II-III; The mean fluid balance was 272.2 mL for group I, 826.6 mL for groups II-II (in general, it has been demonstrated in the clinical practice that 1000 mL is the maximum amount of fluid absorbance before the onset of severe adverse events related to the procedure; anyway, this parameter is variable, depending on several factors such as stature, clinical status and other comorbidities [17]). Moreover, in this study the accuracy to predict the complete or incomplete removal of submucous fibroids was investigated. Similarly to the results of the two previous studies by Lasmar et al. in 2011 [13] and in 2005 [12], all myomas with score <4 were completely removed. By using the STEPW classification, it was noticed that 9 of 11 (82%) major complications occurred in myomas with score > 4; notably, this classification not only correlated with the amount of complications, but also with their severity. Overall, this study showed that a score > 4 was associated with longer operative time, higher level of fluid balance and surgical complications ($p < 0.01$); on the other hand, the ESGE scores did not resulted statistically associated with these variables.

4. The FIGO Staging System for Uterine Fibroids (2011)

In 2011, the FIGO [1] published a revision of myoma staging system in a paper dealing with the causes of AUB in women of reproductive age. In addition to primary and secondary classifications (descripted below), a third classification was added; this was based on the previous ESGE classification (type 0, 1, 2 myomas), but it tends to give a more detailed description of myoma location (Table 6, Figure 1).

Table 6. The FIGO classification systems developed for uterine myomas [1]

Primary classification	Absent or present	
Secondary classification	Submucosal or others	
Tertiary classification	Submucosal	Pedunculated intracavitary ≤50% intramural ≥50% intramural
	Other	Contacts endometrium Intramural Subserosal ≥50% intramural Subserosal ≤50% intramural Subserosal pedunculated Other (for example cervical parasitic)
	Hybrid leiomyomas: interests both endometrium (first number) and serosa (second number)	1-6 (for example, hybrid 1–6 means that the myoma is 50% or more located within the endometrial cavity; less than 50% of the leiomyoma is located subserosally outside the myometrium).

FIGO has proposed three classification:

- Primary classification, defined by presence or absence of 1 or more fibroids, regardless of location, number, and size. Thus, it requires only a sonographic assessment of the presence of the myoma;
- Secondary classification, which considers the specific distinction of submucosal fibroids;

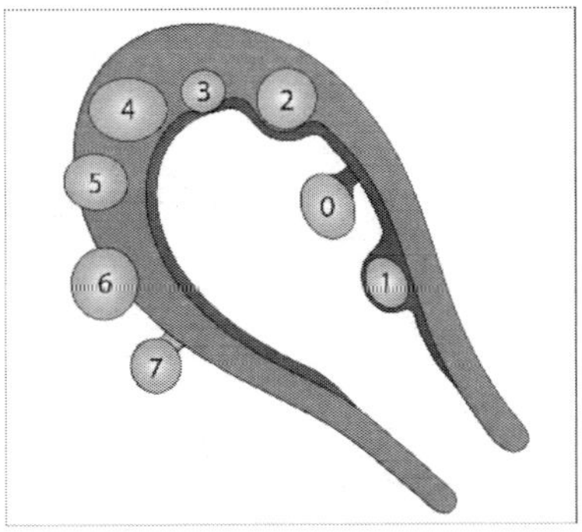

Figure 1. Graphic representation of nodule position into uterine wall according to the FIGO classification system for uterine fibroid.

- Tertiary classification, proposed by Malcolm Munro in 2009 [55], which adopts the ESGE classification system for submucous myomas (type 0, 1, 2) adding also the description of the full spectrum of myoma locations. In fact, the FIGO has added the following subtypes of myomas:
  - type 3, which has direct contact with the endometrium without nevertheless distorting the endometrial cavity;
  - type 4, which is located entirely within the myometrium and it has no direct relation to endometrial cavity or to the serosa;
  - types 5, 6 and 7 (which are equivalent to the three submucous myomas types according to the ESGE classification, but in relation to the serosa instead of the endometrial cavity). Type 5 refers to subserosal myoma with ≥50% of myometrium involved; type 6 to subserosal myoma with ≤50% of myometrium involved; type 7 to subserosal pedunculated myoma;
  - type 8, which represents fibroids with unusual locations (such as cervix) or parasitic myomas. They are described by using a mixed description including the number 8 and a specific location (in written words).

The FIGO classification system allows for using a hybrid nomenclature (to render the description of certain myomas easier). Two numbers are reported and separated by a hyphen: the first number reports the relationship between the myoma and the endometrium;

the second refers to the relationship between the myoma and the mucosa. The theoretical advantage described for this classification is a clear description of myomas, which aims to make the management, the information-sharing and the choice of the best surgical option easier. Recently, to determine the reproducibility of the FIGO classification system for fibroids, Laughlin-Tommaso et al. [56] demonstrated that among 42 myomas, only 14% were classified unanimously whereas 86% were described by using at least two options. In addition, 36% of them had staging discrepancies, which theoretically could impact on the best surgical planning. Thus, additional studies are needed in order to validate the FIGO fibroid classification system.

CONCLUSION

Since 1990, different classifications have been proposed for finding an adequate myoma classification. The work by Wamsteker et al. represents the first attempt to establish a standardized approach in their systematic categorization: this classification tries to predict the surgical outcome for myomas (complete or incomplete hysteroscopic removal) in relation to the degree of intramural extension. This classification has been employed for evaluating the fertility improvement after the removal of myomas: overall, it has been demonstrated a significant improvement of fertility rate for surgically treated type 0 and 1 fibroids, but a reduced benefit for type 2 fibroid (probably due to several mechanisms such as cavity deformation, increased uterine contractility, endometrial inflammation and impaired endometrial blood flow [32]). The major limitation of the Wamsteker/ESGE classification is that it does not describe all fibroid subtypes and it does not suggest the best treatment option for each one. Moreover, over time it has showed a poor correlation with the complexity of the surgical procedure.

As a consequence, in 2005 Lasmar et al. proposed the STEP-W classification: in addition to the intramural extension of myomas, it considered other parameters such as size, position and extension of the myoma on uterine wall. Over time, this classification underwent revision by the same working group in order to improve the accuracy for predicting surgical outcomes. In general, the STEP-W system has shown to be a valid tool for evaluating the likelihood of complete or partial hysteroscopic myoma resection, fluid balance, and length of surgery. Thus, it seems to help the surgeon to plan the best individual treatment. This classification suggests that groups III myomas should be treated with alternatives techniques to the hysteroscopy, even if there is no general agreement on which is the best treatment option in this setting. At the moment, the STEP-W system has been not yet analyzed for predicting important post-surgical outcomes such as improvement of heavy menstrual bleeding or infertility after myoma removal.

In 2011, FIGO published a new fibroid classification system. This classification system is relatively simple to use and it seems to be a useful tool for both researchers and clinicians: it does not consider myoma size, number and the uterine wall location. Thus, although are not part of the classification these additional variables should be considered when describing these benign tumors. Unfortunately, it does not clarify the clinical management of certain myoma types: in fact, guidelines for type 4, 5, 6 and 7 myomas are still under development whereas there is no guideline for symptomatic type 3 myoma [57]. Thus, differently from other classification systems, it necessitates further validation studies because its heterogeneous interpretability, which may negatively impact the treatment choice. Many of the previous limitations have been resolved into the STEP-W classification, specifically designed to have an immediate clinical and surgical utility in selected situations.

In conclusion, at this time, further investigations are needed for accurately classifying myomas. Until now, there are insufficient data to suggest which classification provides the best combination of clinical and research accuracy.

References

[1] Munro MG, Critchley HOD, Broder MS, Fraser IS. FIGO classification system (PALM-COEIN) for causes of abnormal uterine bleeding in nongravid women of reproductive age. *Int J Gynecol Obstet.* 2011;113(1):3-13.

[2] Baird DD, Dunson DB, Hill MC, Cousins D, Schectman JM. High cumulative incidence of uterine leiomyoma in black and white women: Ultrasound evidence. *Am J Obstet Gynecol.* 2003;188(1): 100–7.

[3] Marshall LM, Spiegelman D, Barbieri RL, Goldman MB, Manson JE, Colditz GA, et al. Variation in the incidence of uterine leiomyoma among premenopausal women by age and race. *Obstet Gynecol.* 1997;90(6):967-73.

[4] Myomas and reproductive function. *Fertil Steril.* 2008 Sep;90(5): S111-6.

[5] Wallach EE, Verkauf BS. Myomectomy for fertility enhancement and preservation. *Fertil Steril.* 1992;58(1):1-15.

[6] Hunt, John E and Wallach EE. Uterine factors in infertility—an overview. *Clin Obstet Gynecol.* 1974;17(4):44–64.

[7] Alessandri F, Lijoi D, Mistrangelo E, Ferrero S, Ragni N. Randomized study of laparoscopic versus minilaparotomic myomectomy for uterine myomas. *J Minim Invasive Gynecol.* 2006;13(2):92–7.

[8] Donnez J, Jadoul P. What are the implications of myomas on fertility? A need for a debate?. *Human Reproduction.* 2002;17:1424–30.

[9] Wallach EE, Buttram VC, Reiter RC. Uterine leiomyomata: etiology, symptomatology, and management. *Fertil Steril.* 1981;36(4):433-45.

[10] Olive DL. The Surgical Treatment of Fibroids for Infertility. *Semin Reprod Med.* 2011;29(02):113–23.

[11] Wamsteker K, Emanuel MH, de Kruif JH. Transcervical hysteroscopic resection of submucous fibroids for abnormal uterine bleeding: results regarding the degree of intramural extension. *Obstet Gynecol.* 1993;82(5):736-40.

[12] Lasmar RB, Barrozo PRM, Dias R, De Oliveira MAP. Submucous myomas: A new presurgical classification to evaluate the viability of hysteroscopic surgical treatment - Preliminary report. *J Minim Invasive Gynecol.* 2005;12(4):308-11.

[13] Lasmar RB, Xinmei Z, Indman PD, Celeste RK, Di Spiezio Sardo A. Feasibility of a new system of classification of submucous myomas: A multicenter study. *Fertil Steril.* 2011;95(6):2073-7.

[14] Aydeniz B, Gruber I V., Schauf B, Kurek R, Meyer A, Wallwiener D. A multicenter survey of complications associated with 21 676 operative hysteroscopies. *Eur J Obstet Gynecol Reprod Biol.* 2002;104(2):160–4.

[15] Jansen FW, Vredevoogd CB, Van Ulzen K, Hermans J, Trimbos JB, Trimbos-Kemper TCM. Complications of hysteroscopy: a prospective, multicenter study. *Obstet Gynecol.* 2000;96(2):266–70.

[16] Bradley LD. Complications in hysteroscopy: Prevention, treatment and legal risk. *Current Opinion in Obstetrics and Gynecology.* 2002;14(4):409-15.

[17] AAGL Practice Report: Practice Guidelines for the Diagnosis and Management of Submucous Leiomyomas. *J Minim Invasive Gynecol.* 2012;19(2):152–71.

[18] Cramer SF, Patel A. The frequency of uterine leiomyomas. *Am J Clin Pathol.* 1990;94(4):435–8.

[19] Ferrero S, Abbamonte LH, Giordano M, Parisi M, Ragni N, Remorgida V. Uterine myomas, dyspareunia, and sexual function. *Fertility and Sterility.* 2006;86(5):1504-10.

[20] Lumsden M a, Wallace EM. Clinical presentation of uterine fibroids. *Baillieres Clin Obstet Gynaecol.* 1998;12(2):177-95.

[21] Pritts EA, Parker WH, Olive DL. Fibroids and infertility: an updated systematic review of the evidence. *Fertil Steril.* 2009;91(4):1215-23.

[22] Day Baird D, Garrett TA, Laughlin SK, Davis B, Semelka RC, Peddada SD. Short-term change in growth of uterine leiomyoma: Tumor growth spurts. *Fertil Steril.* 2011;95(1):242-6.

[23] Mavrelos D, Ben-Nagi J, Holland T, Hoo W, Naftalin J, Jurkovic D. The natural history of fibroids. *Ultrasound Obstet Gynecol.* 2010;35(2):238-42.

[24] Farrer???Brown G, Beilby JOW, Tarbit MH. the Vascular Patterns in Myomatous Uteri. *BJOG An Int J Obstet Gynaecol.* 1970;77(11): 967–75.

[25] Bajekal N, Li TC. Fibroids, infertility and pregnancy wastage. *Hum Reprod Update.* 2000;6(6):614–20.

[26] Coutinho EM, Maia HS. The contractile response of the human uterus, fallopian tubes, and ovary to prostaglandins in vivo. *Fertil Steril.* 1971;22(9):539–43.

[27] Marret H, Fritel X, Ouldamer L, Bendifallah S, Brun JL, De Jesus I, et al. Therapeutic management of uterine fibroid tumors: Updated French guidelines. *European Journal of Obstetrics Gynecology and Reproductive Biology.* 2012;165(2):156-64

[28] Clevenger-Hoeft M, Syrop CH, Stovall DW, Van Voorhis BJ. Sonohysterography in premenopausal women with and without abnormal bleeding. *Obstet Gynecol.* 1999;94(4):516–20.

[29] Stewart EA. Uterine fibroids. *Lancet.* 2001;357(9252):293-8.

[30] Wallach EE, Vlahos NF. Uterine myomas: An overview of development, clinical features, and management. *Obstetrics and Gynecology.* 2004;104(2):393-406.

[31] Bendifallah S, Brun J-L, Fernandez H. Myomectomy for infertile women: the role of surgery. *J Gynecol Obstet Biol Reprod.* 2011;40(8):885-901.

[32] Taylor E, Gomel V. The uterus and fertility. *Fertility and Sterility.* 2008; 89(1):1-16.

[33] Hurst BS. Uterine fibroids. *Ultrasound Imaging Reprod Med Adv Infertil Work Treat Art.* 2014;117–31.

[34] Galliano D, Bellver J, Díaz-García C, Simón C, Pellicer A. Art and uterine pathology: How relevant is the maternal side for implantation? *Hum Reprod Update.* 2015;21(1):13–38.

[35] Khaund A, Lumsden MA. Impact of fibroids on reproductive function. *Best Practice and Research: Clinical Obstetrics and Gynaecology.* 2008;22(4):749-60.

[36] Somigliana E, Vercellini P, Daguati R, Pasin R, De Giorgi O, Crosignani PG. Fibroids and female reproduction: a critical analysis of the evidence. *Hum Reprod Update.* 2007;13(5):465-76.

[37] Purohit P, Vigneswaran K. Fibroids and Infertility. *Curr Obstet Gynecol Rep.* 2016;5(2):81–8.

[38] Leone FPG, Lanzani C, Ferrazzi E. Use of strict sonohysterographic methods for preoperative assessment of submucous myomas. *Fertil Steril.* 2003;79(4):998–1002.

[39] Mazzon I, Favilli A, Grasso M, Horvath S, Bini V, Di Renzo GC, et al. Predicting success of single step hysteroscopic myomectomy: A single centre large cohort study of single myomas. *Int J Surg.* 2015;1;22:10–4.

[40] Murakami T, Hayasaka S, Terada Y, Yuki H, Tamura M, Yokomizo R, et al. Predicting Outcome of One-Step Total Hysteroscopic Resection of Sessile Submucous Myoma. *J Minim Invasive Gynecol.* 2008;15(1):74-7.

[41] Emanuel MH. Hysteroscopy and the treatment of uterine fibroids. *Best Pract Res Clin Obstet Gynaecol.* 2015;29(7):920–9.

[42] Casini ML, Rossi F, Agostini R, Unfer V. Effects of the position of fibroids on fertility. *Gynecol Endocrinol.* 2006;22(2):106–9.

[43] Bosteels J, Weyers S, Puttemans P, Panayotidis C, Van Herendael B, Gomel V, et al. The effectiveness of hysteroscopy in improving pregnancy rates in subfertile women without other gynaecological symptoms: A systematic review. *Human Reproduction Update.* 2010;16(1):1-11.

[44] Vercellini P, Zàina B, Yaylayan L, Pisacreta A, De Giorgi O, Crosignani PG. Hysteroscopic myomectomy: Long-term effects on menstrual pattern and fertility. *Obstet Gynecol.* 1999;94(3):341-7.

[45] Ioannis S, Aristotelis A, Antonios T, Panagiotis S, John B. Fertility rates after hysteroscopic treatment of submucous myomas depending on their type. *Gynecol Surg.* 2006;3(3):206–10.

[46] Shokeir TA. Hysteroscopic management in submucous fibroids to improve fertility. *Arch Gynecol Obstet.* 2005 Nov;273(1):50–4.

[47] Namazov A, Karakus R, Gencer E, Sozen H, Acar L. Do submucous myoma characteristics affect fertility and menstrual outcomes in patients underwent hysteroscopic myomectomy? *Iran J Reprod Med.* 2015;13(6):367–72.

[48] Ferrero S, Venturini PL, Remorgida V. Letrozole monotherapy in the treatment of uterine myomas. *Fertility and Sterility.* 2010;93(7):e31.

[49] Tafi E, Scala C, Leone Roberti Maggiore U, Bizzarri N, Candiani M, Venturini PL, et al. Drug safety evaluation of ulipristal acetate in the treatment of uterine fibroids. *Expert Opin Drug Saf.* 2015;14(6):965–77.

[50] Ferrero S, Vellone VG, Barra F. Pharmacokinetic drug evaluation of ulipristal acetate for the treatment of uterine fibroids. *Expert Opinion on Drug Metabolism and Toxicology.* 2018;14(1):107-116.

[51] Bizzarri N, Ghirardi V, Remorgida V, Venturini PL, Ferrero S. Three-month treatment with triptorelin, letrozole and ulipristal acetate before hysteroscopic resection of uterine myomas: prospective comparative pilot study. *Eur J Obstet Gynecol Reprod Biol.* 2015;192:22–6.

[52] Ferrero S, Alessandri F, Vellone VG, Venturini PL, Leone Roberti Maggiore U. Three-month treatment with ulipristal acetate prior to laparoscopic myomectomy of large uterine myomas: a retrospective study. *Eur J Obstet Gynecol Reprod Biol.* 2016;205:43–7.

[53] Leone Roberti Maggiore U, Scala C, Venturini PL, Ferrero S. Preoperative treatment with letrozole in patients undergoing laparoscopic myomectomy of large uterine myomas: A prospective non-randomized study. *Eur J Obstet Gynecol Reprod Biol.* 2014;181:157–62.

[54] Lasmar RB, Lasmar BP, Celeste RK, da Rosa DB, Depes D de B, Lopes RGC. A New System to Classify Submucous Myomas: A Brazilian Multicenter Study. *J Minim Invasive Gynecol.* 2012;19(5):575–80.

[55] Munro MG. *Abnormal Uterine Bleeding*. Cambridge University Press; 2009.

[56] Laughlin-Tommaso SK, Hesley GK, Hopkins MR, Brandt KR, Zhu Y, Stewart EA. Clinical limitations of the International Federation of Gynecology and Obstetrics (FIGO) classification of uterine fibroids. *Int J Gynecol Obstet.* 2017;139(2):143–8.

[57] Capmas P, Voulgaropoulos A, Legendre G, Pourcelot AG, Fernandez H. Hysteroscopic resection of type 3 myoma: a new challenge?. *Eur J Obstet Gynecol Reprod Biol.* 2016;205:165–9.

In: Uterine Fibroids
Editors: Simone Ferrero and Fabio Barra

ISBN: 978-1-53615-046-9

Chapter 3

ULTRASONOGRAPHIC ASSESSMENT OF UTERINE MYOMAS

Fabio Barra[1,2,*]***, MD, Umberto Leone Roberti Maggiore***[1,2]***, MD, Gloria D'Alessandro***[1,2]***, MD, Giulio Evangelisti***[1,2]***, MD, Matteo Tantari***[1,2]***, MD, Franco Alessandri***[3]***, MD and Simone Ferrero***[1,2]***, MD, PhD***

[1]Academic Unit of Obstetrics and Gynecology,
IRCCS Ospedale Policlinico, San Martino, Genoa, Italy
[2]Department of Neurosciences, Rehabilitation, Ophthalmology, Genetics,
Maternal and Child Health (DiNOGMI), University of Genoa, Italy
[3]Unit of Obstetrics and Gynecology, IRCCS Ospedale Policlinico
San Martino, Genoa, Italy

ABSTRACT

Uterine myomas (or fibroids) are the most common form of benign uterine tumors. They occur in 50–60% of women, rising to 70% by the age of 50. Clinically, uterine myomas are mostly asymptomatic, often incidentally found on pelvic examination or by routinely ultrasound evaluation; otherwise, in 30–40% of cases, they cause a large variety of symptoms, which depend on their location and size. The goals of ultrasonographic imaging for myomas include localization, measurement, characterization as well as differential diagnosis from other endometrial and myometrial pathologies. An accurate assessment of their size and location relative to pelvic anatomy is critical to plan the most appropriate therapeutic management. The aim of this chapter in to introduce the role of ultrasonography in the preoperative work-up for uterine myomas.

[*] Corresponding Author's E-mail: fabio.barra@icloud.com.

Keywords: uterine myomas, ultrasound, transvaginal ultrasound, abdominal ultrasound, color Doppler, power Doppler, elastosonography

INTRODUCTION

Uterine myomas (or fibroids) represent the most common form of benign uterine tumors. They occur in 50–60% of women, rising to 70% by the age of 50 [1]. It has been demonstrated that black women have a threefold higher incidence of myomas than white women. Moreover, the prevalence of clinically significant tumors peaks in the perimenopausal years and declines after menopause [1].

In the majority of cases (>50%), myomas are asymptomatic; otherwise, around 30% of women affected may experience multitude of clinical presentations including abnormal bleeding, pelvic masses, pelvic pain, infertility, bulk symptoms and obstetric complications [2, 3].

Currently, the therapeutic options for myomas are medical (hormonal 4-9] and non-hormonal), radiological (uterine fibroid embolization and magnetic resonance-guided focused ultrasound [10, 11]), and surgical (myomectomy 12] and hysterectomy). In particular, with refinement in endoscopic techniques, the laparoscopic surgical management for treating these common benign tumors has gained popularity being characterized by better esthetic outcome, less postoperative pain, and shorter hospital stay in comparison with traditional open surgical methods [13].

Numerous classifications for myomas have been reported in the literature [14]. In general, all of them consider the degree of intramural extension and/or uterine cavity distortion; the classification adopted by the ESGE (European Society for Gynecological Endoscopy) has the advantage of being very understandable (according to it, G0 intends a pedunculated intrauterine myoma, G1 a myomas with largest part (>50%) in the uterine cavity, and G2 with largest part (>50%) in the myometrium); the more recent FIGO classification [15] describes eight types of myomas as well as a hybrid class (association of two types of myomas). This classification is considered more representative for myomas distribution.

Clinically, uterine myomas are often incidentally found on pelvic examination or by routinely ultrasound evaluation. Anyway, they may be suspected when an enlarged uterus or a mass is detected during a pelvic examination or when patients experience heavy menstrual bleeding [3].

In patients with suspicion of uterine myomas, other diagnosis such as adenomyosis, solid tumors of adnexa, and endometrial polyps should be excluded. For this reason, imaging techniques are critical for correctly decting the presence of uterine myomas and thus planning themost appropriate medical or surgical treatment. The diagnostic procedures for investigating these women include ultrasonographic and magnetic resonance imaging (MRI) [12].

Ultrasound is the first-line technique for evaluating uterine myomas, as it is largely available in clinic settings and relatively inexpensive. It can be performed transvaginally or transabdominally; tranvaginal ultrasonography (TVS) provides high resolution imaging and is available in most gynecologic clinics.

Overall, an accurate pre-operative evaluation of myoma size and location is critical to plan the most appropriate therapeutic management [12]; in particular, the goals of ultrasound include localization, measurement, characterization of myomas as well as differential diagnosis from other endometrial and myometrial pathologies.

THE ROLE OF ULTRASOUND

At ultrasound uterine myomas are solid, well-defined, round lesions within the myometrium or attached to it. In general, they are characterized by an inhomogeneous "stripy" or "fasciculate" echo structure with radial shadowing (often referred to as the venetian blind effect) (Figure 1).

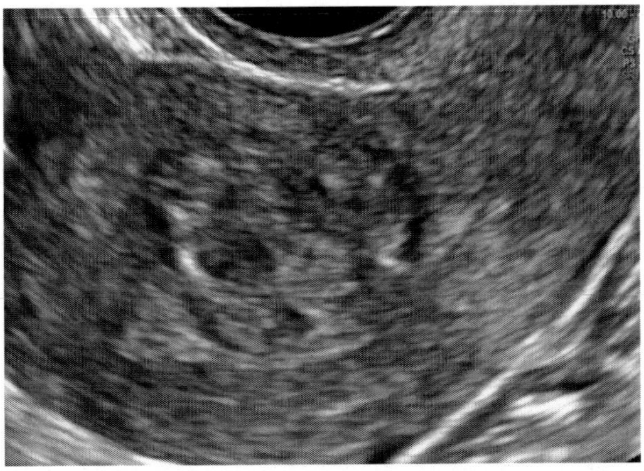

Figure 1. Transvaginal ultrasonography. Intramural FIGO type 2 myoma (largest diameter: 2.4 cm).

Importantly, myomas sonographic texture varies in relation to the different amount of muscle tissue, fibrous stroma, eventual lipomatous or hyaline degeneration and calcification: when fatty tissue is the most prevalent component, their appearance tend to be hyperechoic (Figure 2) [16]; hyperechoic calcification or a hyperechoic capsule due to the deposition of calcium salts may be sometimes detected, especially in postmenopausal women (Figure 3). Anyway, when myomas are small and isoechogenic to the myometrium, the only visible ultrasound sign may be a bulge in the uterine contour [17].

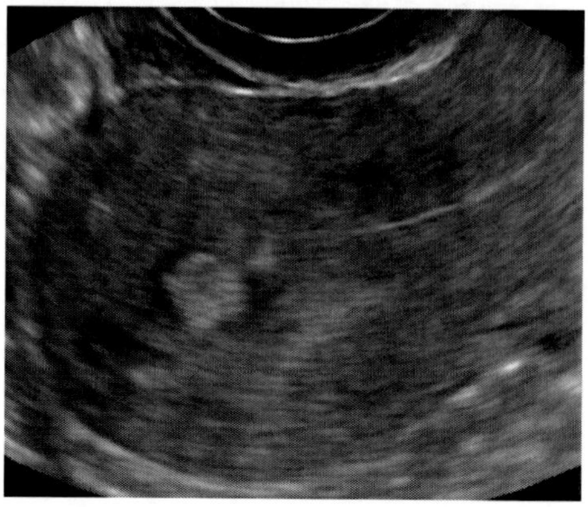

Figure 2. Transvaginal ultrasonography. Small (largest diameter 9 mm) intramural fundal hyperechoic myoma.

In case of relevant size increase, myomas may outgrow their blood supply with subsequent variable degeneration. Moreover, when acute necrosis occurs, myomas tend to present complex heterogeneous internal structures, or internal sonolucent areas; cystic spaces can be sometimes present in cases of central degeneration. In case of fatty degeneration or infiltration, a hyperechoic spherical mass may be detected in the myometrium [18].

The uterus of patients affected by myomas may resulted enlarged with lobular contours, depending on the myomas size and location. Normally, the higher the number of myomas, the greater tends to be the disruption of uterine structure.

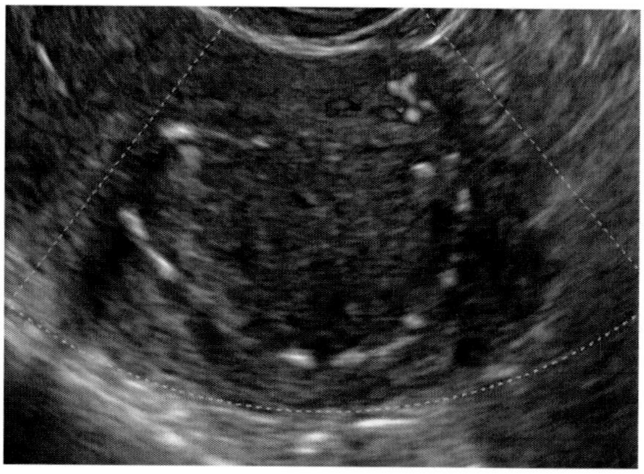

Figure 3. Intramural myoma with peripheral calcifications.

Diameters of myomas should be accurately measured in the three orthogonal planes. In the case of a low number of myomas, it should be recommended to describe each single mass.

Despite of giving accurate resolution and architectural detail, depth penetration of TVS is limited to 10 to 12 cm. Thus, abdominal sonography can be particularly helpful in case of enlarged uterus or whenever the myomas location is not adequately clear at previous TVS. Otherwise, the use of TVS is more accurate in women with large amounts of bowel gas, in those unable to achieve adequate bladder filling and in obese patients, in which the abdominal scan may be very difficult to perform [19].

The ultrasonographic diagnosis of myomas is usually reasonably straightforward; anyway, focal adenomyosis can mimic a myoma as well as a pedunculated myoma can be sometimes mistaken for an adnexal mass [20]. In general, when there is doubt about the origin of a pelvic mass at ultrasound, further evaluation with MRI should be accurately performed [21].

Moreover, large myomas can occasionally lead to obstruction of the ureters, with secondary hydronephrosis. Therefore, ultrasonographic evaluation of the urinary tract should be done whenever a large uterine myomas is detected.

3-dimensional (3D) ultrasound is based on caption of a volume of information, defined as voxels; this technique processes the image evaluating the three orthogonal planes [22].

It has been reported that the addition of 3D multiplanar reconstruction and rendering is able to improve the accuracy of TVS for characterizing myomas [23]. In particular, a more accurate localization of submucous and intramural lesions can be obtained. In a prospective observational cross-sectional study, the diagnostic accuracy of 3D-TVSwas investigated in comparison with that of hysteroscopy for the detection of uterine cavity abnormalities among 69 infertile women. 3D-TVS had 84.1% diagnostic accuracy, 68.2% sensitivity, 91.5% specificity, 79% positive predictive value, and 86% negative predictive value. In particular, this exam successfully succeeded in detecting every case of submucous myoma or other uterine abnormalities [24].

Sonohysterosonography (SHG) is based on TVS during which the additional insertion of contrast agent (such as saline solution) into the endometrial cavity is performed. The distention of the cavity is able to improve visualization of the endometrium as well as delineation of intracavitary lesions (such as submucous myomas and endometrial polyps). This ultrasonographic method also increases the accuracy for determining the degree of penetrance of the myoma into the cavity and myometrium [25]. It has been reported in some studies that the diagnostic accuracy of SHG is comparable to that hysteroscopy with regard to the assessment of endometrial disorders; overall sensitivity and specificity of 96% and 96% for SHG and 100% and 99% for hysteroscopy have been reported in this setting [26]. In a second study, SHG obtained a sensitivity and a specific of 91.38% and of 65.00% whereas hysteroscopy of 98.25% and 85.37%, respectively. Interestingly, the authors found SHG more accurate than TVS but less sensitive and specific than hysteroscopy [27].

Uterine myomas at color and power Doppler tend to demonstrate circumferential flow around the lesion (defined as peri fibroid plexus); otherwise, central flow is not very well represented in these lesions (Figure 4). In general, it has been supposed that centripetal branches can reach the center of this benign tumor via peripheral arteries; thus, the peripheral vascularity of myomas has been demonstrated increased in comparison to normal myometrium and the center portion of the benign tumor [27].

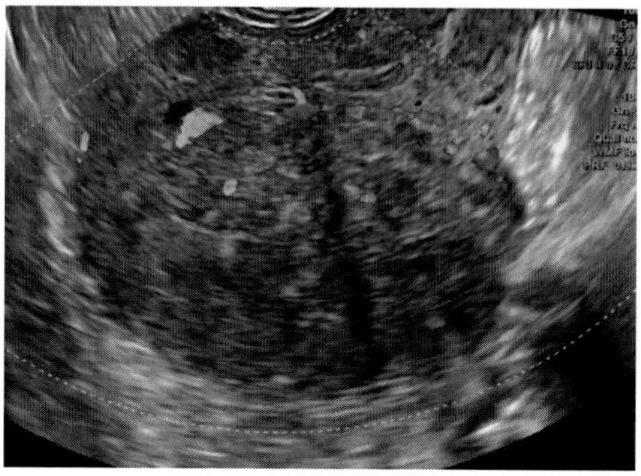

Figure 4. Transvaginal ultrasonography. Intramural FIGO type 5 myoma, peripheral vascularization can be observed (largest diameter: 7.5 cm).

Color flow Doppler imaging completes the myoma ultrasonographic evaluation by estimating location, amount and type of vascular flow to or near the myoma. In particular, it facilitates the operator in distinguishing endometrial polyps that have single feeding vessel from an intracavitary submucosal fibroids and adenomyosis, in which vascularization tends to be characterized by diffusely spread vessels [28, 29].

Additionally, Doppler velocimetry usually attests a decreased resistance index in the peri fibroid plexus of myomas differently from normal myometrium. These indices have been thus largely investigated aiming to differentiate benign from malignant tumors [30]. A statistically significant negative correlation between resistance index parameter and myoma volume has been observed [31]. Moreover, vascular density, ischemic necrosis, and histologic cellular activity score of myomas have been found to be statistically significantly associated with some 3D power Doppler ultrasound parameters. In particular, hyper cellularity, a fibrosclerosis rate less than 25%, and positive Ki-67 staining correlated in a multivariate analysis to high velocimetry index in spherical samples and vascularization flow index; positive CD31 staining (marker of vascularization) was statistically related to high velocimetry index in spherical samples; in contrast, ischemic necrosis was statistically related to low velocimetry index and vascularization flow index [32].

Elastography is an ultrasound-based modality of imaging employed for assessing tissue stiffness. It involves light external tissue compression that provokes strain or displacement within the tissue analyzed. Algorithms calculating the strain profile along the axis of the compression can elaborate the definitive elastographic image: the stiffness of the tissue is graphically represented by colors ranging from red (components with the greatest strain or displacement) to green (components with average strain) to blue (components with no strain). In the literature, it has demonstrated that the mean strain value of elastography differs between uterine myomas (0.08%) and normal myometrium (0.77%) [33].

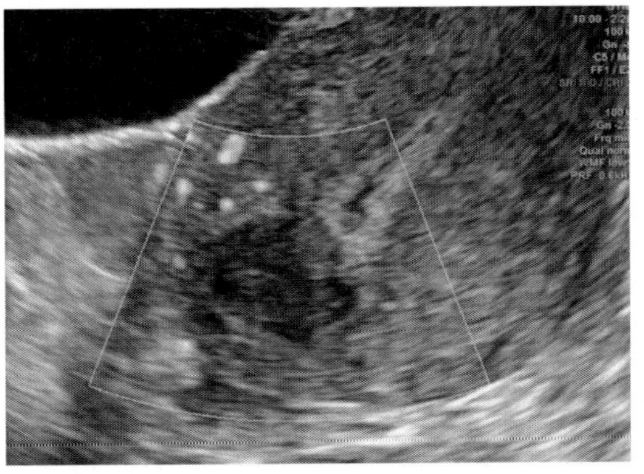

Figure 5. Transvaginal ultrasonography. Intramural FIGO type 3 myoma (largest diameter: 1.8 cm).

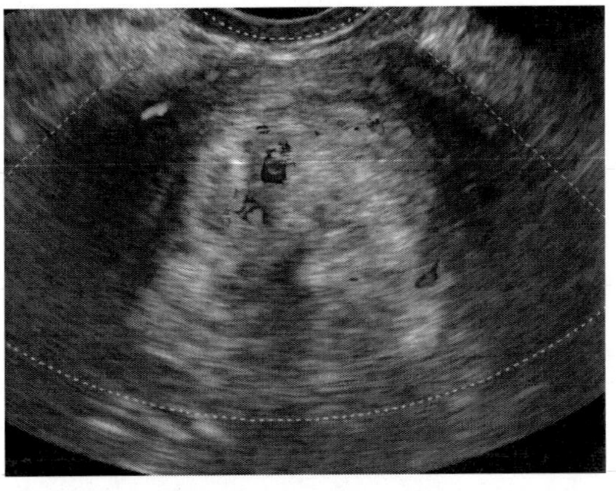

Figure 6. Hyperechoic intramural myoma.

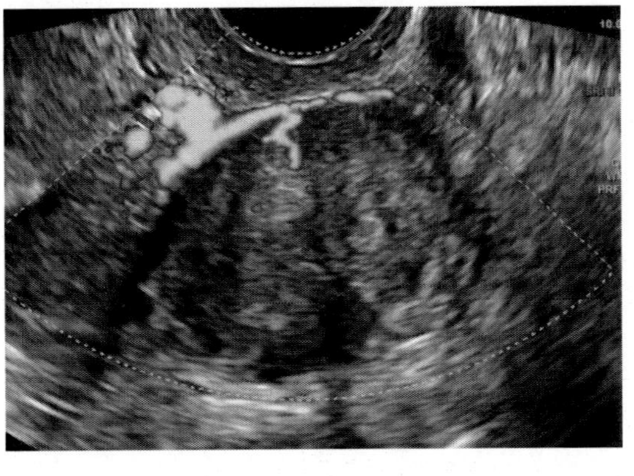

Figure 7. Transvaginal ultrasonography. Sub serous FIGO type 7 myoma, the vascular pedicle can be observed (largest diameter: 4.3 cm).

This may allow for more precise distinction of myomas from the surrounding myometrium. This technique may be helpful for overcoming the commonly observed poor visualization of posterior myoma wall due to acoustic attenuation at conventional ultrasound.

Strain elastography can be also used for better differentiating intrauterine lesions: in fact, due to their histologic structure, it has been assumed that endometrial polyps should appear as soft lesions, whereas submucosal fibroids should appear as hard lesions on this exam.

The accuracy of elastography has been compared with other ultrasonographic techniques in a prospective study; among forty-seven patients underwent hysteroscopy, 18 had submucosal myomas. Overall, the diagnostic accuracy rates for conventional TVS, power Doppler TVS, and strain elastography TVS in distinguishing endometrial polyps and submucosal fibroids resulted to be 70.2%, 65.9%, and 89.4%, respectively [34]. Moreover, in a recent study, Stoelinga et al. demonstrated that elastographic assessment was able to clearly discriminate fibroids from adenomyosis; moreover; this ultrasonographic diagnosis was in excellent agreement with that of MRI [35].

According to their position and association with the uterine wall, myomas are classified as intramural, subserous, or submucous. Ultrasound examination is fondamental to accurately describe type and characteristics of these benign uterine tumors [36].

Overall, intramural myomas are the most commonly found lesions (50%) (Figure 5, 6) [3]. At ultrasound they are usually well demarcated, tending tocompress the sorrounding myometrium and subsequently forming a pseudocapsule. They can be often misdiagnosed as adenomyosis and vice versa; anyway, some ultrasound features, such as cystic anechoic spaces or lakes in the myometrium, subendometrial echoic linear striations and heterogeneous echo texture are usually suggestive of adenomyosis, helping to distinguish these two conditions [37, 38].

Subserosal myomas are localized beneath the peritoneal covering of the uterus, extending into the peritoneal cavity; they may be sessile or pedunculated (Figure 7). In the second case, they are connected to the uterus via a stalk containing vessels. However, the pedicle of a subserous leiomyoma can not be frequently detectable at ultrasound. Nevertheless, the absence of blood flow may characterize necrotic subserous myomas or those undergone torsion [39].

Parasitic myoma is a rare type of pedunculated subserosal myoma partially or completely separated from the uterus; it often receives an alternative blood supply from the omentum and mesenteric vessels [40]. In particular, broad ligament fibroids extend laterally from the uterus and are often confused with adnexal masses [41]. Ultrasound examination may facilitate diagnosis of these type of myomas, allowing a clear visual separation of the uterus and ovaries from this mass as well as the mapping of tumoral vascular supply.

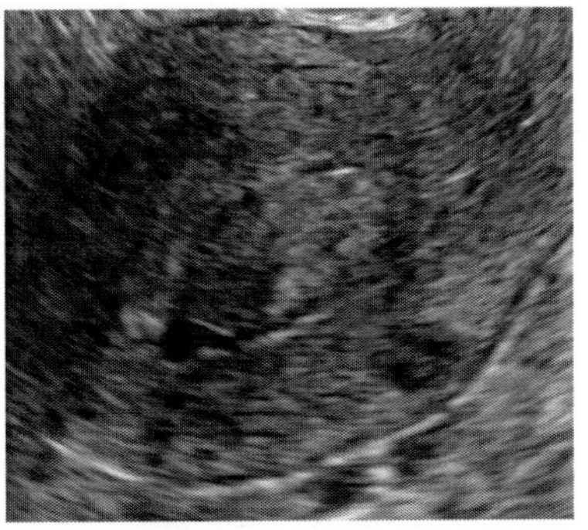

Figure 8a. Transvaginal ultrasonography. Submucosal FIGO type 0 myoma (largest diameter 2.8 cm).

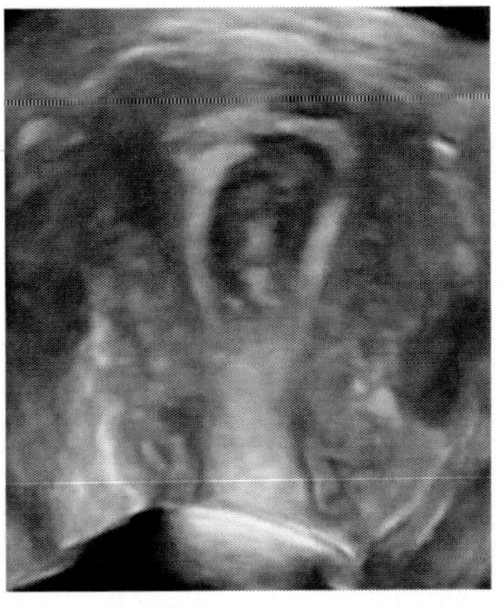

Figure 8b. 3D transvaginal ultrasonography showing the submucosal myoma shown above.

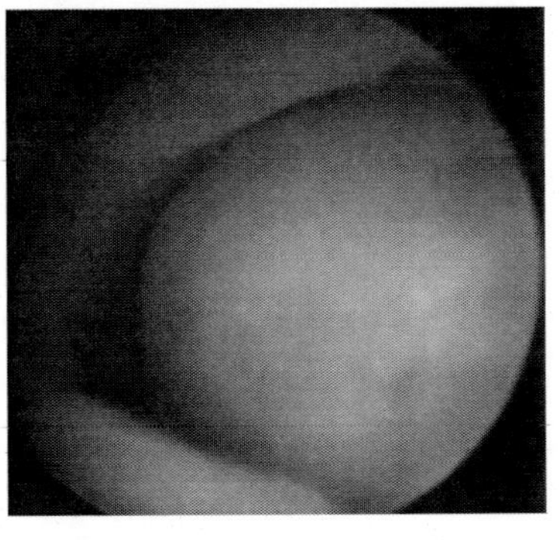

Figure 8c. Hysteroscopic view of the submucosal myoma shown above.

Submucosal myomas, which are located in close proximity to the endometrium, are estimated to represent 5-10% of all myomas; they may be sessile or pedunculated [3]. Submucosal myomas tend to be the most bothersome clinically, often causing relevant symptoms such as menorrhagia (due to the alteration of uterine contractility) and infertility (due to distortion of the endometrium) (Figure 8a-8b-8c). Overall, extending into the uterine cavity, they are evaluated according to the depth of protrusion by standardized classifications.

In general, homogeneous hyperechogenic masses in the uterine cavity at ultrasound are highly suggestive of endometrial polyps; anyway, as discussed before, the myometrial echogenicity of uterine myomas may vary, depending on the size and nature of the myoma. Thus, the distinction of endometrial polyps and submucous myomas can be sometimes difficult.

In case of submucosal fibroids, the distance between the outer margin of the mass and the uterus surface, defined as minimal free myometrial margin, should be measured before performing hysteroscopic resection; in fact, although some studies reported the possibility to remove submucosal myomas with a minimal free margin <5 mm, the recommended margin for the hysteroscopic eligibility ranges between 5 and 10 mm [42, 43].

In terms of the differential diagnosis between endometrial polyps and sub mucous myomas, Tamura-Sadamori et al. reported that if the dimension is above 20 mm, the seconds can be more likely suspected [44]. Moreover, at color Doppler ultrasound myomas tend to have multiple, circular feeding vessels whereas most polyps often present a single feeding artery. Strain elastography complements ultrasound evaluation for assessing these intrauterine lesions as they tend to have different stiffness. SHG allows for accurate delineation of submucosal myomas [45]. From the results published in the literature, it has demonstrated that this procedure presents the same accuracy as hysteroscopy for determining location, breadth of attachment and extent of protrusion into the uterine cavity of submucous myomas [25, 46].

It is extremely difficult to distinguish between benign leiomyoma and malign leiomyosarcoma because the presenting symptoms are very similar.

No imaging technique can reliably differentiate between them because both of them are focal masses within the uterus and both often have central necrosis. Moreover, both may present mixed echogenic and poor echogenic parts, central necrosis; color Doppler appearances of irregular vessel distribution, low impedance to flow, and high peak systolic velocity can be present (Figure 9-10). In these cases, although MRI may be particularly helpful, a definitive diagnosis is only given by histology [21, 47]. In a retrospective study including 13 patients with uterine sarcomas (six leiomyosarcoma and seven carcinosarcoma) and 98 with uterine myomas, ultrasonographic differences at gray scale and at color Doppler were detected between myomas and carcinosarcomas but not between myomas and leiomyosarcomas. Among all, resistance index was significantly different between myomas and carcinosarcomas ($P < .001$) but not between leiomyomas and leiomyosarcomas. Exacoustos C. et al., analyzing the characteristics of eight leiomyosarcomas, reported a median larger size (88% with>8 cm of diameter) and an in homogeneous echo structure characterized by degenerative cystic areas (50%) and rich central vascularization for leiomyosarcomas when compared with the 249 benign myomas [48].

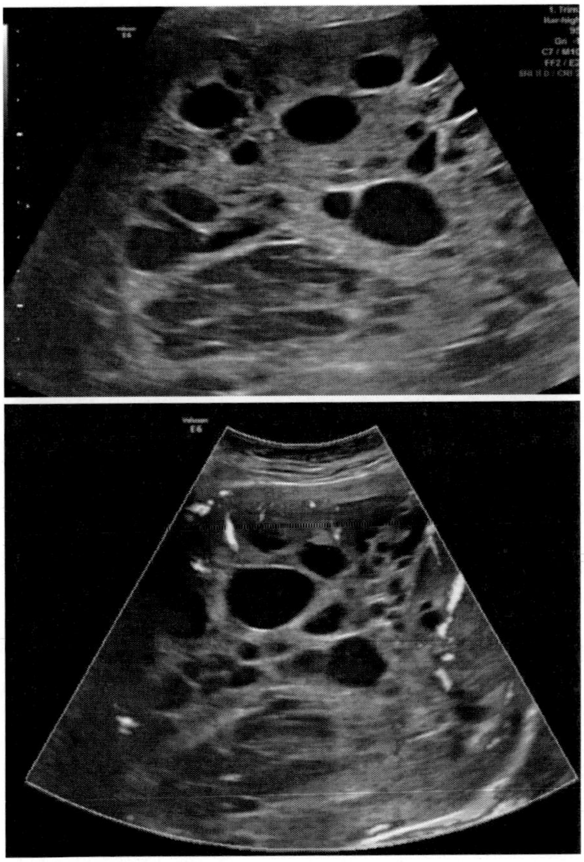

Figure 9-10. Endometrial stromal sarcoma.

CONCLUSION

Nowadays, ultrasonography is the first-line imaging modality for detection and evaluation of uterine myomas, as it is easy, accessible, harmless and inexpensive. Overall, it likely allows the differentiation of these benign uterine tumors from other common gynecological conditions such as adenomyosis or endometrial polyps. Power Doppler blood flow mapping is a useful, practical, and noninvasive ultrasonographic method for the differential diagnosis of these benign intrauterine lesions. Moreover, submucosal myomas can be easily studied by SHG, a simple and well-tolerated procedure that uses saline solution as contrast medium. Results published in the literature show that this procedure presents the same accuracy as hysteroscopy in terms of location, breadth of attachment, and extent of protrusion into the uterine cavity of submucous myomas. Importantly, it is important to under light that MRI provides additional information as a means of further diagnostics in women in whom ultrasound findings are confusing.

References

[1] Sparic R, Mirkovic L, Malvasi A, Tinelli A. Epidemiology of Uterine Myomas: A Review. *International Journal of Fertility & Sterility*. 2016;9(4):424-35.

[2] Vlahos NF, Theodoridis TD, Partsinevelos GA. Myomas and Adenomyosis: Impact on Reproductive Outcome. *Biomed Res Int*. 2017;2017:5926470.

[3] Parker WH. Etiology, symptomatology, and diagnosis of uterine myomas. *Fertil Steril*. 2007;87(4):725-36.

[4] Ferrero S, Racca A, Tafi E, Sozzi F, Leone Roberti Maggiore U, Remorgida V, et al. 3-Month Versus 6-Month Treatment With Ulipristal Acetate Prior to Laparoscopic Hysterectomy of Large Myomatous Uteri. *J Minim Invasive Gynecol*. 2015;22(6S):S108.

[5] Tafi E, Scala C, Leone Roberti Maggiore U, Bizzarri N, Candiani M, Venturini PL, et al. Drug safety evaluation of ulipristal acetate in the treatment of uterine fibroids. *Expert Opin Drug Saf*. 2015;14(6):965-77.

[6] Ferrero S, Vellone VG, Barra F. Pharmacokinetic drug evaluation of ulipristal acetate for the treatment of uterine fibroids. *Expert Opin Drug Metab Toxicol*. 2018;14(1):107-16.

[7] Ferrero S, Vellone VG, Barra F, Scala C. Ulipristal Acetate before Hysteroscopic and Laparoscopic Surgery for Uterine Myomas: Help or Hindrance? *Gynecol Obstet Invest*. 2018:1-13.

[8] Ferrero S, Alessandri F, Vellone VG, Venturini PL, Leone Roberti Maggiore U. Three-month treatment with ulipristal acetate prior to laparoscopic myomectomy of large uterine myomas: a retrospective study. *Eur J Obstet Gynecol Reprod Biol*. 2016;205:43-7.

[9] Ferrero S, Scala C, Barra F. Regarding "Does Ulipristal Acetate Affect Surgical Experience at Laparoscopic Myomectomy?" *J Minim Invasive Gynecol*. 2018;25(3):541.

[10] Silberzweig JE, Powell DK, Matsumoto AH, Spies JB. Management of Uterine Fibroids: A Focus on Uterine-sparing Interventional Techniques. *Radiology*. 2016;280(3):675-92.

[11] Cheung VY. Sonographically guided high-intensity focused ultrasound for the management of uterine fibroids. *J Ultrasound Med*. 2013;32(8):1353-8.

[12] Alessandri F, Lijoi D, Mistrangelo E, Ferrero S, Ragni N. Randomized study of laparoscopic versus minilaparotomic myomectomy for uterine myomas. *J Minim Invasive Gynecol*. 2006;13(2):92-7.

[13] Evans P, Brunsell S. Uterine fibroid tumors: diagnosis and treatment. *Am Fam Physician*. 2007;75(10):1503-8.

[14] Lasmar RB, Barrozo PR, Dias R, Oliveira MA. Submucous myomas: a new presurgical classification to evaluate the viability of hysteroscopic surgical treatment-preliminary report. *J Minim Invasive Gynecol.* 2005;12(4):308-11.

[15] Munro MG, Critchley HO, Fraser IS, Group FMDW. The FIGO classification of causes of abnormal uterine bleeding in the reproductive years. *Fertil Steril.* 2011;95(7):2204-8, 8 e1-3.

[16] Johari B, Koshy M, Sidek S, Hanafiah M. Lipoleiomyoma: a rare benign tumour of the uterus. *BMJ Case Rep.* 2014;2014.

[17] Wilde S, Scott-Barrett S. Radiological appearances of uterine fibroids. *Indian J Radiol Imaging.* 2009;19(3):222-31.

[18] Valentin L. Characterising acute gynaecological pathology with ultrasound: an overview and case examples. *Best Pract Res Clin Obstet Gynaecol.* 2009;23(5):577-93.

[19] Karasick S, Lev-Toaff AS, Toaff ME. Imaging of uterine leiomyomas. *AJR Am J Roentgenol.* 1992;158(4):799-805.

[20] Shwayder J, Sakhel K. Imaging for uterine myomas and adenomyosis. *J Minim Invasive Gynecol.* 2014;21(3):362-76.

[21] Murase E, Siegelman ES, Outwater EK, Perez-Jaffe LA, Tureck RW. Uterine leiomyomas: histopathologic features, MR imaging findings, differential diagnosis, and treatment. *Radiographics.* 1999;19(5):1179-97.

[22] Wong L, White N, Ramkrishna J, Araujo Junior E, Meagher S, Costa Fda S. Three-dimensional imaging of the uterus: The value of the coronal plane. *World J Radiol.* 2015;7(12):484-93.

[23] Dueholm M, Lundorf E, Hansen ES, Ledertoug S, Olesen F. Evaluation of the uterine cavity with magnetic resonance imaging, transvaginal sonography, hysterosonographic examination, and diagnostic hysteroscopy. *Fertil Steril.* 2001;76(2):350-7.

[24] Apirakviriya C, Rungruxsirivorn T, Phupong V, Wisawasukmongchol W. Diagnostic accuracy of 3D-transvaginal ultrasound in detecting uterine cavity abnormalities in infertile patients as compared with hysteroscopy. *Eur J Obstet Gynecol* Reprod Biol. 2016;200:24-8.

[25] Leone FP, Lanzani C, Ferrazzi E. Use of strict sonohysterographic methods for preoperative assessment of submucous myomas. *Fertil Steril.* 2003;79(4):998-1002.

[26] Pasqualotto EB, Margossian H, Price LL, Bradley LD. Accuracy of preoperative diagnostic tools and outcome of hysteroscopic management of menstrual dysfunction. *J Am Assoc Gynecol Laparosc.* 2000;7(2):201-9.

[27] Grimbizis GF, Tsolakidis D, Mikos T, Anagnostou E, Asimakopoulos E, Stamatopoulos P, et al. A prospective comparison of transvaginal ultrasound, saline infusion sonohysterography, and diagnostic hysteroscopy in the evaluation of endometrial pathology. *Fertil Steril.* 2010;94(7):2720-5.

[28] Exacoustos C, Manganaro L, Zupi E. Imaging for the evaluation of endometriosis and adenomyosis. *Best Pract Res Clin Obstet Gynaecol.* 2014;28(5):655-81.

[29] Wozniak A, Wozniak S. Ultrasonography of uterine leiomyomas. *Prz Menopauzalny.* 2017;16(4):113-7.

[30] Pelage JP, Cazejust J, Pluot E, Le Dref O, Laurent A, Spies JB, et al. Uterine fibroid vascularization and clinical relevance to uterine fibroid embolization. *Radiographics.* 2005;25 Suppl 1:S99-117.

[31] Testa AC, Pomini F, Fattorossi A, Battaglia A, Ferrandina G, Mansueto D, et al. Doppler velocimetry and cytofluorimetric analysis in uterine myomas. *Gynecol Obstet Invest.* 2003;56(3):139-42.

[32] Minsart AF, Ntoutoume Sima F, Vandenhoute K, Jani J, Van Pachterbeke C. Does three-dimensional power Doppler ultrasound predict histopathological findings of uterine fibroids? A preliminary study. *Ultrasound Obstet Gynecol.* 2012;40(6):714-20.

[33] Ami O, Lamazou F, Mabille M, Levaillant JM, Deffieux X, Frydman R, et al. Real-time transvaginal elastosonography of uterine fibroids. *Ultrasound Obstet Gynecol.* 2009;34(4):486-8.

[34] Czuczwar P, Wozniak S, Szkodziak P, Kudla MJ, Pyra K, Paszkowski T. Elastography Improves the Diagnostic Accuracy of Sonography in Differentiating Endometrial Polyps and Submucosal Fibroids. *J Ultrasound Med.* 2016;35(11):2389-95.

[35] Stoelinga B, Hehenkamp WJ, Brolmann HA, Huirne JA. Real-time elastography for assessment of uterine disorders. *Ultrasound Obstet Gynecol.* 2014;43(2):218-26.

[36] Donnez J, Dolmans MM. Uterine fibroid management: from the present to the future. *Hum Reprod Update.* 2016;22(6):665-86.

[37] Sakhel K, Abuhamad A. Sonography of adenomyosis. *J Ultrasound Med.* 2012;31(5):805-8.

[38] Ascher SM, Arnold LL, Patt RH, Schruefer JJ, Bagley AS, Semelka RC, et al. Adenomyosis: prospective comparison of MR imaging and transvaginal sonography. *Radiology.* 1994;190(3):803-6.

[39] Roy C, Bierry G, El Ghali S, Buy X, Rossini A. Acute torsion of uterine leiomyoma: CT features. *Abdom Imaging.* 2005;30(1):120-3.

[40] Huang PS, Chang WC, Huang SC. Iatrogenic parasitic myoma: a case report and review of the literature. *Taiwan J Obstet Gynecol.* 2014;53(3):392-6.

[41] Fasih N, Prasad Shanbhogue AK, Macdonald DB, Fraser-Hill MA, Papadatos D, Kielar AZ, et al. Leiomyomas beyond the uterus: unusual locations, rare manifestations. *Radiographics.* 2008;28(7):1931-48.

[42] Ludwin A, Ludwin I, Pitynski K, Basta P, Basta A, Banas T, et al. Transrectal ultrasound-guided hysteroscopic myomectomy of submucosal myomas with a

varying degree of myometrial penetration. *J Minim Invasive Gynecol.* 2013;20(5):672-85.

[43] Pakrashi T. New hysteroscopic techniques for submucosal uterine fibroids. *Curr Opin Obstet Gynecol.* 2014;26(4):308-13.

[44] Tamura-Sadamori R, Emoto M, Naganuma Y, Hachisuga T, Kawarabayashi T. The sonohysterographic difference in submucosal uterine fibroids and endometrial polyps treated by hysteroscopic surgery. *J Ultrasound Med.* 2007;26(7):941-6.

[45] Seshadri S, El-Toukhy T, Douiri A, Jayaprakasan K, Khalaf Y. Diagnostic accuracy of saline infusion sonography in the evaluation of uterine cavity abnormalities prior to assisted reproductive techniques: a systematic review and meta-analyses. *Hum Reprod Update*. 2015;21(2):262-74.

[46] McLucas B. Diagnosis, imaging and anatomical classification of uterine fibroids. *Best Pract Res Clin Obstet Gynaecol.* 2008;22(4):627-42.

[47] Thomassin-Naggara I, Dechoux S, Bonneau C, Morel A, Rouzier R, Carette MF, et al. How to differentiate benign from malignant myometrial tumours using MR imaging. *Eur Radiol.* 2013;23(8):2306-14.

[48] Exacoustos C, Romanini ME, Amadio A, Amoroso C, Szabolcs B, Zupi E, et al. Can gray-scale and color Doppler sonography differentiate between uterine leiomyosarcoma and leiomyoma? *J Clin Ultrasound.* 2007;35(8):449-57.

In: Uterine Fibroids
Editors: Simone Ferrero and Fabio Barra

ISBN: 978-1-53615-046-9

Chapter 4

SURGICAL PATHOLOGY OF UTERINE MYOMAS: FROM USUAL FORMS TO DIFFERENTIAL DIAGNOSIS

Valerio Gaetano Vellone*[1,2,*]*, MD, PhD,
Michele Paudice*[1]*, MD, Chiara Maria Biatta*[1]*, MD,
Leonardo Peñuela*[1,3]*, MD, PhD, Gabriele Gaggero*[4]*, MD,
Fabio Barra*[5,6]*, MD, Simone Ferrero*[5,6]*, MD, PhD
and Bruno Spina*[4]*, MD

[1]Pathology, Department of Integrated Surgical and Diagnostic Sciences (DISC), University of Genoa, Italy
[2]Pathology Academic Unit, IRCCS Ospedale Policlinico San Martino, Genoa, Italy
[3]Fetal, Perinatal and Gynaecologic Pathology Unit, IRCCS Istituto G. Gaslini, Genoa, Italy
[4]Pathology Unit, IRCCS Ospedale Policlinico San Martino, Genoa, Italy
[5]Obstetrics and Gynecology, Department of Neurosciences, Rehabilitation, Ophthalmology, Genetics, Maternal and Child Health (DiNOGMI), University of Genoa, Italy
[6]Academic Unit of Obstetrics and Gynecology, Ospedale San Martino, Genoa, Italy

[*] Corresponding Author's E-mail: vgvellone@gmail.com.

ABSTRACT

Uterine leiomyomas, commonly named fibroids or myomas, represent the most frequent indication for hysterectomy. Hysterectomy, or at least myomectomy, is still the only procedure that – together with consequent histopathological examination – provides sufficient information about the tumor malignancy potential. As a consequence, uterine myomas are common findings in daily practice of gynecological surgical pathologists. These neoplasms generally appear as well-demarcated, solid, whitish elastic masses, often multiple. In most cases there are no issues in their histopathological diagnosis. However, leiomyomas may exhibit a variety of unusual morphology revealing their biological behavior. The malignant counterpart, named leiomyosarcoma and stromal tumors of uncertain malignant potential (STUMP) – in order of malignancy – are much rare but may share the same odd features with otherwise benign lesions, requiring a thorough examination. The description of the morphology of usual leiomyoma and its variants is provided in this chapter.

Keywords: spindle cell leiomyoma, epithelioid leiomyoma, myxoid leiomyoma, surgical pathology, differential diagnosis

1. INTRODUCTION

Uterine leiomyomas, also known as fibroids or simply as myoma, are common findings in daily practice of gynecological surgical pathologists, being the primary indication for hysterectomy in women in reproductive age and accounting for more than 200 000 hysterectomies per year in the USA [1].

Uterine leiomyomas are benign clonal tumors arising from the smooth-muscle cells of the human uterus. They are clinically apparent in about 25% of women [2] and the clinical prevalence may be even higher with the newer imaging techniques. Careful pathological examination of surgical specimens suggests that the prevalence is as high as 77% [3].

Most myomas cause no symptoms, but many women show significant symptoms warranting therapy. Symptoms attributable to myomas can generally be classified in three distinct categories: abnormal uterine bleeding, pelvic pressure and pain, and reproductive dysfunction.

Myomas respond to the gonadal steroid estrogen and progesterone, and their epidemiology reflects the ontogeny and the life-cycle changes of reproductive hormones. They are uncommon in women less than 30 years of age; however, the youngest patient on record was 13 years old. Some leiomyomas apparently shrink after menopause, but their frequency does not decrease. Fibroids are more common in African-American women than in white women [4]. The growth of leiomyomas is affected by the hormonal milieu [5, 6], containing estrogen and progesterone receptors, which can be demonstrated biochemically and immunohistochemically [7]. These tumors remain benign, although they can be numerous, large and responsive to hormones.

During both pregnancy and use of oral contraceptives, concentrations of estrogen and progesterone are high, yet both factors decrease the risk of fibroids. Reproductive factors also affect the risk of myomas. Many studies have shown that being parous (having one or more pregnancies extending beyond 20 weeks) decreases the chance of myoma formation [8, 9]. Thus, influences other than concentrations of steroid hormones are important. The common factor may be the lack of menstrual cyclicity. One hypothesis is that myoma formation may be viewed as a response to injury, potentially from hypoxia in myometrial cells during menstruation [10].

Environmental factors also influence the risk of fibroid formation. Several studies have shown that smoking decreases the risk [11]. Substantial consumption of red meats was associated with an increased relative risk and consumption of green vegetables with a decreased risk [12]. However, there is no evidence that dietary intervention leads to changes in incidence or symptom patterns.

Smooth muscle tumors represent the most common uterine mesenchymal neoplasms that may cause diagnostic dilemmas for the practicing surgical pathologist. In most instances, the clinical behavior of uterine smooth muscle neoplasms can be reliably predicted by application of conventional gross and light microscopic features. Discordance between morphology and clinical outcome may lead to a demanding diagnosis, although these lesions account for a minority of uterine smooth muscle neoplasms.

Benign uterine smooth muscle tumors, especially leiomyoma variants, display a wide spectrum of gross and morphologic appearances becoming often a diagnostic challenge. Correct classification is important as currently prognosis of its malignant counterpart, leiomyosarcoma, is dismal even when confined to the uterus at time of diagnosis [13-15].

A morphological continuity exists between frankly benign nodules with an absolute favorable prognosis and frankly malignant neoplasms with a marked tendency to metastasize to distant sites and to relapse locally with a poor prognosis even in spite of aggressive treatments.

Some rare smooth muscular lesions have peculiar morphological features resulting in an unpredictable clinical course. Such neoplasms are referred to as smooth muscle tumors of unknown malignant potential (STUMP). The designation "uncertain malignant potential" is still warranted, at least until additional experience is accumulated and a better estimate of the potential clinical behavior for these lesions can be obtained.

Leiomyosarcoma represents about 1.3% of uterine malignancies and more than 50% of uterine sarcomas, excluding carcinosarcoma [13]. Approximately 1 of every 800 smooth muscle tumors of the uterus is a leiomyosarcoma, but less than 1% of women thought clinically to have leiomyoma prove to have leiomyosarcoma.

More commonly uterine leiomyomas have typical spindle differentiation but other differentiations do exist. The usual smooth muscle differentiation denotes a pattern of differentiation similar to the constituent cells of the normal myometrium. Usual smooth muscle cells are elongated, possess distinct cell membranes, and have readily apparent eosinophilic, sometimes fibrillar cytoplasm. These cells grow in a fascicular arrangement. Other differentiations, commonly observed in daily practice are epithelioid and myxoid differentiation.

Every differentiation has a malignant counterpart and the differential features for a proper diagnosis are provided in the following sections. Other rarer forms do exist and are illustrated in the following section.

2. Usual Gross Features

These tumors are typically round, well-circumscribed, non-encapsulated myometrial masses (which can be enucleated) with white, whorled, bulging, solid sectioned surfaces.

Leiomyomas are multiple in ~75% of cases and are typically confined to the uterine corpus; <2% are cervical. Leiomyomas are spherical and firm; they bulge above the surrounding myometrium from which they are easily shelled out. The cut surfaces are white to tan, with a whorled trabecular pattern.

Fibroids can be located anywhere in the myometrium, being submucosal, intramural and subserosal. Submucosal leiomyomas compress the overlying endometrium and, as they enlarge, bulge into the endometrial cavity. Rarely, they become pedunculated and prolapse through the cervix. Intramural leiomyomas are the most common. Subserosal leiomyomas can become pedunculated and, if pedicle torsion with subsequent necrosis occurs, the leiomyoma can lose its connection with the uterus. Very rarely, some of them attach to another pelvic structure (parasitic leiomyoma). Rare tumors are confined to the endometrium, but usually these are microscopic.

Despite the variety of histologic subtypes of leiomyoma, all are grossly similar. Multiple leiomyomas are present in two thirds of women with these neoplasms [3]. The appearance of a leiomyoma is commonly altered by degenerative changes. Submucosal leiomyomas are frequently ulcerated and hemorrhagic. The damaged smooth muscle is replaced eventually by firm white or translucent collagenous tissue. Cystic degeneration also occurs, and some leiomyomas become extensively calcified.

3. Usual Microscopic Features: Spindle Cell Leiomyoma

Spindle cell leiomyomas represent, by far, the commonest variant of uterine leiomyoma.

Typical leiomyomas are composed of whorled, anastomosing fascicles of uniform fusiform smooth muscle cells. The spindle-shaped cells have indistinct borders and abundant fibrillar eosinophilic cytoplasm. Nuclei are elongated with blunt or tapered ends, and have finely dispersed chromatin and small nucleoli. Mitotic figures usually are infrequent. Nuclear palisading is occasionally a prominent feature ("schwannoma-like" leiomyoma). Except for leiomyomas more cellular than the surrounding myometrium, typical lesions are identified by their nodular circumscription and by the disorderly arrangement of the smooth muscle fascicles within them, which are out of alignment with the surrounding myometrium. The leiomyomas have a whorled white-tan cut surface that bulges above the surrounding myometrium. Most leiomyomas have a sharp smooth border with the myometrium, but occasionally it is somewhat infiltrative, a finding that is much more common in highly cellular leiomyomas. Degenerative changes are common in leiomyomas. Hyaline fibrosis is present in more than 60%, particularly in postmenopausal women [16]. Variable amounts of collagen that typically increases with age separate the tumor cells, hence the term "fibromyoma" used in older texts. Hyaline change is common and appears as a cellular homogenized collagen that can form bands or plaques or replace large areas of the tumor (Figure 1). Nests and cords of tumor cells can be compartmentalized by collagen, resulting in pseudo-epithelial patterns. Edema is present in about 50% of leiomyomas and, on occasion, marked hydropic change can mimic the appearance of a myxoid smooth muscle tumor or produces a pattern that can be confused with intravenous leiomyomatosis [17, 18]. There are significant areas of hemorrhage, which tend to be zonal and sharply demarcated in enlarged uterus containing multiple leiomyomas. The necrosis found in leiomyomas is typically of infarct type; infarcts consist of necrotic mummified smooth muscle cells and blood vessels, often accompanied by hemorrhage [19]. Some leiomyomas have conspicuous vessels, including large muscular arteries, arterioles, and veins. About 10% of leiomyomas, and cystic degeneration and microcalcification each occur in about 4%. Hemorrhage, edema, myxoid change, hypercellular foci, and cellular hypertrophy occur in leiomyomas in women who are pregnant or taking progestins. Progestational agents are associated with a slight increase in mitotic activity, but not to the level observed in a leiomyosarcoma. The margins of most leiomyomas are microscopically circumscribed, but some benign tumors interdigitate with the surrounding myometrium, occasionally extensively. Submucousal leiomyomas, particularly if they protrude into the endometrial cavity, may display extensive necrosis, often with acute inflammatory cells. Not infrequently, there is increased mitotic activity in tumor cells around areas of necrosis. On the other hand, the coagulative tumor cell necrosis common in leiomyosarcoma is not often associated with acute inflammation. In addition, the outlines of cells are prominent in the latter whereas they are inconspicuous or absent in submucous necrosis. Also, the mitotic figures seen in conjunction with inflammatory necrosis have normal morphology.

Figure 1. Typical uterine spindle cell leiomyoma composed of bland cells with smooth muscle differentiation intermingled with abundant collagenous stroma (hematoxylin/eosin, 200x).

4. Epithelioid Leiomyoma

This category includes tumors formerly classified as leiomyoblastomas, clear cell leiomyomas, and plexiform leiomyomas [20]. Grossly they appear yellow or gray and may contain areas of hemorrhage, tending to be softer than the usual leiomyoma; they are solitary and can occur in any part of the uterus. The median diameter is 6–7 cm. Epithelioid smooth muscle cells are round or polygonal and have eosinophilic to colorless cytoplasm. They may have perinuclear cytoplasmic vacuoles or there may be a perinuclear rim of eosinophilic cytoplasm, although the rest of the cytoplasm is clear. Leiomyoblastoma is composed of round cells with eosinophilic cytoplasm resembling fetal uterine smooth cells. When the cytoplasm is completely clear, the label "clear cell" is used. The cells may contain glycogen, but there is minimal lipid component and mucin is absent. The nucleus sometimes is displaced to the periphery of the cell, resulting in a signet-ring appearance. Plexiform leiomyoma is characterized by cords or nests of round cells with scanty to moderate amounts of cytoplasm. Transition to more typical spindled smooth muscle cells is often identified within an epithelioid leiomyoma. Immunohistochemistry generally demonstrate positivity for smooth muscle markers such as desmin and alpha smooth muscle actin; keratin stains too may be positive. CD1a and HMB45 are usually negative. The behavior of epithelioid smooth muscle neoplasms of the uterus is difficult to predict [21, 22]. Small tumors that lack cytologic atypia, tumor cell necrosis, and an elevated mitotic index can be safely regarded as benign. The behavior of epithelioid leiomyomas with two or more of the following features is not well established: large size (>6 cm), moderate mitotic activity (2–4 MF/10HPF), moderate to severe cytologic atypia, and necrosis. Neoplasms with moderate to severe atypia, without necrosis, and fewer than 5 MF/10HPF should be classified as STUMP because experience is too limited to be certain about their aggressive potential. Careful follow-up is warranted. Neoplasms with 5 MF/10HPF metastasize with sufficient frequency that all should be regarded as epithelioid leiomyosarcomas [20].

5. Myxoid Leiomyoma

Myxoid leiomyomas represent a rare neoplasm with a putative correlation with pregnancy. They usually appear soft and translucent on gross examination, and may have focal or extensive gelatinous appearance. Microscopically, there is abundant amorphous myxoid material between islands of spindled and stellated smooth muscle cells in myxoid connective tissue containing large vessels. Myxoid areas are weakly basophilic and alcianophilic. The nuclei appear small and bland with no atypia and no mitotic activity [23]. The margins of a myxoid leiomyoma are circumscribed, and neither cytologic atypia nor mitotic features are present. Areas of ordinary leiomyoma should be present focally. Large myxoid smooth muscle tumors and those in which an infiltrating margin, cytologic atypia, or mitotic activity are observed microscopically should be regarded with suspicion. Hydropic degeneration of a conventional leiomyoma and myxoid leiomyosarcoma should be considered in differential diagnosis.

6. Rare and Peculiar Variants and Presentations

Spindle cell, epithelioid and myxoid leiomyomas are the most relevant and commonly observed histological forms of uterine leiomyomas but other rare and peculiar variants can be observed in daily practice. Their features can cause some issue concerning the risk of malignancy and relapse. Diagnostic dilemmas may arise due to the presence of cytological atypia (such as in cellular leiomyomas or leiomyomas with bizarre nuclei), for mitotic activity (as in mitotically active leiomyomas) or for clinical and topographic presentation (such as intravascular leiomyomas or metastasizing leiomyomas). Moreover, the hormonal status of the patient and previous medical treatment can change the usual histology of the neoplasm, raising concerns for malignancy.

6.1. Mitotically Active Leiomyoma

These tumors are otherwise typical spindle cell leiomyomas of premenopausal women with more than 5 mitoses/10HPF [24]. The mitotic counts usually 5–9 MF/10HPF, but occasionally 10–20 mitoses/10HPF have been reported. Although mitotically active leiomyomas with >15 mitoses/10HPF and a clinically benign course have been described, they are so rare thus should be considered with suspicion and be labeled as STUMPs. The cellularity may be variable with areas of hypercellularity, but atypia should be absent or mild by definition. Necrosis should be absent in differential diagnosis with leiomyosarcoma. Hormonal factors may have a critical role: leiomyomas removed during the secretory phase of the menstrual cycle have a significantly increased mitotic index compared to those removed during menses or during the proliferative phase [25]. Also, leiomyomas removed from women who are taking progestins have a higher mitotic rate than that observed in women who are taking a combination of estrogen and progestin or who are not taking any exogenous hormones [26].

6.2. Cellular Leiomyoma

Gross examination of these neoplasms does not usually provide any diagnostic cue, showing features similar to the usual leiomyomas but when particularly cellular may have a fleshier, soft, yellow or brown cut surface, sometimes with areas of hemorrhage and/or necrosis. By definition, a cellular leiomyoma shows a cellularity "significantly" greater than the surrounding myometrium (Figure 2). Palisading nuclei, evocative of nuclear pattern in Verocay bodies of a neurilemoma, are present in some cellular leiomyomas [27]. No nuclear atypia, no tumor cell necrosis and <5 mitoses/10HPF should be present.

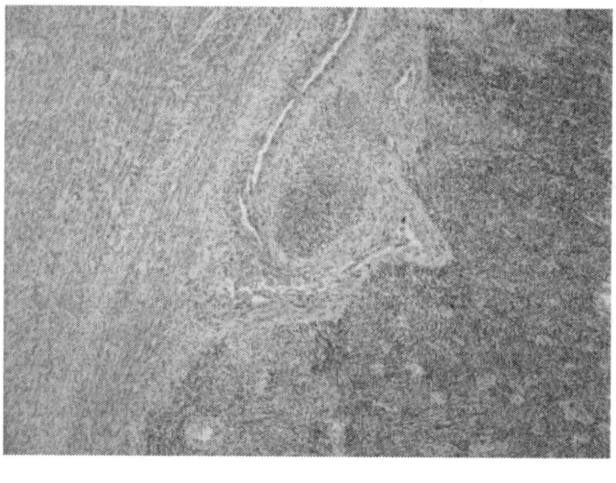

Figure 2. Cellular leiomyoma: tumor cells appear much more tightly packed than the surrounding myometrium (hematoxylin/eosin, 100x).

6.3. Hemorrhagic Cellular Leiomyomas

Hemorrhagic cellular leiomyoma, or "apoplectic" leiomyoma, is a form of cellular leiomyoma found in women who are taking oral contraceptives or who are either pregnant or puerperal [28, 29]. Gross examination typically reveals foci of hemorrhage within one or more leiomyomas. Microscopically, the leiomyoma is cellular and contains patchy areas of hemorrhage and edema. Necrosis generally is not present. Mitotic figures, which may be slightly increased in number, are detected mainly within a narrow zone resembling granulation tissue around areas of hemorrhage. In contrast to leiomyosarcoma, neither atypical mitoses nor significant cytological atypia are present, and the neoplasm has a circumscribed, compressive margin.

6.4. Leiomyoma with Bizarre Nuclei

Leiomyomas with bizarre nuclei are also referred as symplastic leiomyomas, bizarre leiomyomas and atypical leiomyomas. The term "atypical leiomyoma" should be avoided for neoplasms exhibiting features described below and should be reserved to neoplasms with an uncertain malignant potential, to avoid any misunderstanding between pathologists and clinicians. The gross appearance usually resembles that of a typical leiomyoma including a well-circumscribed, pushing border, and in some cases yellow to tan areas, softening and cystic spaces are reported. The most prominent microscopic feature is the presence of large cells with eosinophilic cytoplasm and bizarrely shaped, multilobate or multiple, hyperchromatic, often "smudged" nuclei, but a usual absence of other worrisome histological features. The nuclei often contain cytoplasmic pseudo inclusions (Figure 3).

As an isolated finding, cytologic atypia, even when severe, is an unreliable criterion for the diagnosis of clinically malignant uterine smooth muscle tumors because it can be seen in clinically benign, otherwise banal smooth muscle neoplasms [30, 31]. The atypical cells may be distributed throughout the leiomyoma or they may be focal. By definition, mitotic figures cannot >10 MF/10HPF in a leiomyoma with bizarre nuclei, and tumor cell necrosis must be absent. Leiomyoma with bizarre nuclei can result immunohistochemically positive for p53 and p16, limiting the reliability of this ancillary technique in differential diagnosis [32].

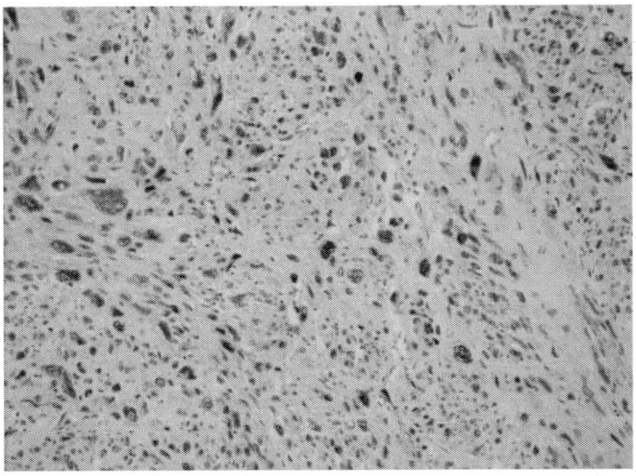

Figure 3. Leiomyoma with bizarre nuclei: severe cellular atypia without evidence of tumor cell necrosis and brisk mitotic activity (hematoxylin/eosin, 100x).

6.5. Hydropic Leiomyomas

Hydropic degeneration is represented by the accumulation of watery edema fluid and is common in leiomyomas and often confused with myxoid degeneration, a much less common finding. The process is usually focal but can replace most or all of tumor, and may lead to cystic degeneration. Hydropic change typically occurs within collagenized areas, the edema fluid separating thin strands or spherical aggregates of collagen. The smooth muscle component is often atrophic and reduced to thin cords. Thick-walled blood vessels are often prominent [33].

6.6. Parasitic Leiomyomas

The older literature suggests that leiomyomas may detach themselves from an initial subserosal location and attach to some other pelvic structure or even grow in the retroperitoneum. This improbable event presumably takes place through the combination of infarction and inflammatory adhesions. A diagnosis of parasitic leiomyoma should be made with great caution because smooth muscle neoplasms that arise in the retroperitoneum and gastrointestinal tract and that have recurring or metastatic potential are notorious for being morphologically bland and having few or no mitotic figures [34].

6.7. Leiomyomatosis Peritonealis Disseminata

Leiomyomatosis peritonealis disseminata (LPD) or disseminated peritoneal leiomyomatosis is characterized by multiple subperitoneal or peritoneal nodules of varying sizes on the omentum and peritoneal surfaces, grossly mimicking disseminated carcinoma. The nodules are usually between 0.5 and 50 mm, firm, and well circumscribed. On cut section, they show white and whorled trabeculations. The histologic features of LPD are similar to those of benign uterine myoma. They show smooth-muscle cell proliferation with no atypia or necrosis (Figure 4). Immunohistochemistry staining is typical of smooth muscle tumors showing positivity for vimentin, desmin, smooth muscle actin, and muscle specific actin. LPD is a rare disease and usually follows a benign course. Its pathophysiology remains unclear. However, it may be due to metaplasia of mesenchymal cells of the peritoneum. In susceptible women, fragments myoma left in the abdominal cavity after morcellation might contribute to the development of LPD [35].

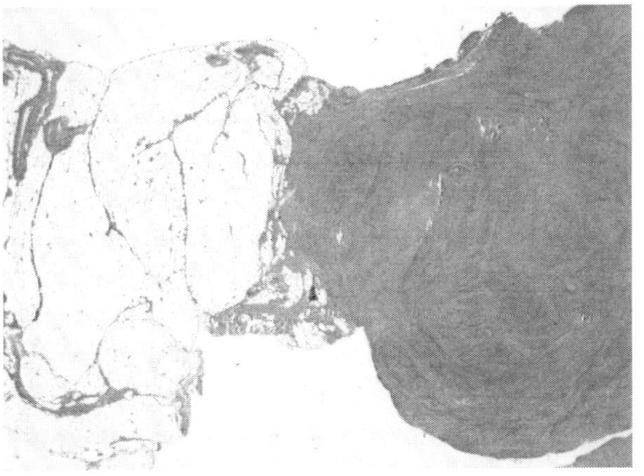

Figure 4. Leiomyomatosis peritonealis: small nodule composed of innocent-looking smooth muscle cells attached to subcutaneous adipose tissue of a port-site track (hematoxylin/eosin, 40x).

6.8. Intravenous Leiomyomatosis and Leiomyoma with Vascular Invasion

Intravenous leiomyomatosis (IVL) is a very rare smooth muscle tumor characterized by nodular masses of histologically benign smooth muscle cells growing within venous channels. Grossly, IVL is a complex coiled or nodular growth within the myometrium with convoluted, wormlike extensions into the uterine veins in the broad ligament or into other pelvic veins. The growth extends into the vena cava in more than 10% of patients, and in some it reaches as far as the heart. The wormlike masses vary from soft and spongy to rubbery and firm, and their color is pink-white or gray; it is important to carefully assess any such growth for features that might signify malignancy (high mitotic rate, significant nuclear atypia, and tumor cell necrosis). Microscopically, tumor is found within venous channels lined by endothelium; arteries are not involved. The histologic appearance is highly variable, even within the same tumor. The cellular composition of some examples of IVL is similar to a leiomyoma, but most contain prominent zones of fibrosis or hyalinization. Smooth muscle cells may be inconspicuous and difficult to identify. The intravenous growth is itself highly frequent and, in some cases, contains so many small and large blood vessels that the process may resemble a vascular tumor. Any type of smooth muscle differentiation that occurs in a leiomyoma can be present in IVL. Sometimes, a morphologically benign uterine smooth muscle tumor may be associated with intravascular growth; in these cases, a solitary unremarkable leiomyoma is associated with a microscopic focus of intravascular neoplasm within the confines of the leiomyoma, often designated as leiomyoma with vascular intrusion, is benign without any implication of recurrence [34].

6.9. Benign Metastasizing Leiomyomas

Benign metastasizing leiomyoma (BML) is a rare, nebulous, disorder that affects women with a history of uterine leiomyoma, which is found to metastasize within extrauterine sites. The disease develops as a proliferation of multiple nodules composed of smooth muscle cells. The most frequent site of metastasis is the lungs, although other areas may also be affected as well, including some atypical locations, e.g., the heart or spinal cord. The majority of case study authors demonstrate the time relation between the patient's primary surgery and BML onset. Cases of BML in women who have not undergone prior surgery are anecdotal. The primary neoplasm, typically removed years before the metastatic deposits are detected, often has been inadequately studied and a few examples may represent deportation metastases from IVL that reach the lungs, where they become implanted and grow as multiple intrapulmonary nodules of smooth muscle [36].

6.10. Hormonal and Therapy-Induced Modifications

Hormonal status and some drugs used in leiomyoma therapy can induce relevant morphological changes. If the administration of drugs or the hormonal status of the patient is not communicated by the clinician to the pathologist, the finding of such induced alterations can lead to incorrect diagnoses. Uterine leiomyomas are well known to be hormone-responsive neoplasms. As stated above they are most common in reproductive years, often regress or decrease in size after the menopause and exhibit positive immunohistochemistry staining with steroid hormone receptors. Red degeneration, which typically occurs in pregnancy or less commonly oral contraceptive (OC) users, results in a beefy red appearance due to infarction and hemorrhage with subsequent hemolysis. Rupture of the tumor may cause acute abdominal signs. Although many uterine leiomyomas do not cause symptoms, some women will develop abnormal bleeding, abdominal distension, urinary symptoms, or pelvic discomfort. Until recently, hysterectomy has been the primary treatment modality for such symptomatic leiomyomas, but new treatment modalities are emerging. Several medical therapies have been proposed during the years with the declared purpose of reducing dimension and related symptoms of leiomyoma; furthermore, leiomyoma can be affected by drugs commonly used to treat atypical uterine bleedings. These iatrogenic alterations can be observed in subsequent surgical specimens. Progestins containing compounds are widely prescribed for a range of indications encompassing the management of endometriosis, of abnormal uterine bleeding, inhibition of ovulation and inhibition of endometrial growth.

Uterine leiomyomas in women who had been treated with oral progestogens or a progestogen containing intrauterine devices are reported to comprise small and/or large areas of infarct-type necrosis (sometimes mimicking coagulative tumor cell necrosis) with surrounding increased cellularity, mitotic activity, nuclear pyknosis, cytoplasmic eosinophilia, epithelioid morphology, stromal edema, hemorrhage, and myxoid change and infiltration by CD56 positive granulated lymphocytes. Sometimes the features resulted in an almost deciduous appearance [37].

Treatment with gonadotropin-releasing hormone agonists (GnRHa) provides a temporary reduction in the size of leiomyomas before their surgical removal and is now used routinely in clinical practice, primarily as a surgical adjunct. The reduction of leiomyoma size during GnRH agonist therapy may be due to both ischemic injury and cellular atrophy. There is a suggestion that leiomyomas subjected to preoperative GnRH agonist treatment showed increased cellularity necrosis. Although necrosis of leiomyomas is associated with GnRH agonist treatment, the lack of significant pleomorphism or mitotic activity distinguishes these altered leiomyomas from leiomyosarcomas [38].

Leuprolide acetate-treated leiomyomata had significantly increased hyalinization and decreased cellularity if compared to conventional leiomyomas; thickening of blood vessel walls with narrowing of the lumen can be frequently observed. A subgroup of leuprolide acetate-treated patients categorized as clinical responders (having >30% reduction in tumor size) more frequently had thickening of vessel walls ($p < 0.05$) and vascular thrombosis ($p < 0.10$) than did non-responders. Our data suggest that a leuprolide acetate-induced hypoestrogenic state may cause vasoconstriction, thickening of blood vessel walls, and thrombosis, leading to ischemia, hyalinization, and atrophy of the leiomyoma [39].

Uterine artery embolization (UAE) for uterine leiomyomas is now emerging as an innovative treatment modality, using particles or microspheres of polyvinyl alcohol (PVA) or tris-acryl gelatin microspheres (TGMs). UAE is becoming an effective alternative to hysterectomy in the treatment of symptomatic uterine leiomyomas in Europe, North America, and Australia thanks to significant uterine volume reductions in excess of 50% and low complication rates.

Microscopic changes within the treated leiomyomas vary with the post-UAE interval. There is typically necrosis of infarct type or less commonly tumor cell or suppurative necrosis. The cardinal finding is the presence of intra- or extravascular embolic material, often with a foreign body granulomatous reaction, and in some cases thrombosis and partial to complete vessel destruction. These changes may occur within, around, or distant from the leiomyomas, including within the cervix, endometrium, tubes, and ovaries. PVA appears on hematoxylin-eosin stained sections as a pale gray–blue fibrillar latticework in its particulate form or as oval structures (microspheres) [40].

Antifibrinolytic agents such as tranexamic acid, used in the treatment of menorrhagia and/or leiomyomas, can also produce thrombosis and infarction within leiomyomas. The infarcts may mimic tumor cell necrosis or necrosis of uncertain type, potentially leading to a misdiagnosis of leiomyosarcoma or smooth muscle tumor of uncertain malignant potential [19].

7. Hints and Pitfalls in Differential Diagnosis

As discussed in the previous sections, most of the leiomuscular lesions of the uterus do not constitute issues in routine diagnostics. However, some cases have morphologic features that can raise doubts of malignancy if the clinicians – pathologist communication is poor, incomplete or missing with disastrous consequences for patient management.

A meticulous macroscopic examination with extensive sampling and observation of conventional histological preparations stained with hematoxylin-eosin still play a key role in the diagnosis of smooth muscle neoplasms of the uterus. Immunohistochemistry (mostly p16 and p53), and molecular tools including MED12 mutations have currently a very limited role in the classification of smooth muscle tumors as benign or malignant [41].

To establish a diagnosis of spindle cell leiomyosarcoma a combination of two of three of the following features are needed: tumor cells necrosis, marked moderate to severe cytologic atypia and/or ≥10 mitoses/10HPF. An epithelioid leiomyosarcoma should show ≥4 mitoses/10HPFs with either tumor cell necrosis or at least moderate cytologic atypia, whereas a myxoid leiomyosarcoma can be diagnosed with the finding of either tumor cell necrosis or marked cytologic atypia; in their absence, ≥2 mitoses/10HPFs is diagnostic of malignancy (Figure 5). Notice that the threshold to establish a diagnosis of myxoid leiomyosarcoma is much lower than that used for the spindle cell variant; thus, it is important to sample extensively any smooth muscle tumor, particularly if myxoid, in order to identify the most mitotically active areas [42].

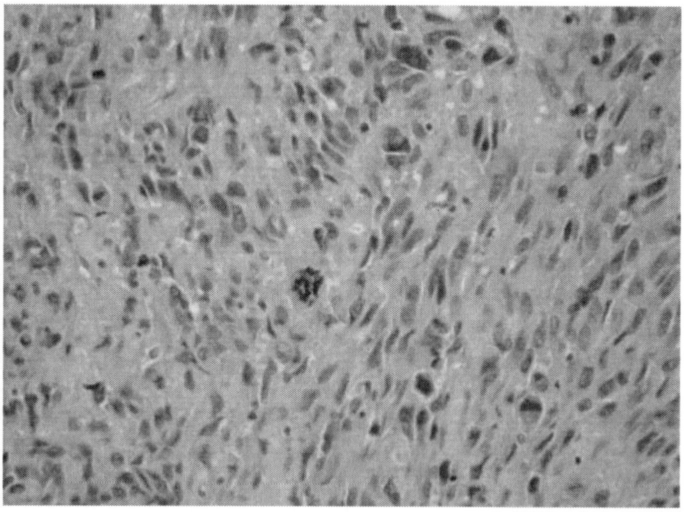

Figure 5. Spindle cell leiomyosarcoma: severe cytological atypia associated to brisk mitotic activity and atypical mitoses (hematoxylin/eosin, 400x).

7.1. Tumor Cell Necrosis ("Coagulative Necrosis")

Three types of necrosis can be encountered in smooth muscle tumors:

1. Ulceration with underlying necrosis if submucosal;
2. Infarct-type necrosis in benign and malignant neoplasms;
3. Tumor cell necrosis which is only seen in leiomyosarcomas.

The latter is defined by an abrupt transition from necrotic to non-necrotic areas without interposed granulation tissue. Viable tumor cells typically have a perivascular distribution [42].

The term tumor cell necrosis (TCN) should be preferred to "coagulative tumor cell necrosis" as the latter term leads to confusion with infarct-type necrosis [19].

7.2. Cytologic Atypia

Evaluation of cytologic atypia is subjective and may vary greatly among pathologists. There are several grading systems that could be applied to uterine leiomyosarcomas as they are used in soft tissues including the Broders system and the French classification (FNCLCC). However, all of these systems fail in identifying bona fide low-grade leiomyosarcomas. On the basis of the Stanford criteria for malignancy in smooth muscle tumors, the vast majority of leiomyosarcomas are also by definition high grade. If low-grade leiomyosarcomas exist, they are rare and criteria to recognize this subset of tumors is currently lacking and patient outcome was basically identical to that of high-grade tumors
[43-46].

7.3. Mitotic Index

Even though mitotic index is important in establishing the diagnosis of leiomyosarcoma, this finding in isolation is not enough to render such diagnosis as some leiomyoma variants may occasionally have brisk mitotic activity. As mentioned above, a cutoff of 10, ≥4, and ≥2 mitoses/10HPFs is used for spindle, epithelioid or myxoid leiomyosarcomas, respectively. Thus, objective mitotic count is crucial but at the same time it is often difficult to be certain about it as apoptotic cells with karyorrhectic nuclei can be easily misinterpreted as mitoses [47].

Conclusion

The diagnosis of uterine tumors with smooth muscle differentiation accounts for a demanding task for the gynecological pathologist. Most cases do not pose problems, but some diagnoses may be challenging. There are many variants to the conventional spindle cell morphology, each with a malignant counterpart that must be considered in the differential diagnosis. Macroscopic and microscopic examination remains the cornerstone of this activity with ancillary methods that are not yet crucial.

References

[1] Mauskopf J, Flynn M, Thieda P, Spalding J, Duchane J. The economic impact of uterine fibroids in the United States: a summary of published estimates. *J Womens Health* (Larchmt). 2005;14(8):692-703.

[2] Buttram VC Jr, Reiter RC. Uterine leiomyomata: etiology, symptomatology, and management. *Fertil Steril*. 1981 Oct;36: 433–45;36:433–45.

[3] Cramer SF, Patel A. The frequency of uterine leiomyomas. *Am J Clin Pathol*. 1990;94(4):435-8.

[4] Kjerulff KH, Langenberg P, Seidman JD, Stolley PD, Guzinski GM. Uterine leiomyomas. Racial differences in severity, symptoms and age at diagnosis. *J Reprod Med*. 1996;41(7):483-90.

[5] Andersen J. Factors in fibroid growth. *Baillieres Clin Obstet Gynaecol*. 1998;12(2):225-43.

[6] Marsh EE, Bulun SE. Steroid hormones and leiomyomas. *Obstet Gynecol Clin North Am*. 2006;33(1):59-67.

[7] Viville B, Charnock-Jones DS, Sharkey AM, Wetzka B, Smith SK. Distribution of the A and B forms of the progesterone receptor messenger ribonucleic acid and protein in uterine leiomyomata and adjacent myometrium. *Hum Reprod*. 1997;12(4):815-22.

[8] Ross RK, Pike MC, Vessey MP, Bull D, Yeates D, Casagrande JT. Risk factors for uterine fibroids: reduced risk associated with oral contraceptives. *Br Med J* (*Clin Res Ed*). 1986;293(6543):359-62.

[9] Parazzini F, La Vecchia C, Negri E, Cecchetti G, Fedele L. Epidemiologic characteristics of women with uterine fibroids: a case control study. *Obstet Gynecol*. 1988;72(6):853-7.

[10] Stewart EA, Nowark RA. New concepts in the treatment of uterine leiomyomas. *Obstet Gynecol*. 1998 Oct;92(4 Pt 1):624-7.

[11] Parazzini F, Negri E, La Vecchia C, Rabaiotti M, Luchini L, Villa A, Fedele L. Uterine myomas and smoking: results from an Italian study. *J Reprod Med.* 1996;41(5):316-20.

[12] Chiaffarino F, Parazzini F, La Vecchia C, Chatenoud L, Di Cintio E, Marsico S. Diet and uterine myomas. *Obstet Gynecol.* 1999;94(3):395-8

[13] Abeler VM, Royne O, Thoresen S, Danielsen HE, Nesland JM, Kristensen GB. Uterine sarcomas in Norway. A histopathological and prognostic survey of a total population from 1970 to 2000 including 419 patients. *Histopathology.* 2009;54(3):355-64.

[14] Wang WL, Soslow R, Hensley M, Asad H, Zannoni GF, de Nictolis M, Branton P, Muzikansky A, Oliva E. Histopathologic prognostic factors in stage I leiomyosarcoma of the uterus: a detailed analysis of 27 cases. *Am J Surg Pathol.* 2011;35(4):522-9.

[15] Mayerhofer K, Obermair A, Windbichler G, Petru E, Kaider A, Hefler L, Czerwenka K, Leodolter S, Kainz C. Leiomyosarcoma of the uterus: a clinicopathologic multicenter study of 71 cases. *Gynecol Oncol.* 1999;74(2):196-201.

[16] Cramer SF, Horiszny J, Patel A, Sigrist S. The relation of fibrous degeneration to menopausal status in small uterine leiomyomas with evidence for postmenopausal origin of seedling myomas. *Mod Pathol.* 1996;9(7):774-80.

[17] Clement PB, Young RH, Scully RE. Diffuse, perinodular, and other patterns of hydropic degeneration within and adjacent to uterine leiomyomas. Problems in differential diagnosis. *Am J Surg Pathol.* 1992;16(1):26-32.

[18] Coad JE, Sulaiman RA, Das K, Staley N. Perinodular hydropic degeneration of a uterine leiomyoma: a diagnostic challenge. *Hum Pathol.* 1997;28(2):249-51.

[19] Clement FP, Young RH. Mesenchymal and Mixed Epithelial–Mesenchymal Tumors of the Uterine Corpus and Cervix. In Clement FP, Young RH (Eds): *Atlas of Gynecologic Surgical Pathology*. 2014.

[20] Kurman RJ, Norris HJ. Mesenchymal tumors of the uterus. VI. Epithelioid smooth muscle tumors including leiomyoblastoma and clear cell leiomyoma: a clinical and pathological analysis of 26 cases. *Cancer.* 1976;37(4):1853-65.

[21] Clement PB. The pathology of uterine smooth muscle tumors and mixed endometrial stromal-smooth muscle tumors: a selective review with emphasis on recent advances. *Int J Gynecol Pathol*. 2000;19(1):39-55.

[22] Prayson RA, Goldblum, Hart WR. Epithelioid smooth-muscle tumors of the uterus – A clinicopathologic study of 18 patients. *Am J Surg Pathol*. 2012;21(4):383–391

[23] Mazur MT, Kraus FT. Histogenesis of morphologic variations in tumors of the uterine wall. *Am J Surg Pathol*. 1980;4(1):59-74.

[24] Prayson RA, Hart WR. Mitotically active leiomyomas of the uterus. *Am J Clin Pathol*. 1992;97(1):14-20

[25] Kawaguchi K, Fujii S, Konishi I, Nanbu Y, Nonogaki H, Mori T. Mitotic activity in uterine leiomyomas during the menstrual cycle. *Am J Obstet Gynecol.* 1989;160(3):637-41.

[26] Tiltman AJ. The effect of progestins on the mitotic activity of uterine fibromyomas. *Int J Gynecol Pathol.* 1985;4(2):89-96.

[27] Gisser SD, Young I. Neurilemoma-like uterine myomas: an ultrastructural reaffirmation of their non-Schwannian nature. *Am J Obstet Gynecol.* 1977;129(4):389-92.

[28] Myles JL, Hart WR. Apoplectic leiomyomas of the uterus. A clinicopathologic study of five distinctive hemorrhagic leiomyomas associated with oral contraceptive usage. *Am J Surg Pathol.* 1985;9(11):798-805.

[29] Norris HJ, Hilliard GD, Irey NS. Hemorrhagic cellular leiomyomas ("apoplectic leiomyoma") of the uterus associated with pregnancy and oral contraceptives. *Int J Gynecol Pathol.* 1988;7(3):212-24.

[30] Bell SW, Kempson RL, Hendrickson MR. Problematic uterine smooth muscle neoplasms: a clinicopathologic study of 213 cases. *Am J Surg Pathol.* 1994;18(6):535-58.

[31] Downes KA, Hart WR. Bizarre leiomyomas of the uterus: a comprehensive pathologic study of 24 cases with long-term follow-up. *Am J Surg Pathol.* 1997;21(11):1261-70.

[32] Sung CO, Ahn G, Song SY, Choi YL, Bae DS. Atypical leiomyomas of the uterus with long-term follow-up after myomectomy with immunohistochemical analysis for p16INK4A, p53, Ki-67, estrogen receptors, and progesterone receptors. *Int J Gynecol Pathol.* 2009;28(6):529-34.

[33] Ceyhan K, Simşir C, Dölen I, Calýşkan E, Umudum H. Multinodular hydropic leiomyoma of the uterus with perinodular hydropic degeneration and extrauterine extension. *Pathol Int.* 2002;52(8):540-3.

[34] Kempson RL, Hendrickson MR. Smooth muscle, endometrial stromal, and mixed Müllerian tumors of the uterus. *Mod Pathol.* 2000;13(3):328-42.

[35] Al-Talib A, Tulandi T. Pathophysiology and possible iatrogenic cause of leiomyomatosis peritonealis disseminata. *Gynecol Obstet Invest.* 2010;69(4):239-44.

[36] Barnaś E, Książek M, Raś R, Skręt A, Skręt- Magierøo J, Dmoch- Gajzlerska E. Benign metastasizing leiomyoma: A review of current literature in respect to the time and type of previous gynecological surgery. *PLoS One.* 2017;12(4):e0175875.

[37] Boyd C, McCluggage WG. Unusual morphological features of uterine leiomyomas treated with progestogens. *J Clin Pathol.* 2011;64(6):485-9.

[38] Colgan TJ, Pendergast S, LeBlanc M. The histopathology of uterine leiomyomas following treatment with gonadotropin-releasing hormone analogues. *Hum Pathol.* 1993;24(10):1073-7.

[39] Demopoulos RI, Jones KY, Mittal KR, Vamvakas EC. Histology of leiomyomata in patients treated with leuprolide acetate. *Int J Gynecol Pathol.* 1997;16(2):131-7.

[40] Colgan TJ, Pron G, Mocarski EJ, Bennett JD, Asch MR, Common A. Pathologic features of uteri and leiomyomas following uterine artery embolization for leiomyomas. *Am J Surg Pathol.* 2003;27(2):167-77.

[41] Chiang S, Oliva E. Recent developments in uterine mesenchymal neoplasms. *Histopathology.* 2013;62(1):124-37.

[42] Oliva E. Practical issues in uterine pathology from banal to bewildering: the remarkable spectrum of smooth muscle neoplasia *Mod Pathol.* 2016;29 Suppl 1:S104-20.

[43] Giuntoli RL 2nd, Metzinger DS, DiMarco CS, Cha SS, Sloan JA, Keeney GL, Gostout BS. Retrospective review of 208 patients with leiomyosarcoma of the uterus: prognostic indicators, surgical management, and adjuvant therapy. *Gynecol Oncol.* 2003;89(3):460-9.

[44] Akhan SE, Yavuz E, Tecer A, Iyibozkurt CA, Topuz S, Tuzlali S, Bengisu E, Berkman S. The expression of Ki-67, p53, estrogen and progesterone receptors affecting survival in uterine leiomyosarcomas. A clinicopathologic study. *Gynecol Oncol.* 2005;99(1):36-42.

[45] Pautier P, Genestie C, Rey A, Morice P, Roche B, Lhommé C, Haie-Meder C, Duvillard P. Analysis of clinicopathologic prognostic factors for 157 uterine sarcomas and evaluation of a grading score validated for soft tissue sarcoma. *Cancer.* 2000;88(6):1425-31.

[46] Veras E, Zivanovic O, Jacks L, Chiappetta D, Hensley M, Soslow R. "Low-grade leiomyosarcoma" and late-recurring smooth muscle tumors of the uterus: a heterogenous collection of frequently misdiagnosed tumors associated with an overall favorable prognosis relative to conventional uterine leiomyosarcomas. *Am J Surg Pathol.* 2011;35(11):1626-37.

[47] Oliva E, Carcangiu ML, Carinelli S et al. Mesenchymal tumours In: Kurman RJ, Carcangiu ML, Herrington CS et al. (eds). *WHO Classification of Tumours of Female Reproductive Organs.* IARC Press: Lyons, France, 2014;p 135–147.

In: Uterine Fibroids
Editors: S. Ferrero and F. Barra

ISBN: 978-1-53615-046-9

Chapter 5

PRESURGICAL HORMONAL TREATMENT FOR UTERINE MYOMAS

Gloria D'Alessandro, MD, Fabio Barra, MD, Giulio Evangelisti, MD, Carolina Scala, MD and Simone Ferrero*, MD, PhD

Obstetrics and Gynecology, Department of Neurosciences, Rehabilitation, Ophthalmology, Genetics, Maternal and Child Health (DiNOGMI), University of Genoa, Italy
Academic Unit of Obstetrics and Gynecology, IRCCS Ospedale San Martino, Genoa, Italy

ABSTRACT

Preoperative treatment of uterine fibroids aims to improve iron-deficiency anemia, decrease the volume of fibroids and potentially facilitate surgery (mainly decreasing the intraoperative blood loss). Several drugs have been used in this setting including gonadotrophin releasing hormone analogues (GnRH-a), aromatase inhibitors (AIs) and selective progesterone receptor modulator (SPRMs). Over the last 20 years, among these, GnRH-a have been the most widely used drugs; however, their administration is associated with relevant adverse effects caused by the hypoestrogenism (such as hot flushes and insomnia). AIs have been only used in clinical studies, demonstrating to facilitate surgery; however, these agents too may be responsible for several adverse effects (such as myalgia and arthralgia) and currently they are not approved for treating uterine fibroids. SPRMs have recently been introduced in the market for the preoperative treatment of uterine fibroids. In particular, several randomized controlled trials showed that ulipristal acetate rapidly controls the heavy menstrual bleeding and it is well tolerated. Moreover, several

* Corresponding Author's E-mail: simoneferrero@me.com.

studies showed that it may even facilitate both hysteroscopic and laparoscopic myomectomy. Vilaprisan is currently under investigation for the preoperative treatment of uterine fibroids. Overall, the benefits of preoperative administration of hormonal therapies should always be balanced with cost of the treatment, delay in the surgical procedures and safety.

Keywords: uterine fibroids, gonadotropin releasing hormone-analogues, presurgical therapy

INTRODUCTION

One of the most frequently investigated question in daily practice concerns whether preoperative treatment actually is able to make fibroids surgery easier. Based on large amount of clinical observation and epidemiologic data, it is known that sex hormones play a critical role on the development and maintenance of uterine myomas [1]; thus, hormonal therapy, reducing the gonadal steroids levels, may constitute an important option for the treatment of these benign tumors.

Since the treatment reduces estrogen secretion, it is possible to observe a myoma shrinkage. Moreover, acting through modulation of progesterone pathway, it can add a better control of bleeding symptoms and a restore higher hemoglobin levels [2]. Medical therapy before hysterectomy can be a suitable option to treat anemia before surgery, to reduce blood loss during surgery. Moreover, it can theoretically make the procedure less invasive increasing the ratio of vaginal hysterectomy and hysteroscopicor laparoscopic myomectomy [3, 4]. In fact, after preoperative therapy, surgeon can change the surgical approach based on response. Conservative surgery is an option also for women wishing to preserve their fertility. In a systematic review regarding to the impact of leiomyomas on fertility, the authors under lighted how submucous myomas may low fertility rates and their removal may enhance conception and live births [5].

However, compared with hysterectomy, myomectomy is affected by more technical difficulties, postoperative complications (fever and pelvic hematoma formation and intraoperative hemorrhage requiring eventual blood transfusion); all these complications do not generally occur during hysteroscopic surgery, available for submucous myomas. Moreover, preoperative treatments are able to reduce the risk of intraoperative blood loss and can guarantee an easier surgical procedure, a better anatomical reconstruction and the possibility of transverse incision (pfannenstiel type) rather than vertical midline at laparotomy. On the other hand, the fibroid capsule may become less evident or totally missing, with the result of a more complicated excision or a difficult 'shelling out' of the myoma [6].

Most women with fibroids are asymptomatic only necessitating a clinical observation and follow-up [1]. However, symptoms such as anemia caused by heavy menstrual bleeding (HMB), pelvic pain, pressure symptoms, dysmenorrhea, infertility and low quality of life (QoL) affected up to 50% of women; these patients require some medical treatments [6]. The choice of treatment depends on multiple factors such as patient's age and preference, reason for treatment, fertility preservation 1].

The treatment of myomas has become multidisciplinary in the past 20 years [1]. In fact, it includes various possibilities such as an expectant management, medical therapy, surgery, uterine artery embolization or other radiologic ablative techniques. Medical therapy represents an option for symptomatic women who prefer avoiding surgery, desire conserve their fertility, or wait for a less aggressive surgical procedure after shrinkage of the uterine volume 1]. The aim of using medical therapies before surgery is to reduce the difficulty of the surgical procedure. However, these therapies are expensive. As fibroids constitute a major public health cost, an economic analysis should be done for drawing conclusion on this topic [6].

GnRH analogues and, more latterly, other types of medical therapy, have been investigated to be used before surgery for treating uterine fibroids. The aim this chapter is to describe the specific advantages and disadvantages of preoperative options for myomas and their direct surgical management [6].

Steroid Hormones Role

It is essential to understand the role of sex hormones in fibroid pathogenesis; this mechanism supports the use of hormonal therapies in this setting.

Estradiol (E2) and progesterone on the female reproductive system are interrelated, involving in their action receptors, transcription factors, kinase proteins, growth factors and numerous autocrine and paracrine factors (such as gonadotropins, adipokines, ovarian peptides) [7].

The main targets of progesterone are the endometrium cells and smooth muscle cells in the myometrium [8, 9]; its role may be critical for the development and proliferation of leiomyoma. In fact, it regulates proliferation, apoptosis (upregulating antiapoptotic protein Bcl-2 expression as well as decreasing tumor necrosis factor-α expression) [10], collagen deposition in the extracellular matrix (ECM) [11]; moreover, it induces the epidermal growth factor (EGF) [1, 7]. On the other hand, it also inhibits myomas growth via the downregulation of insulin-like growth factor-1(IGF-1) expression [12]. Overall, its action is mediated by two isoforms of progesterone receptors (PRs), PR-A and PR-B, which have been found at different concentrations in normal myometrium and uterine myoma [13]. Their expression is stimulated by E2, whose role is to increase tissue sensitivity to progesterone [7]. Progesterone can act stimulating growth of myomas as well as inhibiting growth of the endometrium due to differential balance of PR [14]. Thus, PR is an attractive therapeutic target.

Moreover, mitogenic stimuli released by mature leiomyoma cells on myoma stem cells (SC), which are poor in estrogen receptors (ERs) and PRs, are critical for the development of myomas [15]. Cytokines, like IL-1, IL-6, IL-11, IL-13, IL-15, IFN-γ, TNF-α, GM-CSF, are important for leiomyoma formation, having a key role in regulation of inflammation, angiogenesis, ECM remodeling and fibrosis [16]. These autocrine and paracrine factors have to be more explored, being potential pharmacological strategies in the future for the treatment of uterine fibroids.

Medical Therapy

The aim of preoperative medical therapy is to make surgery easier and less aggressive thanks to the fibroid shrinkage. Current medical treatments are non-hormonal (non-steroidal anti-inflammatory drugs, tranexamic acid) and hormonal [1]. Hormonal treatments include:

- GnRH-a;
- progestins;
- selective estrogen receptor modulators (SERMs);
- dopamine agonists;
- prostaglandin analogues;
- selective progesterone receptor modulators (SPRMs) [6];
- aromatase inhibitors (AIs) [17].

Each of these agents is able to reduce uterine and leiomyoma volume as well as provokes amenorrhea with the result of restoring hemoglobin and iron stores [17–19]. Clinical Practice Guideline, written by Society of Obstetricians and Gynecologists of Canada (SOGC), suggests correcting anemia prior to proceed with elective surgery (level of evidence and grade of recommendations II-2A) for myomas; in particular, SPRMs and GnRH-a are effective for this purpose and, thus, they should be considered preoperatively in anemic patients (level of evidence and grade of recommendations I-A); moreover, these two compounds are effective also for the treatment of bulk symptoms associated with fibroids (level of evidence I) [20].

An important contraindication of receiving medical treatment is represented by presence of concomitant or suspicious of malignant uterine tumor; thus, the gynecologists have to determine whether the uterine sarcomas could be suspected in these patients [1]. However, in women under the age of 50, the incidence of sarcomas is extremely low [17]; therefore, the final clinical decision should be made considering this awareness.

GONADOTROPHIN RELEASING HORMONE ANALOGUES

GnRH-a have been studied for treating uterine fibroids since the 1980s and nowadays are considered a suitable preoperative option (Table 1). GnRH-a are synthetic analogues of endogenous GnRH; their therapeutic effect is based on the suppression of pituitary ovarian function that causes a state of hypoestrogenism (Figure 1) [6]. Median E_2 levels are reduced to a range included between 80 to 180 pmol/L during the therapy with GnRH-a [21].

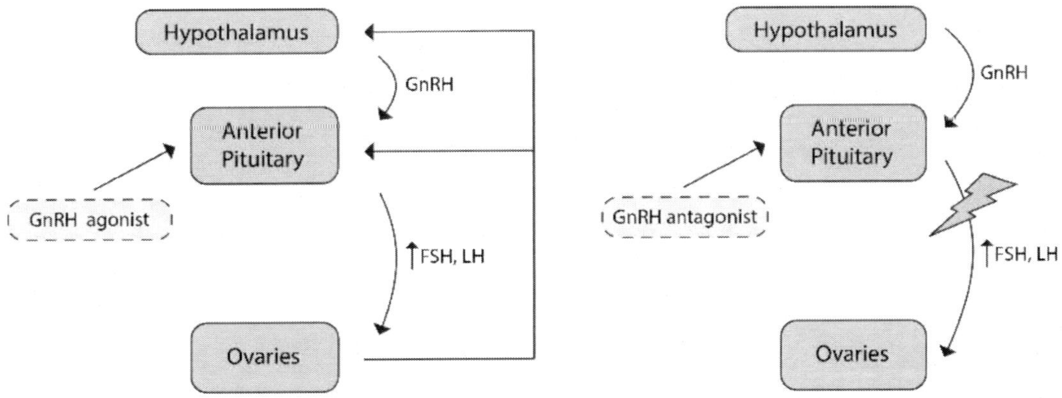

Figure 1. GnRH agonist and GnRH antagonist act on pituitary GnRH receptors. GnRH agonists show an initial increase of sex hormones secretion, known as "flare-up effect," that leads to a negative feedback on hypothalamus and pituitary gland. GnRH agonists directly provoke a desensitisation and a downregulation of pituitary receptors at a later stage.

Their action is due to the reduction of gonadotropin levels, which limit the growth of leiomyomas [22]. The unphysiologically long stimulation of GnRH receptors provokes their downregulation and desensitization. Consequently, the level of LH and FSH decreases and the production of ovarian hormones is suppressed [21, 23]. This endocrinological status causes a transient menopausal condition [1].

It has been proposed also a treatment with GnRH antagonist, concomitantly developed. Cetrorelix, ganirelix and abarelix belong to this class. While GnRH-a act by desensitization of GnRH-R, GnRH antagonists directly compete with endogenous GnRH for pituitary binding sites, suppressing gonadotropin release quicker than GnRH-a (within 4 to 8 hours, although the ovarian suppression is observed within 48 hours [24, 25]) in absence of an initial "flare-up" effect, which is typical of the use of GnRH-a (Figure 1). Moreover, action of GnRH antagonists is dose-dependent. GnRH-a showed to be more reliable in myoma shrinkage while GnRH antagonists frequently led to a lack of response [26]. Currently, GnRH antagonists are licensed for others indications, such as premature luteinizing hormone surge prevention in controlled ovarian hyperstimulation and the palliative treatment of advanced prostate cancer [1].

Table 1. GnRH analogues characteristics

Posology and Route of Administration	Pharmacodynamics	Pharmacokinetics	Side Effects and Controindications	Special Considerations
Buserelin s.c. 200 μg/die i.n. 300 μg × 4/die **Goserelin** implants.c. 3,6 mg/month 10,8 mg/3 months **Leuprolide** s.c. 500-1000 μg/die i.n. 400 μg × 4/die i.m. depot 3,75-7,5 mg/month 10,25 mg/3 months **Nafarelin** i.n. 200 μg × 2/die (?) i.m. depot 3 mg/ month	Bind pituitary GnRH-R ↓ Downregulation GnRH-R ↓ Soppression release of FSH, LH ↓ Hypoestrogenism state	Ka, Ke, EBA depend on formulation (higher in suspension than solution form). After administration of goserelin implant 10.8 mg: C_{max} = 8-10 ng/mL reached within 2 h (t_{max}) with a second peak plasma concentration after 7 weeks. Volumes of distribution = 20 ± 4 L (into total body water). Plasma protein binding low (20-30% forgoserelin).	**Side effect:** -Hot flushes -Vaginal dryness -↓Libido -Osteoporosis -↑Cardiovascular risk -Headache -Dizziness -Vaginitis -Change in breast size -Sweating -Insomnia -Depression **Contraindications:** -Pregnancy -Breastfeeding -Post-menopausal age -Renal failure -Liver failure -Ipersensitivity	Beginning and duration of therapy: it should start within the first 5 days of the menstrual cycle. The length of a course is 12 weeks. Frequent bleeding episodes in the second week after the beginning (flare-up effect) Consider add-back therapy if young (<45y). Contraceptive effect: no.
Triptorelina i.m. depot 3,75 mg/ month 11,25 mg/3 months **Triptorelina** s.c. 0,1 mg/die i.m. 3,75 mg/month **Leuprorelina (Enantone®)** i.m. depot 3,75 mg/month 11,25 mg/3 month s.c. 0,2 ml/die		Rapid clearance: >90% excreted by urine, 2% by feces. >75% of the dose is excreted within 12h $T_{1/2}$ = 4.2 h		

Ka = absorption rate constant; Ke = elimination rate constant; EBA = Extent of Biological Availability; h = hours; C_{max} = maximum concentration; $T_{1/2}$= half-life; T_{max} = time taken to reach the maximum concentration.

Leuprolide, buserelin, nafarelin, histrelin, goserelin, deslorelin, and triptorelin are GnRH-a. The drugs are available in nasal spray, subcutaneous or intramuscular injections.

The main advantage of this class of compounds is the temporary control of bleeding and the shrinkage of fibroids and uterine volume, with the effect of simplifying the surgical procedure and decreasing operative morbidity. However, their use is associated to some hypoestrogenism-related side effects, especially during a long-term therapy [6]. The main symptoms experienced are hot flushes, vaginal dryness and decreased libido; moreover, they can cause a decrease of bone mineral density and an increase of cardiovascular risk. To avoid postmenopausal climacteric disturbances, it has been proposed a reduction of dose therapy or the use of an add-back therapy. These strategies aim to maintain the beneficial effects on myoma size and the cycle suppression. The add-back therapy consists in the administration of progestins alone, estrogens alone, combined estrogen plus progestins, veralipride, tibolone and raloxifene. It has been reported that ceralipride administration, a benzamide derivative, can reduce the vasomotor symptoms [27]; raloxifene or tibolone help to prevent bone loss; anyway, raloxifene does not act on vasomotor symptoms whereas tibolone show a significant impact against hot flushes [28, 29]. The Food and Drug Administration (FDA) approved the use of GnRH-a without add-back therapy only for 6-9 months and with add-back therapy for longer durations [30–32].

The reduction of myoma size is obtained through several mechanisms although the exact process is still controversial. An induction of cellular atrophy (due to a decrease in myoma myofilaments) [33], cell necrosis and apoptosis [34], an increase of deoxyribonucleic acid damage and repair [35], a decrease in cell proliferation, a reduction of trophic mediators and of uterine blood flow by vasoconstriction have been hypothesized as possible mechanisms involved [18].

Symptoms such as menorrhagia, bleeding or anemia are controlled in women after the first month of treatment. The exact diminution of myoma volume is variable, ranging from 27% to 70% [36]; the shrinkage by up to 50% can occur within 3 or 6-months interval [20]; the maximal reduction is achieved within the first 12 weeks of therapy [37]. The direct clinical consequence by reducing the uterine and myoma size consists in a relief of symptoms (such as pain and pressure sense) in the first 2 months [1]. However, the effect of GnRH agonists on the myoma volume is transient and after the therapy is stopped. Thus, a re-growth of fibroids and a re-increase of uterus size and a reappearance of associated symptoms is predictable. In particular, it has been supposed that estrogen levels can return to pretreatment levels in about 4 weeks [20]. Moreover, myoma volume return again to its pretreatment size within about 6 months [1]. The rate of enlargement is quicker than the natural fibroid growth [38].

The evidence of fibroids shrinkage and improvement of hemoglobin levels in patients treated with GnRH-a before surgery results from randomized controlled trials (RCTs). These clinical studies showed a reduction of vertical incisions and blood loss in women undergoing hysterectomy or myomectomy, an increase in vaginal procedures and a decrease of postoperative complications after hysterectomy. However, there is inadequate evidence to support the use of GnRH-a for all women with fibroids undergoing these surgical procedures. The main indications for the use of preoperative therapy are women with greatly enlarged uteri, preoperative anemia or where a midline rather than transverse incision has been planned whereas there is not sufficient evidence of benefit for other patients. Moreover, the reduction of surgery time or hospital stay have not been demonstrated after the therapy [6].

In a randomized prospective study [39] focused on the impact of GnRH-a before myomectomy, emerged that the only advantage of administering GnRH-a preoperatively was a higher hemoglobin level prior to surgery among the women who received the drug thrice-monthly instead of twice-monthly or no preoperative treatment; there were no significant differences between the three groups about intraoperative blood loss, preoperative and postoperative blood transfusion, length of hospital stays.

Two main systematic reviews evaluated the administration of GnRH-a before laparoscopic myomectomy. The first one [40], showed a preoperative shrinkage of fibroids with an increase of hemoglobin levels, a reduction of the chance of a vertical incision, an intensification of vaginal procedure, without any increase in postoperative complications. The second review [41] showed a reduction in intraoperative blood loss.

Another review [42] examined the role of GnRH-a before hysteroscopic myomectomy for treating submucous fibroids. Anyway, there was the lack of evidence to support the routine use of GnRH-a.

The Advancing Minimally Invasive Gynecology Worldwide published in 2012 a practice guideline [17] analyzed the evidence regarding to the use of GnRH-a before hysteroscopic resection. There was concluded that:

- GnRH-a are effective in facilitating the treatment of anemia before the hysteroscopic procedure (recommendation level A);
- GnRH-a allow a complete resection of larger myomas in one-step procedure because there are able to obtain a 35% reduction of the endometrial cavity area after 2 months of treatment;
- It has not been established the role of GnRH-a for reducing operating time, the amount of systemic absorption of distention media and the risk of incomplete resection (recommendation level B).

Aromatase Inhibitors

Aromatase is an enzyme belonging to cytochrome P450 superfamily that catalyzes the conversion of androgens to estrogens through a hydroxylation process [43]. AIs are able to suppress the activity of this enzyme causing an anti-estrogenic effect with the purpose of limiting the growth of uterine fibroids [20].

17b-hydroxysteroid dehydrogenase (17b-HSD) type I takes part in the chemical reaction leading to the estrogens production: in fact, in myoma cells circulating androstenedione is converted by aromatase into estrone and this latter into the active form

E_2 by dehydrogenase [44]. Aromatase and 17b-HSD are overexpressed in tumor myometrial cells compared with normal myometrium; Bulun et al. [45] found aromatase mRNA in more than 90% of myoma cells [46]. However, this enzyme is not only expressed in endometrium and myometrium but also in ovary, breast, adipose tissue, brain, skin, bone, vascular endothelium and other organs [47]. The vast presence of aromatase allows for the investigation of a specific inhibitor. These compounds were firstly used on wide-scale for the treatment of metastatic breast cancer; after the development of the 'third-generation', AIs became a standard adjuvant endocrine therapy for estrogen receptor-positive postmenopausal breast cancer [48]. AIs has been proposed as medical treatment for endometriosis, anovulatory cycle and polycystic ovary syndrome in infertile women (Table 2) [49, 50].

AIs are classified into two groups; first group (for example exemestane holds *irreversible steroidal inhibitors*, as these compounds) form a permanent bond with the aromatase enzyme complex. The second group (for example, anastrozole and letrozole) consists of *reversible non-steroidal inhibitors.*

Table 2. Aromatase inhibitors features

Posology and Route of Administration	Pharmacodynamics	Pharmacokinetics	Side Effects and Controindications	Special Considerations
Anastrozole Orally 1 mg/day **Letrozole** Orally 2.5 mg/day **Exemestane** Vorozole, Formestane, Fadrozole Testolactone	Bond with aromatase enzyme and suppression its activity ↓ No conversion of androgens in estrogens ↓ Anti-estrogenic effect	Both letrozole and anastrozole are rapidly absorbed after oral administration. Clearance: by liver T1/2: almost 45 h. Clinical effects decrease after 10 days, on average.	**Side effects:** -Hot flushes -Osteoporosis -Headache -Back pain -Leg cramps -Arthralgia -Myalgia -Tiredness -Vaginal dryness -Nausea **Contraindications:** -Pregnancy -Breastfeeding -Pre-menopausal age -Ipersensitivity	Beginning of therapy: their assumption is independent from menstrual cycle Different sites of actions (endometrium, myometrium, ovary, breast, adipose tissue, brain, skin, bone, vascular endothelium)

H = hours; $T_{1/2}$ = half-life.

Additionally, AIs are divided in:

1. *First-generation compounds* (for example, aminoglutethimide and testolactone) [51];

2. *Second generation compounds* (for example, formestane and fadrazole);
3. *Third generation compounds* (for example, anastrozole, letrozole, eximestane and vorozole).

Table 3. Selective progesterone receptor modulator features

Posology and Route of Administration	Pharmacodynamics	Pharmacokinetics	Side Effects and Controindications	Special Considerations
ASOPRISNIL, MIFEPRISTONE, ULIPRISTAL Oral route 5mg/day **Telapristone** **CP-8947** **Onapristone** **Lonaprisan** **Vilaprisan**	Bind with PRs ↓ Competition with natural progesterone (agonist/antagonist properties) + Alternative mechanisms of post-receptor signaling: - Pro-apoptotic activity: ↑caspase 3, TRAIL ↓Bcl-2 - Suppression of growth factors: ↓Activin A, VEGF, ADM - Collagen degradation: ↑MMPs, ↓TIMPs -Modulation of inflammatory mediators: ↓IL-15 pathway, NK cells	Rapidly absorbed. C_{max} : 23.5 ± 14.2 ng/ml after 1h:50.0 ± 34.4 ng/ml $T_{1/2}$ (after 30mg of ulipristal):32.4 ± 6.3 h Bind to plasma proteins: albumin, a-1-acid glycoprotein, globulins, Cholesterol binding proteins. Bio transformed by liver. Clearance: 90% by feces, 10% by urines.	**Side effects:** -Headaches -Hot flushes -Breast discomfort (but these symptoms decrease by continuing the treatment) -Increase of transaminases. **Contraindications:** -Pregnancy -Breastfeeding -Ipersensitivity	Beginning and duration of therapy: it should start within the first week of the menstrual cycle. The length of a course is 3 months. Possible appearance of PAEC. Contraceptive effect: no.

C_{max} = maximum concentration; $T_{1/2}$ = half-life.

Interestingly, letrozole and anastrozole, in spite of their reversible binding to aromatase enzyme, suppress up to 97% of aromatase activity [52] with a consequent high reductions of estrogen levels [53]. With especial regard to their pharmacokinetics, these compounds have a high adsorption rate after oral administration, are cleared by the liver. They have an average half-life of 45 hours; anyway, their clinical action lasts about 10 days [43].

AIs are well tolerated in premenopausal women and are effective to reduce the symptoms and fibroid volume [54], however, in patients treated some side effects have been reported, and they are particularly related to the induced hypoestrogenic state. The most common are hot flushes and bone mineral density loss in prolonged treatment; other less common (usually of mild intensity) are headache, back pain, leg cramps, arthralgia for joint disorders [55], myalgia, tiredness, vaginal dryness, nausea. The FDA has reported also cases of infertility, aggressive behavior, adrenal insufficiency, kidney failure and liver dysfunction in women who ate food illegally containing AIs [56].

Despite of the rapid decrease of circulating estrogens by using AIs, systemic side effects are less pronounced than expected as these drugs provides a complete estrogen suppression in the fibroids as well as a partial suppression in the ovary [43].

From different clinical trials conducted with the purpose to evaluate the role of AIs in the treatment for uterine fibroids, it was found that letrozole significantly succeed in obtaining fibroid shrinkage and controlling bleeding symptoms without changing bone mineral density [57]; anastrozole shows similar effectiveness in reducing their volume and in controlling symptoms (it may be correlated also to a reduction of endometrial thinning obtained with this drug), nevertheless without changing circulating FSH or E2 levels [54, 58]. Finally, it has emerged that AIs acquire a strategic significance among the postmenopausal women through an *in situ* estrogen inhibition considering that GnRH agonists are ineffective in this age group [59].

However, further studies are requested to establish more systematically advantages and risks of this class of compounds and to evaluate their economic impact; in fact, no study has reported yet a cost-effectiveness analysis related to AIs treatment in women with uterine fibroids [43] and they are not currently approved for the treatment of this condition.

Selective Progesterone Receptor Modulator

Progesterone exerts its action by selectively binding to PR-A and PR-B, which play an essential role in leiomyoma pathogenesis; thus, these receptors represent attractive therapeutic targets.

Selective progesterone receptor modulators (SPRMs) are a class of synthetic steroids with agonist, antagonist or mixed activity on PRs that is different among targeted tissues (Table 3). This class of compounds constitutes an option for the treatment of hormone dependent diseases like uterine fibroids, endometriosis. Moreover, it has an important role in emergency contraception, termination of pregnancy, premenstrual syndrome, assisted reproduction [60]. However, the exact mechanism of action of SPRMs still remains to be established [61].

The Story

The evolution of SPRMs accidently started in 1992, thanks to the clinical attention given to a woman with HMB associated to uterine fibroids. She used levonorgestrel-intrauterine system (LNG-IUS) as contraceptive method; she showed a significant relief of bleeding episodes. This observation allowed considering LNG-IUS as a potential treatment of menorrhagia in women with myomas. However, following studies on magnetic resonance (MR) revealed that a third of the women with the IUS presents an increment in fibroids volume, another third an unchanged volume and the last third a reduction in their size [62]. Further *in vitro* studies about the impact of progesterone on myoma cells revealed remarkable results [63]. In particular, there was demonstrated the joint action of progesterone and E2 on leiomyoma growth and the increment of cell proliferation in cultured leiomyoma cells, under the influence of progesterone, differently from cultured normal myometrial cells. These evidences led to awareness of researching new compounds that can act selectively on leiomyoma cells without affecting the normal myometrium [64].

Compounds

SPRMs include asoprisnil (J-867), mifepristone (RU-486), ulipristal acetate (CDB-2914), telapristone (CDB-4124), CP-8947, onapristone, lonaprisan, vilaprisan, CP8863, CP8947.

Mifepristone was the first discovered PR antagonist; since this compound other steroidal progesterone ligands have been developed [65]. Telapristone has been investigated for the treatment of endometriosis and uterine myomas nevertheless showing a significant increase in AST and ALT enzymes [66]. Lonaprisan was developed for acting against breast cancer, asoprisnil was experimentally employed for endometriosis, uterine fibroids and dysfunctional uterine bleeding, whereas onapristone for both breast cancer and endometriosis [63, 67]. In 2012, ulipristal acetate (UPA) has been authorized by the European Medicines Agency for 3-month preoperative treatment of uterine fibroids (5 mg daily).

Asoprisnil, UPA and mifepristone have been largely investigated in clinical trials; among these, mifepristone showed a pure antagonistic effect reducing the activity of PRs in the normal myometrium and in leiomyoma. Asoprisnil showed similar antagonist properties on leiomyoma cells, endometrium, ovary, and breast but with different tissue selectivity [68]. UPA exerts its action by mixed agonist and antagonist features [20].

Pharmacodynamics

The cellular mechanisms by which SPRMs control bleeding episodes [61] is still largely unknown.

These drugs act specifically on the PRs, not only by competing with natural progesterone for binding the receptor, but also by alternative mechanisms of post-receptor signaling [7].

Several pathways may be involved in the action of these compounds, which may be responsible for the agonist/antagonist features of these compounds. One of non-genomic progesterone pathways is represented by SRC-1, a steroid receptor coactivator that modulates phosphorylation signaling pathways like proliferative RAS/RAF/MEKK/

MAPK kinase [61]. Wardell et al. [69] tried to investigate the partial agonist properties of mifepristone proving that it is able to bind to both the coactivator SRC-1 and the co-repressor SMRT (silencing mediator for retinoid and thyroid hormone receptor); thus, its action is influenced by the relative availability/abundance of these factors [61].

Later, Afhuppe et al. [70] compared the efficacy of different SPRMs, evaluating also their interaction with PR and other co-regulators. They demonstrated that lonaprisan, which has antagonistic properties, did not induce interactions with the LX-H10 peptide (containing a motif of coactivators) whereas mifepristone and asoprisnil presented the recruitment of PR coactivators *in vitro* [61].

Some other pathways explain how SPRMs are able to induce the shrinkage of uterine fibroids. Mifepristone and UPA, in different studies, were capable to inhibit proliferation of cultured fibroid cells by starting apoptosis: in fact, these drugs act up-regulating the expression of caspase 3, a proapoptotic protein, down-regulating that of Bcl-2, an antiapoptotic protein [71–73] and activating TRAIL (mitochondrial and tumor necrosis factor-related apoptosis-inducing ligand)-dependent pathways [74]. Moreover, UPA modulates the ratio of PR isoforms (in particular, increasing PR-A expression and decreasing PR-B expression) [74] with the result of reducing cell viability as well as suppressed expression of growth factors, angiogenic factors and their receptors [64]. In particular, UPA decreases the expression of VEGF (vascular endothelial growth factor) and ADM (adrenomedullin), which are normally induced by progesterone; this results in a decrement of angiogenesis in the leiomyoma cells [75]. Moreover, it inhibits activin A, a growth factor that belongs to the TGF-β (tumor growth factor beta) superfamily, thus contributing to reduce fibroid volume [76].

Furthermore, since uterine fibroids are characterized by qualitative and quantitative abnormalities in several ECM components; SPRMs reduce the strong deposition of ECM that characterizes fibroids suppressing the collagen synthesis (type I and III) and modulating matrix metalloproteinase s (MMPs) and tissue inhibitor of metalloproteinases (TIMPs) [77, 78].

Finally, the regulation of endometrial bleeding by assumption of SPRMs may be explained by another molecular mechanism consisting in the interleukin-15 (IL-15) pathway. This pathway has a key role for uterine NK (natural killer) cells development and function; the reduction of NK cells and their interaction on endometrial stromal cells and spiral arteries have a positive clinical effect [61]. By performing various experiments, some evidences have been reported with specific regard to asoprisnil. A significant reduction of inflammatory genes, the suppression of IL-15, a marked endometrium reduction in number of uterine NK cells have been described [79]. These drug-induced characteristics may explain the stopping of HMB.

Progesterone Receptor Modulator Associated Endometrial Changes

All the SPRMs have been associated to morphological and histological endometrium changes known as "progesterone receptor modulator associated endometrial changes" (PAECs), as described by Mutter et al. [80]. These entities are a new morphologic category [81], not been described before in any physiological state neither subsequently to the administration of any drugs.

Williams et al. [82] described that the following features characterize PAECs: cystic glandular dilatation, apoptosis, low mitotic activity in the glands and stroma, absence of stromal breakdown and glandular crowding.

PAECs consist only in a temporary endometrial alteration that tend to regress at the end of the treatment with SPRMs [83]; they are considered to be a pattern of benign, non-physiological, non-proliferative histologic features of the endometrium. They should not be confused with endometrial hyperplasia; therefore, it is important to inform the pathologist about the use of SPRMs in order to be confused by the suspicion of a malignant diagnosis. On the contrary, SPRMs have been shown to be characterized by an antiproliferative effect that leads to reducing mitotic activity of the endometrial glandular epithelium. Anyway, an extensive cystic glandular dilatation is seen despite of progesterone antagonism and maintenance of circulating E_2levels. However, the mechanisms by which these endometrial features develop under SPRM treatment are poorly understood [61, 84–86].

SPRMs have demonstrated a reduction in markers of endometrium proliferation in macaques [87]. In another study, the assumption of a low-dose of mifepristone showed similar results [88]. Endometrial hyperplasia was not reported neither after administration of asoprisnil for 12 weeks or in a long-term oral administration of UPA [89]. In general, there were no reports of cytological atypia associated with the use of SPRMs considering a normal endometrial biopsy prior to treatment [61].

Ulipristal Acetate

UPA is a SPRM licensed in 2012 by the European Medicines Agency (EMA) for the treatment of moderate-to-severe symptoms related to uterine fibroids in women of reproductive age [6, 64]. It has been approved for preoperative treatment of these benign tumors. Each course consists in a daily administration of a single 5 mg dose by oral route; it can used for up to 3 months and it may be eventually repeated by doing breaks between each course.

UPA is a synthetic steroid developed from 19-norprogesterone; it is an active antagonist of PR and a competitive antagonist of glucocorticoid receptor (GR) [90-91]. Its chemical structure is shown in Figure 2.

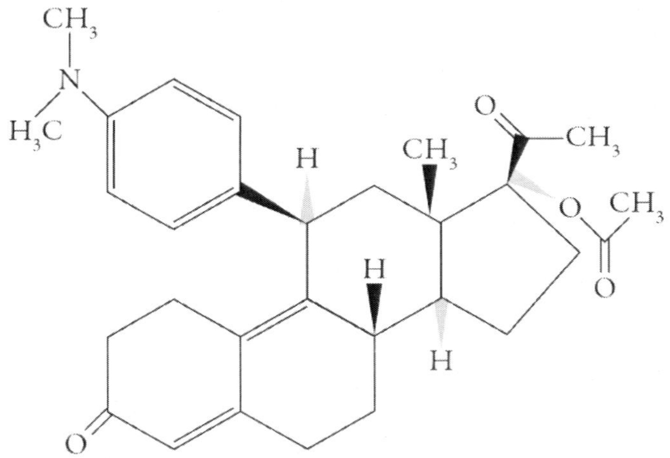

Figure 2. Chemical structure of Ulipristal acetate (17-acetoxy-11β-[4-N,N-dimethylaminophenyl]-19-norpregna-4,9-diene-3,20-dione) [64].

Similarly to other SPRMs, UPA is able to improve bleeding discomfort and to positively act on fibroid volume [2, 92]. In fact, it shows an anti-proliferative activity on leiomyoma cells and on the endometrium [93].

Clinical Studies

One of the first studies on the preoperative use of UPA for uterine fibroids was performed by Levens et al. [94]; anyway, the main publications supporting its use derived from the PEARL studies.

The PEARL I and II studies showed that UPA was effective in controlling uterine bleeding related to myomas, in reducing their size. This drug demonstrated also a good safety profile. The PEARL III and IV studies focused their attention on long-term safety of this drug. All of these studies have multicenter, randomized, double bind, parallel-group design. They received pharmaceutical company funding.

The PEARL I study compared UPA versus placebo before surgical treatment of symptomatic fibroids. The results showed the myoma shrinkage after 13 weeks of treatment (21.2% in the 5 mg UPA group and 12.3% in the 10 mg UPA group). The placebo group had a median 3% growth of myoma volume ($P < 0.01$)). In addition, a great decrease of bleeding symptoms was detected after treatment [2].

In the PEARL II study, UPA was compared with leuprolide acetate. The results showed similar effectiveness in controlling HMB (90% of patients in the 5 mg UPA group and 98% of gem in the 10 mg UPA group experienced controlled bleeding symptoms versus 89% in the GnRH-a group). No differences were found in hemoglobin at the end of each treatment.

However, leuprolide acetate obtained a greater reduction in uterine volumes (47% in the leuprolide acetate group versus 20% in the 5 mg UPA group and 22% in the 10 mg UPA group). Vasomotor symptoms were observed in 11% of patients in the UPA 5 mg and 10% in the 10 mg UPA groups ($P < 0.001$) [95]. Moreover, PEARL I and II studies found UPA-related PAEC, previously described.

The PEARL III study and its extension showed the effectiveness and the tolerability of a long-term intermittent treatment with UPA (10 mg/day for 3 months with drug-free intervals) [92].

The PEARL IV study investigated the safety and efficacy of the long-term repeated intermittent treatment with four 12-week treatment courses of UPA (the results from the first two treatment courses had previously been published in the previous PEARL III) of daily oral administration of different doses of UPA, 5 and 10 mg (women were divided into two groups). This is the first full clinical trial concerning the use of the authorized dose of UPA at 5 mg in a long-term repeated intermittent regimen [96].

The tolerability of UPA administration in the long-period makes necessary the comparative evaluation with GnRH agonists, since these compounds can be used only for a limited period due to their side-effects and rapid fibroids regrowth after the treatment cessation.

In a trial, UPA was administered to premenopausal women during their first 4 days of menses. The study design predicted a drug-free interval between each treatment course during which the menstruation appeared. Subsequent courses started with the beginning of the period. A final follow-up of 3-month drug-free was conducted after the last course. The outcomes examined were: amenorrhea, episodes of heavy bleeding, fibroid volume, pain, QoL and safety. All of these did not present any important differences between the 5mg and 10mg UPA groups. The UPA effectiveness confirmed previous data with regards to controlling bleeding symptoms, shrinking fibroid volume and improving pain and QoL. Amenorrhea was obtained in a high percentage of subjects (>70%) during each course and was reached, on average, within 1 week. A high percentage of subjects were in amenorrhea for all four courses. After the therapy, women presented a significant reduction of HMB (>73%) compared with pretreatment bleeding.

The volume of the three largest fibroids was decreased after the first treatment course and showed a further decrease after each subsequent treatment. The reduction in size was maintained until the end of the follow-up. Moreover, over 73% of women presented a reduction >25% in fibroid volume at the end of the last course. Pain and QoL got better during the treatment. Regarding safety, the authors focused their attention on endometrial thickness, laboratory parameters and side-effects and they did not notice any important differences between the 5-mg and 10-mg groups. They found that all cases of hyperplasia observed after the first course (7.4% of women presented an endometrial thickness >16 mm) returned to benign endometrium during the subsequent courses or during the follow-up period. Hemoglobin level increased reaching a peak at the end of the last course; levels of E2 remained well above postmenopausal levels, suggesting that bone mineral density will not be adversely impacted by repeated intermittent use of UPA, and cholesterol and triglyceride values had a little increased but below the cardiovascular risk. However, some sporadic increases of AST and ALT were found in some subjects. The majority of side-effects (97.6%) were mild or of moderate severity in both groups, the most frequent of which were headaches and hot flushes but these symptoms decreased by continuing the treatment. Breast pain or discomfort was detected in 3% of cases but also this effect decreased with successive courses. The results of this study finally demonstrated the efficacy and safety in a repeated intermittent treatment of symptomatic fibroid with UPA [83, 96].

Despite UPA has been approved for the preoperative treatment of fibroid, a multicenter, prospective, non-interventional study, study PREMYA, showed the potential application of this drug also for postponing or avoiding surgical procedures. The trial included 1473 eligible women who underwent pre-operative treatment with UPA. During 15 months of the whole study (3-months treatment course plus 12 months of drug-free interval), only 38.8% of patients underwent surgery after medical treatment; most of those underwent a minimally invasive procedure. Interestingly, the majority of patients did not undergo surgery immediately after the therapy, because symptoms, QoL and pain improved and remained better than baseline during the follow up period [97]

However, in terms of evaluating the facilitation of surgery after UPA administration, a retrospective, multicenter cohort study showed controversial results. In this study, two gynecologists had to watch laparoscopic/robotic myomectomy videos (Canadian Task Force Classification III) and compare surgical experience of patients pretreated with UPA versus absence of hormonal pretreatment, valuating 6 points (depth of myometrial incision, ease of myoma-myometrium cleavage plane identification, ease of myoma detachment, blood loss during myoma detachment, myometrial blood loss after myoma detachment, and myoma consistency). The operators were blinded about which patients received pretreatment with the SPRM. The results showed no differences in surgical experience between the 2 groups of patients [98]. Other studies investigated the use of UPA before performing laparoscopic or hysteroscopic myomectomy, showing positive outcomes [99-102].

With respect to economic effects of UPA, two analyses have been conducted. The first one demonstrated that the addition of a course of UPA before surgery rather than immediate hysterectomy is able to obtained an incremental cost effectiveness ratio of EUR 3575 per quality-adjusted life year in women with moderate to severe bleeding [103]. The second one, conducted in Netherlands, compared UPA versus leuprolide; the authors concluded that UPA represented a cost-saving option for preoperative treatment of moderate and severe symptoms related to fibroids [104].

Safety

After the commercial approval of UPA in 2012, four cases of serious liver disease that conduced to hepatic transplantation were recorded. However, no information concerning hepatic disorders is currently included in the warning label of UPA. Now European Medicines Agency (EMA) is reviewing benefits and risks related to the use of UPA.A new advice on its use of UPA has been published by the EMA and the Medicines and Healthcare products Regulatory Agency (MHRA) [105-108]. The temporary safety measures are:

- UPA treatment should not be initiated in new patients or in patients who have finalized a previous treatment course;
- for patients on current treatment with UPA, liver function should be monitored at least monthly, and 2-4 weeks after stopping treatment;
- if a patient shows signs or symptoms compatible with liver injury (nausea, vomiting, right hypochondrial pain, anorexia, asthenia, jaundice, etc.), it should be investigated immediately and liver function tests performed.

Patients developing transaminase levels >2 times the upper limit of normal during UPA treatment should stop treatment and be closely monitored.

Patients should be advised about specific actions to take in case of signs and symptoms of liver injury as described above.

Comparison between Preoperative Medical Options for Myomas

Several clinical trials have been conducted for evaluating the efficacy of hormonal therapy before surgery for fibroids (Table 4) (Figure.3).

A Cochrane Review [6], published in 2017 (an update of previous Cochrane Reviews published in 2000 and 2001), considered 3623 women with symptomatic fibroids from 38 RCTs. The patients underwent any type of surgery for uterine fibroids. The following pre-surgical therapies were evaluated:

- GnRH-a versus no presurgical treatments or placebo;
- GnRH-a versus other presurgical treatments (progestins, SPRMs, SERMs, dopamine agonists, estrogen receptor antagonists);
- SPRMs versus placebo.

The study aims to evaluate several preoperative intraoperative and postoperative outcomes.

Table 4. Comparison between GnRH-a, AIs, SPRMs

	GnRH-a	SPRMs	AIs
Fibroid shrinkage	-32-47% (6)/-27-70% [36] Up to 50% within 3- 6-months interval [20] The maximal reduction within the first 12 weeks of therapy [37]. Re-growth after the therapy is stopped: myoma volume returns to its pretreatment size within about 6 months [1].	-20% [6] after 3 months and further size decrease after subsequent courses. The reduction in volume seems maintained after 3 months of follow-up drug-free [83].	-46% [43]
Reduction of bleeding episodes; hemoglobin levels increment	Yes, after the first month of treatment.	Yes, amenorrhea is reached within 1 week on overage. Episodes of heavy bleeding are reduced >73% during each course and post-treatment menstrual bleeding are markedly reduced compared with pretreatment bleeding. Hemoglobin levels increase ever more after each course [83].	Yes
Relief of symptoms like pain and pressure sense	Yes, in the first 2 months [1]	Yes	Insufficient conclusions
Others	Flare-up effect in the second week, climacteric disturbance	Liver dysfunction to evaluate	Joint disorders

GnRH-a = GnRH-analogue; SPRM = selective progesterone receptor modulator; AI = aromatase inhibitor.

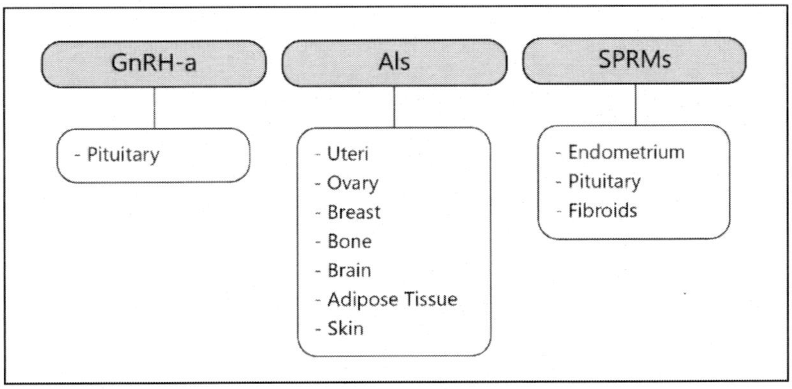

Figure 3. GnRH-analogues, aromatase inhibitors and selective progesterone receptor modulators play their action on different tissues.

Concerning the use of GnRH-aversus no treatment or placebo, preoperative use of GnRH-a was associated with:

- a reduction of both uterine (MD -175 mL) and fibroid volume (MD 5.7 mL);
- an increment of preoperative hemoglobin levels (median 0.88 g/dL);
- a higher incidence of hot flushes, headache, dizziness, vaginitis, change in breast size and sweating;
- a reduction of mean operation time (-9.59 minutes), fever incidence and complication rates during hysterectomy;
- a reduction of intraoperative blood loss (MD 22 mL to 157 mL) and blood transfusions;
- no significant difference operation time, intraoperative blood transfusions, duration of hospital stay, recurrence of fibroids and postoperative hemoglobin levels during and after myomectomy;
- a reduction of duration of surgery (-5.4 minutes) without evidence that pretreatment negatively influenced the difficulty of the surgical technique and the recurrence of fibroids after hysteroscopic myomectomy.

In the second comparison, GnRH-a compared with UPA had:

- greater reduction in uterine volume (-47% with GnRH-a compared to -20% and -22% with 5 mg and 10 mg UPA);
- more incidence of hot flushes;
- no significant difference in improving bleeding symptoms and hemoglobin rate.

With specific regard to this comparison, another Cochrane review (85) compared the treatment with SPRMs versus that with leuprolide. There was no difference between the two groups for improving the QoL and pelvic pain; in the SPRMs group some endometrial changes (PAEC) was observed.

Finally, SPRMs therapy with different compounds belonging to this class (mifepristone, CDB-2914, UPA and asoprisnil) was compared versus placebo with the following results. The SPRMs group showed:

- a greater reduction in both uterine and fibroid size;
- an increment of preoperative hemoglobin rate (MD 0.93 g/dL);
- a greater reduction in bleeding symptoms before surgery;
- a greater QoL;
- no significant differences in preoperative complications.

AIs, compared with GnRH-a, present the advantage of a direct action on both fibroids and ovary, suppressing locally androgen conversion in estrogen. Differently, GnRH-a act indirectly on pituitary gland downregulating GnRH-R. As said before, AIs have a more role among postmenopausal-age where GnRH-a are ineffective [59].

Moreover, even if both drug classes are generally equally effective, AIs do not present the bleeding often occurring in the second week after initiation of the therapy with GnRH-a [17].

A Cochrane systematic review [43], published in 2014, compared GnRH-a with letrozole (AI). Data have been obtained by only one trial [19] on 70 premenopausal women; the results showed that letrozole was more effective in fibroid shrinkage (46% in letrozole group versus 32% in GnRH-a group) after 12 weeks of treatment, although these conclusions were not statistically significant. Moreover, in letrozole group there was a lower incidence of hot flushes (0/33 in letrozole group versus 26/27 in GnRH-a group, $P < 0.05$). The trial did not demonstrate enough evidence to support relief of fibroids symptoms by using AIs. Thus, the authors concluded that the current use of AIs needs to more evidence about safety and side effects.

REFERENCES

[1] Cheng MH, Chao HT, Wang PH. Medical treatment for uterine myomas. *Taiwan J Obstet Gynecol.* 2008;47(1):18-23.

[2] Donnez J, Tatarchuk TF, Bouchard P, Puscasiu L, Zakharenko NF, Ivanova T, et al. Ulipristal Acetate versus Placebo for Fibroid Treatment before Surgery. *N Engl J Med.* 2012;366(5):409-20.

[3] West CP, Lumsden MA, Baird DT. Goserelin (Zoladex®) in the treatment of fibroids. *BJOG An Int J Obstet Gynaecol.* 1992.

[4] Stovall TG, Ling FW, Henry LC, Woodruff MR. A randomized trial evaluating leuprolide acetate before hysterectomy as treatment for leiomyomas. *Am J Obstet Gynecol.* 1991;99 Suppl 7:27-30.

[5] Pritts EA, Parker WH, Olive DL. Fibroids and infertility: an updated systematic review of the evidence. *Fertil Steril.* 2009;91(4):1215-23.

[6] Lethaby A, Puscasiu L, Vollenhoven B. Preoperative medical therapy before surgery for uterine fibroids. Vol. 2017, *Cochrane Database of Systematic Reviews.* 2017;11:CD000547.

[7] Reis FM, Bloise E, Ortiga-Carvalho TM. Hormones and pathogenesis of uterine fibroids. *Best Pract Res Clin Obstet Gynaecol.* 2016;34:13-24.

[8] Critchley HOD, Saunders PTK. Hormone receptor dynamics in a receptive human endometrium. In: *Reproductive Sciences.* 2009;16(2):191-9.

[9] Mesiano S. Myometrial progesterone responsiveness. Vol. 25, *Seminars in Reproductive Medicine.* 2007;25(1):5-13.

[10] Kurachi O, Matsuo H, Samoto T, Maruo T. Tumor necrosis factor-alpha expression in human uterine leiomyoma and its down-regulation by progesterone. *J Clin Endocrinol Metab.* 2001;86(5):2275-80.

[11] Islam MS, Protic O, Stortoni P, Grechi G, Lamanna P, Petraglia F, et al. Complex networks of multiple factors in the pathogenesis of uterine leiomyoma. *Fertil Steril.* 2013;100(1):178-93.

[12] Lee EJ, Kong G, Lee SH, Rho S, Park CS, Kim BG, et al. Profiling of differentially expressed genes in human uterine leiomyomas. *Int J Gynecol Cancer.* 2005;15(1):146-54.

[13] Rein MS, Barbieri RL, Friedman AJ. Progesterone: A critical role in the pathogenesis of uterine myomas. *Am J Obstet Gynecol.* 1995;172(1 Pt 1):14-8.

[14] Hagan CR, Knutson TP, Lange CA. A common docking domain in progesterone receptor-B links DUSP6 and CK2 signaling to proliferative transcriptional programs in breast cancer cells. *Nucleic Acids Res.* 2013; 41(19): 8926.

[15] Ono M, Qiang W, Serna VA, Yin P, Coon JS, Navarro A, et al. Role of stem cells in human uterine leiomyoma growth. *PLoS One.* 2012;7(5):e36935.

[16] Chegini N. Proinflammatory and profibrotic mediators: Principal effectors of leiomyoma development as a fibrotic disorder. Vol. 28, *Seminars in Reproductive Medicine.* 2010;28(3):180-203.

[17] AAGL Practice Report: Practice Guidelines for the Diagnosis and Management of Submucous Leiomyomas. *J Minim Invasive Gynecol.* 2012;19(2):152-71.

[18] Stovall TG, Muneyyirci-Delale O, Summ1tt RL, Scialli AR. GnRH agonist and iron versus placebo and iron in the anemic patient before surgery for leiomyomas: A randomized controlled trial. *Obstet Gynecol.* 1995;86(1):65-71.

[19] Parsanezhad ME, Azmoon M, Alborzi S, Rajaeefard A, Zarei A, Kazerooni T, et al. A randomized, controlled clinical trial comparing the effects of aromatase inhibitor (letrozole) and gonadotropin-releasing hormone agonist (triptorelin) on uterine leiomyoma volume and hormonal status. *Fertil Steril.* 2010;93(1):192-8.

[20] Vilos GA, Allaire C, Laberge PY, Leyland N. The Management of Uterine Leiomyomas. *J Obs Gynaecol Can.* 2015;37(2):157-178.

[21] Lethaby A, Vollenhoven B, Sowter M. Efficacy of Pre-Operative Gonadotropin Hormone Releasing Analogues for Women With Uterine Fibroids Undergoing Hysterectomy or Myomectomy: A Systematic Review. *BJOG.* 2002 Oct;109(10):1097-108.

[22] Plewka D, Marczyński J, Morek M, Bogunia E, Plewka A. Receptors of hypothalamic-pituitary-ovarian-axis hormone in uterine myomas. *Biomed Res Int.* 2014; 2014:521313.

[23] David Adamson G. Treatment of uterine fibroids: Current findings with gonadotropin-releasing hormone agonists. *Am J Obstet Gyneco*l. 1992;166(2):746-51.

[24] Kettel LM, Murphy AA, Morales AJ, Rivier J, Vale W, Yen SSC. Rapid regression of uterine leiomyomas in response to daily administration of gonadotropin-releasing hormone antagonist. *Fertil Steril.* 1993;60(4):642-6.

[25] Felberbaum RE, Germer U, Ludwig M, Riethmüller-Winzen H, Heise S, Buttge I, et al. Treatment of uterine fibroids with a slow-release formulation of the gonadotrophin releasing hormone antagonist Cetrorelix. *Hum Reprod.* 1998;13(6):1660-8.

[26] Flierman PA, Oberyé JJL, Van Der Hulst VPM, De Blok S. Rapid reduction of leiomyoma volume during treatment with the GnRH antagonist ganirelix. *BJOG An Int J Obstet Gynaecol*. 2005;112(5):638-42.

[27] Vercellini P, Sacerdote P, Trespidi L, Manfredi B, Panerai AE, Crosignani PG. Veralipride for hot flushes induced by a gonadotropin-releasing hormone agonist: a controlled study. *Fertil Steril.* 1994;62(5):938-42.

[28] Palomba S, Orio F, Russo T, Falbo A, Cascella T, Doldo P, et al. Long-term effectiveness and safety of GnRH agonist plus raloxifene administration in women with uterine leiomyomas. *Hum Reprod.* 2004;19(6): 1308–1314.

[29] Palomba S, Affinito P, Di Carlo C, Bifulco G, Nappi C. Long-term administration of tibolone plus gonadotropin-releasing hormone agonist for the treatment of uterine leiomyomas: Effectiveness and effects on vasomotor symptoms, bone mass, and lipid profiles. *Fertil Steril.* 1999;72(5):889-95.

[30] Hoellen F, Griesinger G, Bohlmann MK. Therapeutic drugs in the treatment of symptomatic uterine fibroids. *Expert Opin Pharmacother*. 2013;14(15):2079-85.

[31] Mclaren JS, Rymer J, Morris E. Gonadotrophin receptor hormone analogues in combination with add-back therapy: An update. Vol. 18, *Menopause International.* 2012;18(2):68-72.

[32] DiVasta AD, Laufer MR. The use of gonadotropin releasing hormone analogues in adolescent and young patients with endometriosis. *Curr Opin Obs Gynecol.* 2013;25(4):287-92.

[33] Ito F, Kawamura N, Ichimura T, Tsujimura A, Ishiko O, Ogita S. Ultrastructural comparison of uterine leiomyoma cells from the same myoma nodule before and after gonadotropin-releasing hormone agonist treatment. *Fertil Steril*. 2001; 75(1):125–130.

[34] Mizutani T, Sugihara A, Nakamuro K, Terada N. Suppression of cell proliferation and induction of apoptosis in uterine leiomyoma by gonadotropin-releasing hormone agonist (leuprolide acetate). *J Clin Endocrinol Metab*. 1998;83(4):1253-5.

[35] Huang SC, Chou CY, Lin YS, Tsai YC, Hsu KF, Liu CH, et al. Enhanced deoxyribonucleic acid damage and repair but unchanged apoptosis in uterine

leiomyomas treated with gonadotropin-releasing hormone agonist. *Am J Obstet Gynecol.* 1997;177(2):417-24.

[36] Chia CC, Huang SC, Chen SS, Kang JY, Lin JC, Lin YS, et al. Ultrasonographic evaluation of the change in uterine fibroids induced by treatment with a GnRH analog. *Taiwan J Obstet Gynecol.* 2006 45(2):124-8.

[37] AJF, MD, M JN, MSR. Predictors of uterine volume reduction in women with myomas treated with a gonadotropin-releasing hormone agonist. Vol. 58, *Fertility and Sterility.* 1992;58(2):413-5.

[38] Rein MS, Friedman AJ, Stuart JM, MacLaughlin DT. Fibroid and myometrial steroid receptors in women treated with gonadotropin-releasing hormone agonist leuprolide acetate. *Fertil Steril.* 1990; 53: 1018–1023.

[39] Bassaw B, Mohammed N, Jaggat A, Singh-Bhola M, Ramkissoon A, Singh P, et al. Experience with a gonadotrophin-releasing hormone agonist prior to myomectomy-comparison of twice-vs thrice-monthly doses and a control group. *J Obstet Gynaecol* (Lahore). 2014;34(5):415-9.

[40] Zhang Y, Sun L, Guo Y, Cheng J, Wang Y, Fan S, et al. The Impact of Preoperative Gonadotropin-Releasing Hormone Agonist Treatment on Women With Uterine Fibroids. *Obstet Gynecol Surv.* 2014;69(2):100-8.

[41] Chen I, Motan T, Kiddoo D. Gonadotropin-Releasing Hormone Agonist in Laparoscopic Myomectomy: Systematic Review and Meta-Analysis of Randomized Controlled Trials. Vol. 18, *Journal of Minimally Invasive Gynecology.* 2011;18(3):303-9.

[42] Kamath MS, Kalampokas EE, Kalampokas TE. Use of GnRH analogues pre-operatively for hysteroscopic resection of submucous fibroids: A systematic review and meta-analysis. Vol. 177, *European Journal of Obstetrics Gynecology and Reproductive Biology.* 2014;177:11-8.

[43] Song H, Lu D, Navaratnam K, Shi G. Aromatase inhibitors for uterine fibroids. *Cochrane database Syst Rev.* 2013;(10):CD009505.

[44] Sumitani H, Shozu M, Segawa T, Murakami K, Yang HJ, Shimada K, et al. In situ estrogen synthesized by aromatase P450 in uterine leiomyoma cells promotes cell growth probably via an autocrine/intracrine mechanism. *Endocrinology.* 2000;141(10):3852-61.

[45] Bulun SE, Simpson ER, Word RA. Expression of the cyp19 gene and its product aromatase cytochrome p450 in human uterine leiomyoma tissues and cells in culture. *J Clin Endocrinol Metab.* 1994;78(3):736-43.

[46] Shozu M, Sumitani H, Segawa T, Yang HJ, Murakami K, Kasai T, et al. Overexpression of aromatase P450 in leiomyoma tissue is driven primarily through promoter I.4 of the Aromatase P450 gene (CYP19). *J Clin Endocrinol Metab.* 2002; 87: 2540-8.

[47] Simpson ER. Sources of estrogen and their importance. In: *Journal of Steroid Biochemistry and Molecular Biology*. 2003;86(3-5):225-30.

[48] Results of the ATAC (Arimidex, Tamoxifen, Alone or in Combination) trial after completion of 5 years' adjuvant treatment for breast cancer. *Lancet*. 2005;365(9453):60-2.

[49] Franik S, Kremer JAM, Nelen WLDM, Farquhar C. Aromatase inhibitors for subfertile women with polycystic ovary syndrome. *Cochrane Database Syst Rev*. 2014;(2):CD010287.

[50] Pavone ME, Bulun SE. Aromatase inhibitors for the treatment of endometriosis. Vol. 98, *Fertility and Sterility*. 2012; 98(6):1370–1379.

[51] Gershanovich M, Chaudri HA, Campos D, Lurie H, Bonaventura A, Jeffrey M, et al. Letrozole, a new oral aromatase inhibitor: Randomised trial comparing 2.5 mg daily, 0.5 mg daily and aminoglutethimide in postmenopausal women with advanced breast cancer. *Ann Oncol*. 1998; 9: 639-645.

[52] Goss PE, Strasser K. Aromatase inhibitors in the treatment and prevention of breast cancer. *J Clin Oncol*. 2001;19(3):881-94.

[53] Buzdar AU, Robertson JFR, Eiermann W, Nabholtz JM. An overview of the pharmacology and pharmacokinetics of the newer generation aromatase inhibitors anastrozole, letrozole, and exemestane. *Cancer*. 2002;95(9):2006-16.

[54] Hilário SG, Bozzini N, Borsari R, Baracat EC. Action of aromatase inhibitor for treatment of uterine leiomyoma in perimenopausal patients. *Fertil Steril*. 2009;91(1):240-3.

[55] Felson DT, Cummings SR. Aromatase inhibitors and the syndrome of arthralgias with estrogen deprivation. Vol. 52, *Arthritis and Rheumatism*. 2005;52(9):2594-8.

[56] *Alert: Aromatase inhibitors in products marketed as dietary supplements: recall* [Internet]. [cited 2010 Dec 25]. Available from: Drugs.com.

[57] Gurates B, Parmaksiz C, Kilic G, Celik H, Kumru S, Simsek M. Treatment of symptomatic uterine leiomyoma with letrozole. *Reprod Biomed Online*. 2008;17(4):569-74.

[58] Kaunitz AM. Aromatase inhibitor therapy for uterine bleeding in a postmenopausal woman with leiomyomata. *Menopause*. 2007;14:941–943.

[59] Varelas FK, Papanicolaou AN, Vavatsi-Christaki N, Makedos GA, Vlassis GD. The effect of anastrazole on symptomatic uterine leiomyomata. *Obstet Gynecol*. 2007;110(3):643.

[60] Chabbert-Buffet N, Meduri G, Bouchard P, Spitz IM. Selective progesterone receptor modulators and progesterone antagonists: Mechanisms of action and clinical applications. Vol. 11, *Human Reproduction Update*. 2005;11(3):293-307.

[61] Wagenfeld A, Saunders PTK, Whitaker L, Critchley HOD. Selective progesterone receptor modulators (SPRMs): progesterone receptor action, mode of action on the

endometrium and treatment options in gynecological therapies. Vol. 20, *Expert Opinion on Therapeutic Targets.* 2016; 20(9): 1045–1054.

[62] Lähteenmäki P, Haukkamaa M, Puolakka J, Riikonen U, Sainio S, Suvisaari J, et al. Open randomised study of use of levonorgestrel releasing intrauterine system as alternative to hysterectomy. *BMJ.* 1998;317(7167):1250.

[63] Spitz IM. Clinical utility of progesterone receptor modulators and their effect on the endometrium. Vol. 21, *Current Opinion in Obstetrics and Gynecology.* 2009;21(4):318-24.

[64] Talaulikar VS, Manyonda IT. Ulipristal acetate: A novel option for the medical management of symptomatic uterine fibroids. Vol. 29, *Advances in Therapy.* 2012;29(8):655-63.

[65] Melis GB, Piras B, Marotto MF, Orru' MM, Maricosu G, Pilloni M, et al. Pharmacokinetic evaluation of ulipristal acetate for uterine leiomyoma treatment. *Expert Opin Drug Metab Toxicol.* 2012;8(7):901-8.

[66] Luo X, Yin P, Coon V. JS, Cheng Y-H, Wiehle RD, Bulun SE. The selective progesterone receptor modulator CDB4124 inhibits proliferation and induces apoptosis in uterine leiomyoma cells. *Fertil Steril.* 2010;93(8):2668-73.

[67] Bouchard P, Chabbert-Buffet N, Fauser BCJM. Selective progesterone receptor modulators in reproductive medicine: Pharmacology, clinical efficacy and safety. Vol. 96, *Fertility and Sterility.* 2011;96(5):1175-89.

[68] Girish C, Jayanthi M, Sivaraman G. Asoprisnil: A selective progesterone receptor modulator. Vol. 37, *Indian Journal of Pharmacology.* 2005; 37(4): 266-267.

[69] Wardell SE, Narayanan R, Weigel NL, Edwards DP. Partial Agonist Activity of the Progesterone Receptor Antagonist RU486 Mediated by an Amino-Terminal Domain Coactivator and Phosphorylation of Serine ^{400}. *Mol Endocrinol.* 2010;24(2):335-45.

[70] Afhüppe W, Sommer A, Müller J, Schwede W, Fuhrmann U, Möller C. Global gene expression profiling of progesterone receptor modulators in T47D cells provides a new classification system. *J Steroid Biochem Mol Biol.* 2009;113(1-2):105-15.

[71] Hammoud AO, Asaad R, Berman J, Treadwell MC, Blackwell S, Diamond MP. Volume change of uterine myomas during pregnancy: Do myomas really grow? *J Minim Invasive Gynecol.* 2006;13(5):386-90.

[72] Sivin I, Stern J. Health during prolonged use of levonorgestrel 20 micrograms/d and the copper TCu 380Ag intrauterine contraceptive devices: a multicenter study. International Committee for Contraception Research (ICCR). *Fertil Steril.* 1994;61(1):70-7.

[73] Kim JJ, Sefton EC. The role of progesterone signaling in the pathogenesis of uterine leiomyoma. Vol. 358, *Molecular and Cellular Endocrinology.* 2012; 358(2): 223–231.

[74] Malik M, Britten J, Cox J, Patel A, Catherino WH. Gonadotropin-releasing hormone analogues inhibit leiomyoma extracellular matrix despite presence of gonadal hormones. *Fertil Steril.* 2016;105(1):214-24.

[75] Maruo T, Ohara N, Yoshida S, Nakabayashi K, Sasaki H, Xu Q, et al. Lessons learned from the preclinical drug discovery of asoprisnil and ulipristal for non-surgical treatment of uterine leiomyomas. *Expert Opin Drug Discov.* 2011;6(9):897-911.

[76] Ciarmela P, Carrarelli P, Islam MS, Janjusevic M, Zupi E, Tosti C, et al. Ulipristal acetate modulates the expression and functions of activin A in leiomyoma cells. *Reprod Sci.* 2014;21(9):1120-5.

[77] Morikawa A, Ohara N, Xu Q, Nakabayashi K, DeManno DA, Chwalisz K, et al. Selective progesterone receptor modulator asoprisnil down-regulates collagen synthesis in cultured human uterine leiomyoma cells through up-regulating extracellular matrix metalloproteinase inducer. *Hum Reprod.* 2008;23(4):944-51.

[78] Xu Q, Ohara N, Liu J, Amano M, Sitruk-Ware R, Yoshida S, et al. Progesterone receptor modulator CDB-2914 induces extracellular matrix metalloproteinase inducer in cultured human uterine leiomyoma cells. *Mol Hum Reprod.* 2008;14(3):181-91.

[79] Wilkens J, Male V, Ghazal P, Forster T, Gibson DA, Williams ARW, et al. Uterine NK Cells Regulate Endometrial Bleeding in Women and Are Suppressed by the Progesterone Receptor Modulator Asoprisnil. *J Immunol.* 2013;191(5):2226-35.

[80] Mutter GL, Bergeron C, Deligdisch L, Ferenczy A, Glant M, Merino M, et al. The spectrum of endometrial pathology induced by progesterone receptor modulators. *Mod Pathol.* 2008;21(5):591-8.

[81] Ioffe OB, Zaino RJ, Mutter GL. Endometrial changes from short-term therapy with CDB-4124, a selective progesterone receptor modulator. *Mod Pathol.* 2009;22(3):450-9.

[82] Williams ARW, Bergeron C, Barlow DH, Ferenczy A. Endometrial morphology after treatment of uterine fibroids with the selective progesterone receptor modulator, ulipristal acetate. *Int J Gynecol Pathol.* 2012;31(6):556-69.

[83] Donnez J, Donnez O, Matule D, Ahrendt HJ, Hudecek R, Zatik J, et al. Long-term medical management of uterine fibroids with ulipristal acetate. *Fertil Steril.* 2016;105(1):165-173.e4.

[84] Donnez J, Donnez O, Dolmans M-M. Safety of treatment of uterine fibroids with the selective progesterone receptor modulator, ulipristal acetate. *Expert Opin Drug Saf.* 2016;15(12):1679-1686.

[85] Murji A, Horne AW, Whitaker L, Sobel ML, Critchley HOD. Selective progesterone receptor modulators (SPRMs) for uterine fibroids. *Cochrane Database Syst Rev.* 2017;4:CD010770.

[86] Whitaker LHR, Williams ARW, Critchley HOD. Selective progesterone receptor modulators. *Curr Opin Obstet Gynecol.* 2014;26(4):237-42.

[87] Brenner RM, Slayden OD, Nath A, Tsong YY, Sitruk-Ware R. Intrauterine administration of CDB-2914 (Ulipristal) suppresses the endometrium of rhesus macaques. *Contraception.* 2010;81(4):336-42.

[88] Baird DT, Brown A, Critchley HOD, Williams AR, Lin S, Cheng L. Effect of long-term treatment with low-dose mifepristone on the endometrium. *Hum Reprod.* 2003;18(1):61-68.

[89] Pohl O, Williams AR, Bergeron C, Gotteland JP. A 39-week oral toxicity study of ulipristal acetate in cynomolgus monkeys. *Regul Toxicol Pharmacol.* 2013;66(1):6-12.

[90] Tafi E, Scala C, Leone Roberti Maggiore U, Bizzarri N, Candiani M, Venturini PL, et al. Drug safety evaluation of ulipristal acetate in the treatment of uterine fibroids. *Expert Opin Drug Saf.* 2015;14(6):965-77.

[91] Ferrero S, Vellone VG, Barra F. Pharmacokinetic drug evaluation of ulipristal acetate for the treatment of uterine fibroids. *Expert Opin Drug Metab Toxicol.* 2018;14(1):107-16.

[92] Donnez J, Vázquez F, Tomaszewski J, Nouri K, Bouchard P, Fauser BCJM, et al. Long-term treatment of uterine fibroids with ulipristal acetate. *Fertil Steril.* 2014;101(6):1565-73.e1-18.

[93] Chabbert-Buffet N, Pintiaux-Kairis A, Bouchard P, Grp VS. Effects of the progesterone receptor modulator VA2914 in a continuous low dose on the hypothalamic-pituitary-ovarian axis and endometrium in normal women: A prospective, randomized, placebo-controlled trial. *J Clin Endocrinol Metab.* 2007;92(9):3582-9.

[94] Levens ED, Potlog-Nahari C, Armstrong AY, Wesley R, Premkumar A, Blithe DL, et al. CDB-2914 for uterine leiomyomata treatment: A randomized controlled trial. *Obstet Gynecol.* 2008; 111(5): 1129–1136.

[95] Donnez J, Tomaszewski J, Vázquez F, Bouchard P, Lemieszczuk B, Baró F, et al. Ulipristal Acetate versus Leuprolide Acetate for Uterine Fibroids - Supplementary Appendix. *N Engl J Med.* 2012; 366:421-432.

[96] Donnez J, Hudecek R, Donnez O, Matule D, Arhendt HJ, Zatik J, et al. Efficacy and safety of repeated use of ulipristal acetate in uterine fibroids. *Fertil Steril.* 2015;103(2):519-27.e3.

[97] Fernandez H, Schmidt T, Powell M, Costa APF, Arriagada P, Thaler C. Real world data of 1473 patients treated with ulipristal acetate for uterine fibroids: Premya study results. *Eur J Obstet Gynecol Reprod Biol.* 2017;208:91-96.

[98] Luketic L, Shirreff L, Kives S, Liu G, El Sugy R, Leyland N, et al. Does Ulipristal Acetate Affect Surgical Experience at Laparoscopic Myomectomy? *J Minim Invasive Gynecol.* 2017;24(5):797-802.

[99] Ferrero S, Alessandri F, Vellone VG, Venturini PL, Leone Roberti Maggiore U. Three-month treatment with ulipristal acetate prior to laparoscopic myomectomy of large uterine myomas: a retrospective study. *Eur J Obstet Gynecol Reprod Biol.* 2016;205:43-7.

[100] Ferrero S, Racca A, Tafi E, Alessandri F, Venturini PL, Leone Roberti Maggiore U. Ulipristal Acetate Before High Complexity Hysteroscopic Myomectomy: A Retrospective Comparative Study. *J Minim Invasive Gynecol.* 2016;23(3):390-5.

[101] Ferrero S, Scala C, Barra F. Regarding "Does Ulipristal Acetate Affect Surgical Experience at Laparoscopic Myomectomy?". *J Minim Invasive Gynecol.* 2018;25(3):541.

[102] Ferrero S, Vellone VG, Barra F, Scala C. Ulipristal Acetate before Hysteroscopic and Laparoscopic Surgery for Uterine Myomas: Help or Hindrance? *Gynecol Obstet Invest.* 2018:1-13.

[103] Nagy B, Timár G, Józwiak-Hagymásy J, Kovács G, Merész G, Vámossy I, et al. The cost-effectiveness of ulipristal acetate tablets in treating patients with moderate to severe symptoms of uterine fibroids. *Eur J Obstet Gynecol Reprod Biol.* 2014;175:75-81.

[104] Zakiyah N, van Asselt ADI, Postma MJ. Ulipristal acetate for pre-operative treatment of moderate-to-severe uterine fibroids in women of reproductive age in The Netherlands: cost minimization analysis and budget impact analysis. *J Med Econ.* 2017;20(3):280-287.

[105] Inn E. INN/active substance: *Ulipristal acetate.* 2018.

[106] Annex Scientific conclusions *Scientific conclusions.* 2016.

[107] PRAC. Women taking Esmya for uterine fibroids to have regular liver tests while EMA review is ongoing. *Eur Med Agency.* 2018.

[108] *FSRH CEU response to European Medicines Agency recommendations regarding use of ulipristal acetate for management of uterine fibroids – Use of ulipristal acetate for emergency contraception.* 2018.

In: Uterine Fibroids
Editors: S. Ferrero and F. Barra

ISBN: 978-1-53615-046-9

Chapter 6

MINILAPAROTOMIC MYOMECTOMY

Davide Lijoi[1], MD, Fabio Barra[2,3], MD and Simone Ferrero[2,3,*], MD, PhD

[1]Unit of Obstetrics and Gynecology, Galliera Hospital, Genoa, Italy
[2]Department of Neurosciences, Rehabilitation, Ophthalmology, Genetics, Maternal and Child Health (DiNOGMI), University of Genoa, Italy
[3]Academic Unit of Obstetrics and Gynecology, IRCCS Ospedale San Martino, Genoa, Italy

ABSTRACT

In this chapter, several therapeutic options are described for the management of symptomatic uterine myomas. Laparotomic myomectomy represents the gold standard conservative procedure for the treatment of symptomatic intramural and subserosal fibroids in women planning pregnancy. A minilaparotomic transverse incision can reduce postoperative pain as well as the risk of wound dehiscence and development of hernia when compared with traditional abdominal access. This technique requires a transverse skin incision of 4-7 cm that allows the removal of fibroids for a uterine size of 16-weeks pregnancy or smaller. Available literature recommends, where it is possible, to perform a single anterior uterine incision in order to reduce the post-operative formation of adhesions; the closure of myoma bed must be done with multiple layers in order to reduce the risk of uterine rupture in subsequent pregnancies. Recent evidence demonstrates that the use of barbed sutures could guarantee many advantages in terms of surgical outcomes and surgical difficulty.

At the present, myomectomy performed via laparoscopic route is associated with lower hemoglobin drop, lower morbidity, lower post-operative pain, and shorter hospital stay in respect with laparotomic myomectomy. No studies are able to demonstrate a

* Corresponding Author's E-mail: simoneferrero@me.com.

significant difference between the two surgical techniques regarding pregnancy rate, abortion rate, and live-birth rate.

The advantages reported for minilaparotomic myomectomy are the ability to remove multiple or large fibroids, and the possibility for the surgeon to directly palpate the uterus. The learning the curve of minilaparotomic myomectomy is shorter compared to laparoscopic one.

Keywords: myomectomy, uterine fibroids, myomas, minilaparotomy

1. Introduction

Uterine fibroids are the most common uterine neoplasm [1]. They are the leading cause of hysterectomy in the United States, accounting for one third of all hysterectomies performed nationally [2].

Abdominal myomectomy was described for the first time in 1931 [3] and it has rapidly become the gold standard conservative surgical procedure for uterine fibroids, especially for women who wish to preserve their childbearing potential. Despite nonsurgical interventions have been developed for the management of uterine fibroids, also today surgery continues to be the mainstay of treatment for symptomatic patients with fibroids [2].

Uterine fibroids are most frequently asymptomatic. However, women may present with several symptoms due to fibroids location, dimension, and number. In general, the most frequent symptoms associated with fibroids are metrorrhagia, abdominopelvic pain and dysmenorrhea, bulk-related symptoms, subfertility, and pregnancy-related complications [4].

Currently, the optimal management of fibroids is uncertain. Indeed, only a few randomized trials have compared different surgical and not surgical therapies and their comparative effectiveness in terms of future fertility [5].

In particular, regarding surgical management, myomectomy may be performed by several different methods. Currently, the surgical modalities available for myomectomy include hysteroscopic, laparoscopic, laparoscopic-assisted with minilaparotomy, robotic-assisted laparoscopic, or open myomectomy.

2. Indication to Surgical Myomas Removal

According to many guidelines, surgical myomectomy is the preferred option for the treatment of symptomatic intramural and subserosal fibroids in women planning pregnancy [5, 6, 7, 8]. However, myomectomy carries potential risks regarding fertility and of developing postoperative adhesions. Moreover, an intraoperative conversion to hysterectomy may be sometimes required during myomectomy (in about 3 to 4% of cases) [9]. For those reasons, treatment of asymptomatic intramural fibroids is not recommended [6], especially in woman who wish future pregnancy. Furthermore, an extensive literature review has not been able to demonstrate strong evidence to recommend performing myomectomy to improve fertility [8].

Currently, the most important criteria in the clinical practice to evaluate the decision of performing a myomectomy are the desire of future pregnancy and clinical symptoms. Thus, asymptomatic fibroids do not usually require treatment [10].

Fibroids can affect women's fertility producing anatomic distortion of uterus, fallopian tubes, and ovaries. Furthermore, fibroids can lead to pathological changes of endometrial function thus compromising fertility. However, fibroids are the only responsible cause of infertility in < 3% of cases [11].

The location of fibroid (submucosal, intramural, or subserosal) is the most important feature in relation to the alteration of fertility: in fact, submucous fibroids have the greatest impact on fertility while almost no effect is exercised by subserosal fibroids; moreover, there are no clear evidence about the effect of intramural fibroids on fertility. Anyway, it seems that these latter distorting the uterine cavity may significantly decrease implantation rates [12]. Moreover, it has been demonstrated that fibroids are associated with negative obstetrical outcomes such as preterm delivery, abnormal presentation, primary cesarean section and lower birth weight newborns [13]. The decision of surgical removal of fibroids with the aim to improve fertility should be extensively discussed with each patient. Particularly, other non-surgical options should be also offered.

As evidenced before, the majority of fibroids tend to remain asymptomatic. Nevertheless, they can cause profuse menstrual bleeding with subsequent anemia onset. Moreover, large fibroids causing an enlargement of the uterus can lead to bowel and bladder dysfunction as well as pelvic pain. These symptoms often resolve or decrease at menopause; then, the indication to surgical treatment of fibroids should be proposed also considering the expected time at menopause.

The type of fibroids according to the FIGO classification [14] correlates with specific symptoms and can be used to decide the management. This classification describes 8 types of fibroids. Submucosal and intracavitary fibroids (types 0, 1, 2) distorting the uterine cavity may lead to greater bleeding. However, increased menstrual bleeding can also be due to intramural and subserosal fibroids (types 3 to 7), which may inhibit myometrial contractility. These last two types of fibroids can also lead to a great enlargement of the uterus, which may compress adjacent structures, thus causing bulk-related bladder (urinary urgency, frequency and incontinence) and bowel (constipation and tenesmus) symptoms. At least, relevant distension of the abdominal cavity due to their presence can also lead to hydronephrosis or pelvic veins compression.

3. Choosing the Right Surgical Route for Myomas

Surgical management of fibroids should consider the presence of symptoms and the quality of life and the desire for future pregnancy of each patient. In order to choose the appropriate surgical management, it is extremely important to obtain an accurate description of fibroids size, number and location. Moreover, appropriate imaging techniques should be performed to improve optimal surgical planning [15]. At present time, there is agreement about using a minimally invasive surgical approach for performing myomectomy [2]. Hysteroscopic myomectomy is the best surgical route for submucosal fibroids (no more than 5 cm), which are type 0 or type 1 according to the 2011 FIGO classification [14, 16]. Broadly, the best approach for intramural and subserosal fibroids is that laparoscopic. Overall, the different laparoscopic techniques (laparoscopic, laparoscopic-assisted with minilaparotomy, robotic-assisted laparoscopic) can be contraindicated for uterus size >16 weeks, more than 5 fibroids or single fibroid more than 15 cm [17]. However, the indications about minimally invasive approaches should change in case of less experienced surgeons. In fact, there is no doubt that laparoscopic techniques need a longer learning curve and an extensive surgical experience. Furthermore, particular attention is due to posterior fibroids that are hardly removable using laparoscopic techniques. For example, when the fibroids are located in the posterior uterine wall, the laparoscopic suture is difficult and requires a dedicated surgical skill [18].

4. Minilaparotomic Myomectomy

4.1. Surgical Technique

Minilaparotomic transverse incision reduces postoperative pain as well as the risks of wound dehiscence and of developing hernia when compared with traditional laparotomy. Moreover, an optimal esthetic result is almost always obtained when performing it. This surgical access should be avoided when a particularly great operating field is needed.

Traditionally, minilaparotomic myomectomy is performed under general anesthesia. However, for many years, regional anesthesia has been proposed to perform minilaparotomic this surgical procedure.

Currently, minilaparotomic myomectomy requires a transverse skin incision of 4-7 cm, according to the number, size, and position of the fibroids (Figure 1). The distance between the skin incision and the pubic symphysis may differ in relation to leiomyoma dimension and localization (from 2 to 4 cm). Some authors [19] described the positioning of two sutures at the ends of the skin incision in order to avoid extension of minilaparotomy. The skin incision should be longer and further from pubic symphysis in case of great posterior fibroids. Usually, a transverse minilaparotomy of 4-7 cm allows for the removal of fibroids for a uterine size of 16-weeks pregnancy or smaller. In the case of a bigger uterine size, a midline vertical incision can be considered also according to the surgeon skill.

After opening skin and subcutaneous tissues, the anterior rectus fascia is incised transversely in the midline. The anterior rectus fascia is then separated from the below rectus abdominis muscle. The abdominal muscle and the peritoneum are longitudinally opened on the midline. After opening peritoneum and entering the abdominal cavity, the inspection of the uterus and the palpation of its surface help the surgeon to plan the optimal uterine incision. A midline vertical uterine incision as much as possible far from tubal origin is to prefer. When possible, in order to avoid the postoperative formation of adhesions, the surgeon should perform a single anterior incision. In fact, the risk of their subsequent formation is higher for multiple serosal incisions and in case of posterior uterus wall incision. The length of incision should be the most comfortable possible in order to remove the largest fibroid. After the removal of the first fibroid, the same incision should be used to reach the site of other benign tumors.

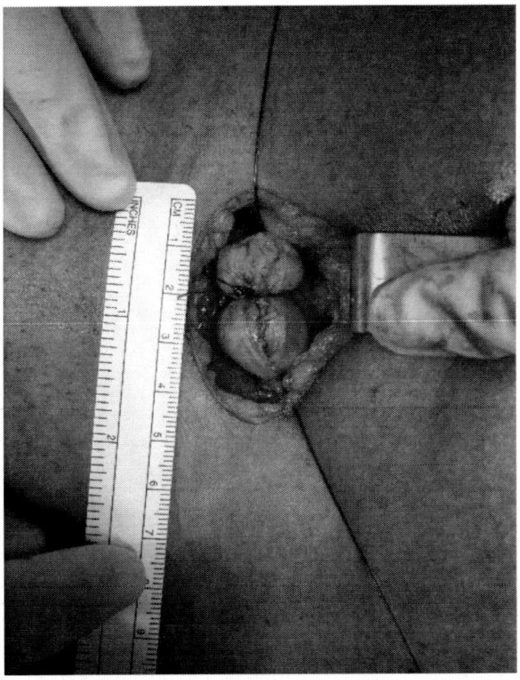

Figure 1. Minilaparotomic abdominal transverse incision for myomectomy.

After the serosal and myometrial incision, the fibroid is exposed and grasped with double-tooth forceps. The traction on the forceps leads to achieve an accurate dissection between the myometrium and the fibroid. Moreover, whenever is possible, the fibroid vessels should be sealed before dissection.

After the removal of all fibroids, particular attention should be made for the eventual lesion of the endometrial cavity. In case of an endometrial lesion, the cavity of the uterus should be closed using a single layer 3-0 or 4-0 absorbable suture. Subsequently, the myometrial incision should be promptly closed. The myometrial suture must be done in multiple layers. This technique is essential in order to reduce the risk of uterine rupture in subsequent pregnancies, thus providing the best fertility outcome. Multiple layers absorbable suture 0 gauge are usually employed, also ensuring adequate hemostasis. Recent evidence demonstrated that the use of barbed sutures could guarantee many advantages. In particular, barbed sutures are expected to reduce the time required for suturing the uterine wall defect and to prevent a higher intraoperative blood loss. Also, the degree of surgical difficulty when using barbed sutures seems to be significantly lower. However, this evidence has been obtained during laparoscopic myomectomy or after caesarian section [20, 21, 22]. In our opinion, barbed sutures could lead to similar advantages also during minilaparotomic myomectomy.

The rate of postoperative adhesion after myomectomy is high and it seems to be associated with the presence of sutures [23]. Their prevention is strictly essential to preserve future women' fertility. Posterior fibroids removal leads to postoperative adhesion more frequently. As demonstrated by Canis et al. [24], absorbable adhesion barriers (as oxidized cellulose) could help in reducing the adhesion formation after myomectomy. The use of these barriers should be strongly considered at the end of the uterus wall reconstruction.

4.2. Comparison with Laparoscopic Myomectomy

In the opinion of several authors, laparoscopy should be the standard approach for myomectomy [25]. Therefore, only a little number of studies compared laparoscopic myomectomy with abdominal myomectomy; moreover, only some of them are prospective and randomized. In recent times, a new increased interest concerning minilaparotomic myomectomy has been demonstrated by many authors, especially since minilaparotomy started being considered a minimally invasive alternative to conventional laparotomy or laparoscopy [18, 26].

At present, in the comparison between laparoscopic and laparotomic myomectomy, it seems that laparoscopic one is associated with lower hemoglobin drop, lower morbidity, lower post-operative pain and shorter hospital stay [18, 27]. However, authors who support minilaparotomic myomectomy underline that this surgical technique allows to remove multiple or large fibroids and enables the surgeon to directly palpate the uterus (removing less detectable fibroids, thus subsequently reducing the disease recurrence). Furthermore, learning the curve of minilaparotomic myomectomy is certainly shorter if compared with laparoscopic one and it does not need specific surgical equipment or advanced surgical skills (for example, for suturing the uterus).

It is quite proven that laparoscopic myomectomy results in better short-term outcomes when compared with minilaparotomic technique [18]. Regarding long-term results, the comparison between the two surgical technique leads to no clear evidence. Postoperative adhesions seem to be more frequent after minilaparotomic route, but also laparoscopy cannot entirely prevent adhesions formation [28, 29]. Uterine rupture during pregnancy or labor after myomectomy is a very important issue for the potential maternal and fetal consequences. This is a rare event mainly related to the strength of the myomectomy scar. Factors that can increase the risk of uterine rupture after myomectomy are the use of electrocoagulation on the myometrium wall and the hematoma formation in the context of the surgical suture. In the past, many publications underlined an increased risk of uterine rupture after laparoscopic myomectomy because of inadequate suturing of the myometrial wall. Nevertheless, it is known that uterine rupture after myomectomy seems to be an exceptional event either after laparoscopic or laparotomic surgical access [30, 31]. Overall, only few studies compared fertility outcomes after laparoscopic and abdominal myomectomy. Among them, the best designed series were not able to demonstrate a significant difference between the two surgical techniques regarding pregnancy rate, abortion rate and live-birth rate [32, 33]. Another important matter of controversy is the recurrence rate of fibroids after surgery. As already mentioned, the possibility of direct palpation of the uterus during minilaparotomic myomectomy could ensure the detection of small intramural fibroids thus reducing cumulative fibroids recurrence rate when compared with laparoscopic one. However, the available data in the literature on this topic are not conclusive and accurate (also considering that fibroids recurrence rate is often evaluated using different definitions.

Different costs characterized the two procedures. Actually, there is a common opinion about the higher direct costs of laparoscopy. A more detailed analysis should account that the indirect costs of laparoscopy are probably lower and might partly compensate for the higher direct costs. Additionally, the total cost of these surgical procedures should be estimated in the view of the health care system also considering the cost of untreated fibroids, the alternative treatments or the subsequent investigations for patients untreated.

Finally, we have to remember that, in order to avoid laparotomic access, fibroids morcellation is often indispensable when performing laparoscopy. During 2014, the FDA published a literature review to assess the prevalence of uterine sarcomas in women who underwent surgery (myomectomy or hysterectomy) to treat supposed benign fibroids [34]. Subsequent, well conducted cohort study assessed an incidence of uterine sarcoma that was estimated to be 1/278 (3.60 for 1000 hysterectomies) [35]. These data cannot be omitted because uterine and fibroids morcellation could importantly aggravate the prognosis of patients with an undiagnosed sarcoma by disseminating malign cells in the abdomen. Based on these data, in the past years, fibroids morcellation was criticized by many authors. Thus, it has been proposed to decrease to perform laparoscopic myomectomy and to subsequently return to perform more often laparotomic myomectomy. Nowadays, several scientific societies proposed various decision algorithm to guide clinicians on using morcellation or not [36]. Further studies are needed to obtain a high level of scientific evidence in order to propose official recommendations.

Conclusion

The management of uterine fibroids requires surgical and/or medical therapy considering the severity of symptoms, age, wish to preserve the uterus and the childbearing potential of each patient [37-40]. Many authors proposed guidelines to ease the clinician choice. It is important to remember that the risks and benefits of each option should be discussed with the patient [41]. It should be underlined that different factors must be considered: not last the skill of the surgeons and the experience of different centers in the available techniques.

Overall, the minilaparotomic myomectomy is a quite simple surgical technique to be considered as a valid alternative to conventional laparotomic or laparoscopic myomectomy, especially in case of multiple and/or large fibroids. The learning curve of the minilaparotomic myomectomy is relatively short if compared to that of other surgical therapies proposed for the treatment of uterine fibroids (laparoscopic or robotic-assisted laparoscopic myomectomy).

References

[1] Walker CL, Stewart EA. Uterine fibroids: the elephant in the room. *Science.* 2005;308:1589–1592.

[2] Flyckt R, Coyne K, Falcone T. *Clin Obstet Gynecol* 2017;60(2): 252–272;60(2): 252–272.

[3] Bonney V. The techniques and results of myomectomy. *Lancet.*1931;220:171–107.

[4] Wallach EE, Vlahos NF. Uterine myomas: an overview of development, clinical features, and management. *Obstet Gynecol.* 2004;104:393–406.

[5] Stewart EA. Clinical practice. Uterine fibroids. *N Engl J Med.* 2015;372:1646–1655.

[6] Marret H, Fritel X, Ouldamer L, et al. Therapeutic management of uterine fibroid tumors: updated French guidelines. *Eur J Obstet Gynecol Reprod Biol* 2012;165:156-64.

[7] American College of Obstetricians and Gynecologists. ACOG practice bulletin: alternatives to hysterectomy in the management of leiomyomas. *Obstet Gynecol.* 2008; 112: 387-400.

[8] Metwally M, Cheong YC, Horne AW. Surgical treatment of fibroids for subfertility. *Cochrane Database Syst Rev* 2012; 11:CD003857.

[9] Practice Committee of American Society for Reproductive Medicine in collaboration with Society of Reproductive Surgeons. Myomas and reproductive function. *Fertil Steril* 2008; 90: Suppl: S125-S130.

[10] Donnez J and Dolmans MM. Uterine fibroid management: from the present to the future. *Hum Reprod Update* 2016;22(6): 665–686.

[11] Farquhar C. Do uterine fibroids cause infertility and should they be removed to increase fertility? *BMJ.* 2009;16:338.

[12] Pritts EA, Parker WH, Olive DL. Fibroids and infertility: an updated systematic review of the evidence. *Fertil Steril.* 2009;91:1215–1223.

[13] Blitz MJ, Rochelson B, Augustine S, et al. Uterine fibroids at routine second-trimester ultrasound survey and risk of sonographic short cervix. *J Matern Fetal Neonatal Med.* 2016;14:1–7.

[14] Munro MG, Critchley HO, Broder MS, et al. FIGO Working Group on Menstrual Disorders. FIGO classification system (PALM-COEIN) for causes of abnormal uterine bleeding in nongravid women of reproductive age. *Int J Gynaecol Obstet.* 2011;113:3–13.

[15] Vilos GA, Allaire C, Laberge PY, et al. The management of uterine leiomyomas. *J Obstet Gynaecol Can.* 2015;37:157–181.

[16] Donnez J, Jadoul P. What are the implications of myomas on fertility? A need for a debate? *Hum Reprod.* 2002;17:1424–1430.

[17] Chen CC, Falcone T. Robotic gynecologic surgery: past, present, and future. *Clin Obstet Gynecol.* 2009;52:335.e43

[18] Alessandri F, Lijoi D, Mistrangelo E, et al. Randomized study of laparoscopic versus minilaparotomic myomectomy for uterine myomas. *J Minim Invasive Gynecol.* 2006;13:92–97.

[19] Prapas, Y., Kalogiannidis, I., Prapas, N. Laparoscopy vs. laparoscopically assisted myomectomy in the management of uterine myomas: a prospective study. *Am J Obstet Gynecol* 2009;200,144, e1-6.

[20] Naval S, Naval R, Naval S, Rane J. Tips for Safe Laparoscopic Multiple Myomectomy. *J Minim Invasive Gynecol.* 2017;24(2):193.

[21] Zayed MA, Fouda UM, Elsetohy KA, Zayed SM, Hashem AT, Youssef MA. Barbed sutures versus conventional sutures for uterine closure at cesarean section; a randomized controlled trial. *J Matern Fetal Neonatal Med.* 2017. 29:1-8

[22] Alessandri F, Remorgida V, Venturini PL, Ferrero S. Unidirectional barbed suture versus continuous suture with intracorporeal knots in laparoscopic myomectomy: a randomized study. *J Minim Invasive Gynecol.* 2010;17(6):725-9.

[23] Dubuisson JB, Fauconnier A, Chapron C, et al. Second look after laparoscopic myomectomy. *Hum Reprod.* 1998;13:2102–2106.

[24] Canis MJ, Triopon G, Daraı E, et al. Adhesion prevention after myomectomy by laparotomy: a prospective multicenter comparative randomized single-blind study with second-look laparoscopy to assess the effectiveness of PREVADHTM. *Eur J Obstet & Gynecol Reprod Biol* 2014;178:42–47.

[25] Herrmann A, De Wild RL. Laparoscopic myomectomy - The gold standard. *Gynecol and Min Inv Ther* 2014;3:31-38.

[26] Glasser MH. Minilaparotomy myomectomy: a minimally invasive alternative for the large fibroid uterus. *J Minim Invasive Gynecol.* 2005;12: 275-283.

[27] Marret H, Chevillot M, Giraudeau B. A retrospective multicentre study comparing myomectomy by laparoscopy and laparotomy in current surgical practice. What are the best patient selection criteria? *Eur J Obstet Gynecol Reprod Biol.* 2004;117:82-86.

[28] Tinelli A, Malvasi A, Guido M, et al. Adhesion formation after intracapsular myomectomy with or without adhesion barrier. *Fertil Steril.* 2011;95:1780-1785.

[29] Kubinova K, Mara M, Horak P, Kuzel D, Dohnalova A. Reproduction after myomectomy: comparison of patients with and without second-look laparoscopy. *Minim Invasive Ther Allied Technol.* 2012;21:118-124.

[30] Golan D, Aharoni A, Gonen R, Boss Y, Sharf M. Early spontaneous rupture of the post myomectomy gravid uterus. *Int J Gynecol Obstet.* 1990;31:167-170.

[31] Hurst BS, Matthews ML, Marshburn P. Laparoscopic myomectomy for symptomatic uterine myomas. *Fertil Steril.* 2005;83:1-23.

[32] Seracchioli R, Rossi S, Govoni F, et al. Fertility and obstetric outcome after laparoscopic myomectomy of large myomata: a randomized comparison with abdominal myomectomy. *Hum Reprod Update.* 2000;15:2663-2668.

[33] Palomba S, Zupi E, Russo T, et al. A multicenter randomized, controlled study comparing laparoscopic versus minilaparotomic myomectomy: short-term outcomes. *Fertil Steril.* 2007;88:942-951.

[34] FDA. Quantitative Assessment of the Prevalence of Unsuspected Uterine Sarcoma in Women Undergoing Treatment of Uterine Fibroid. *FDA*; 2014, April, Retrieved from: http://www.fda.gov/downloads/MedicalDevices/Safety/AlertsandNotices/UCM393589.pdf [13.09.15].

[35] Raine-Bennett. et al. Occult uterine sarcoma and leiomyosarcoma: incidence of and survival associated with morcellation. *Obst Gynecol* 2016;127:29–39.

[36] Brolmann H, et al. Options on fibroid morcellation: a literature review. *Gynecol Surg* 2015;12:3–15.

[37] Petraglia F. Uterine fibroid: from pathogenesis to clinical management. *Best Pract Res Clin Obstet Gynaecol.* 2016;34:1-2.

[38] Leone Roberti Maggiore U, Scala C, Venturini PL, Ferrero S. Preoperative treatment with letrozole in patients undergoing laparoscopic myomectomy of large uterine myomas: a prospective non-randomized study. *Eur J Obstet Gynecol Reprod Biol.* 2014;181:157-62.

[39] Tafi E, Scala C, Leone Roberti Maggiore U, Bizzarri N, Candiani M, Venturini PL, et al. Drug safety evaluation of ulipristal acetate in the treatment of uterine fibroids. *Expert Opin Drug Saf.* 2015;14(6):965-77.

[40] Ferrero S, Alessandri F, Vellone VG, Venturini PL, Leone Roberti Maggiore U. Three-month treatment with ulipristal acetate prior to laparoscopic myomectomy of large uterine myomas: a retrospective study. *Eur J Obstet Gynecol Reprod Biol.* 2016;205:43-7.

[41] Ferrero S, Abbamonte LH, Giordano M, Parisi M, Ragni N, Remorgida V. Uterine myomas, dyspareunia, and sexual function. *Fertil Steril.* 2006;86(5):1504-10.

In: Uterine Fibroids
Editors: S. Ferrero and F. Barra

ISBN: 978-1-53615-046-9

Chapter 7

LAPAROSCOPIC MYOMECTOMY

Matteo Tantari, MD, Fabio Barra, MD and Simone Ferrero*, MD, PhD

Obstetrics and Gynecology, Department of Neurosciences,
Rehabilitation, Ophthalmology, Genetics,
Maternal and Child Health (DiNOGMI), University of Genoa, Italy
Academic Unit of Obstetrics and Gynecology,
Ospedale San Martino, Genoa, Italy

ABSTRACT

Uterine myomas tend to have a serious impact on physical and psychological well-being of women affected. The major clinical presentations of these benign tumors include pelvic pain, abnormal uterine bleeding and infertility.

After the failure of medical therapies or the impossibility to perform hysteroscopic resection, abdominal myomectomy represents an adequate surgical procedure for women desiring to preserve fertility.

The aim of this chapter is to describe the use of laparoscopic myomectomy. We describe the various step of this procedure including port placement, enucleation, tissue extraction and closure of the uterine breach. We also resume the surgical outcomes of this minimally invasive technique with particular attention on fertility outcomes.

Keywords: laparoscopic myomectomy, uterine myoma, single-port surgery, robotic-assisted laparoscopic myomectomy, blood loss, myomectomy procedure, infertility outcomes, surgical outcomes

* Corresponding Author's E-mail: simoneferrero@me.com.

1. Indications

Patients with uterine fibroids may be asymptomatic or may present several clinical symptoms such as heavy uterine bleeding with subsequent anemia, pelvic discomfort and bulk symptoms [1, 2]. For this reason, the recurs to surgery is sometimes necessary in order to ameliorate quality of life of patients affected.

Laparoscopic myomectomy is a minimally invasive procedure for the treatment of symptomatic fibroids in patients desiring to preserve their fertility. Although performing it is technically more complex than performing traditional laparotomy, laparoscopic myomectomy provides numerous advantages such as post-surgical fast recovery, lower postoperative pain when compared with mini-laparotomic myomectomy. Moreover, it has overlapping results with regard to post-surgical fertility outcomes and disease recurrence risk [3–5]. Other advantages of laparoscopic myomectomy are reduction of intraoperative blood loss and lower number of needed transfusion in comparison with traditional laparotomic myomectomy [6, 7]. Furthermore, the incidence of postoperative adhesions seems to be lower for patients undergoing laparoscopic myomectomy [8–11].

Overall, an accurate selection of patients for this minimally invasive procedure seems to allow for low incidence of complications and conversion to laparotomy [12].

1.1. Patients Selection for Laparoscopic Myomectomy

Overall, a laparoscopic myomectomy should be proposed in women with myoma-related symptoms with desire of childbearing [13]. In general, the principle criteria for choosing laparoscopy are dimension and localization of the main myoma [3, 16–18].

Whereas hysteroscopic resection is indicated for small submucosal myomas (with size <5 cm, typically intracavitary or protruding in uterine cavity for more than 50% of the total volume) [14], laparoscopic myomectomy is indicated for women with a number of total fibroids lower than 5, no single myoma > 15 cm and a uterus <16 weeks in size [15].

Following the current management strategies proposed in a literature review by Donnez et al., laparoscopic myomectomy is contraindicated in women having intramural myomas with a maximum diameter >10 cm or multiple fibroids (>4) with different locations, as it can became particularly challenging; for this reason, in these cases, the use of the laparotomic approach tends to be more frequently done [1].

However, some cases of laparoscopic myomectomy for myomas with maximum diameter >20 cm have been reported in the literature [19].

In patients with suspected malignancy, any type of myomectomy should be cautiously performed. In particular, it must be avoided in women with proven malignant disease.

2. Surgical Technique

The type of laparoscopic approach should be selected in relation to the patient's surgical history. In women with previous uncomplicated procedures and small myomas, traditional umbilical entry can be suitable. Instead, in women who underwent previous laparotomy or with large uterine fibroids, intra-abdominal adhesions, large ovarian cysts and hernias, the entry at Palmer's point in the left quadrant below the subcostal margin along the mid-clavicular line can be safer [20].

Current different laparoscopic approaches are available:

- *traditional laparoscopic approach.* The traditional entry is usually performed by using an 11 mm umbilical port for the laparoscope and two or three 5 to 10 mm ancillary ports, which are placed under direct endoscopic visualization after careful gas insufflation of the abdominal cavity [5, 12].
- *single-port laparoscopic approach.* It is performed by a single umbilical incision using specific tools such as curved and articulated cameras [21, 22].
- *laparoscopic-assisted approach with mini-laparotomy.* It is similar to the traditional one, requiring a 5 or 10mm umbilical access and 2 accessory 5 mm trocars. A suprapubic incision of approximately 4 cm is performed in order to facilitate myoma enucleation, suture uterine defects and morcellation [15].

Overall, laparoscopic-assisted myomectomy have showed to reduce hospital stay and operative time when compared with traditional laparotomy [23, 24].

The robotic-assisted laparoscopic myomectomy is a recent innovative surgical option. A 12 mm umbilical access is required (compared to the conventional 5-10 mm for laparoscopic approach) in order to allow the insertion of a 3-dimensional camera. The camera can be placed in the umbilical access or in another supraumbilical access, thus improving the range of visual movement. Due to the size of the robotic arms, further two 8 mm trocars are placed at 8-10 cm from the umbilical port. Moreover, a 12-mm port is located in the lower quadrant of the abdomen to allow manual exchange of needles and other tools under direct observation. The surgical console is situated in the same room of the patient, allowing the surgeon to control by natural hand motions the laparoscopic arms during the procedure under vision by the 3-dimensional camera [25].

To facilitate the laparoscopic myomectomy, the insertion of a trans cervical uterine manipulator is suggested for mobilizing the uterus, allowing correct positioning during surgery. Furthermore, through the uterine manipulator it is possible to directly inject methylene blue or other dyes into the endometrial cavity, thus visualizing eventual perforations during surgery as well as helping the surgeon to repair them [26].

3. Minimization of Blood Loss

It is well established that fibroids are benign tumors with reduced vascular tissue. However, recent research showed that the myoma vascularization is microscopically abnormal [27]. This is one of the causes that make myomectomy a procedure susceptible to eventual hemorrhagic complications. Numerous pharmacological and surgical strategies have been investigated to overcome this aspect.

A study conducted by Lin et al. compared various techniques for reducing the blood loss during laparoscopic intramural myomectomy. This prospective study was performed on 280 patients with symptomatic fibroids who underwent laparoscopic myomectomy with the addition of one of the following hemostatic actions: myoma pedicle ligation, injection of diluted vasopressin (12 IU) around the myoma, injection of oxytocin (20 IU) combined with pedicle ligation and injection of vasopressin (12 IU) combined with pedicle ligation. This study demonstrated that the injection of vasopressin in the pericapsular space during laparoscopic myomectomy was associated with a reduced blood loss; moreover, this reduction was greater if associated with the pedicle ligation [28]. However, the use of vasopressin plus pedicle ligation showed a lower length of hospital stay. The injection of oxytocin demonstrated to be not effective in reducing intraoperative blood loss [29].

The use of vasopressin is not free from complications: hypotension, bradycardia, cardiac arrest and pulmonary edema were sometimes observed in several studies on healthy patients receiving vasopressin at 2-6 u/ml [30–32]. Thus, the therapeutic dose of vasopressin should be 0.5-3 u/ml [31].

The use of prostaglandins is another evaluable option to reduce intraoperative blood loss: the use vaginal dinoprostone (20 mg), which provided a significant reduction of blood loss, transfusion rate and higher level of postoperative hemoglobin during laparotomic myomectomy [33], was not unfortunately tested before laparoscopic myomectomy. A significant reduction of estimated blood loss and of number of postoperative transfusions was shown by the use of a single dose of vaginal misoprostol (400 μg) one hour before laparoscopic myomectomy [34].

Oxytocin infusion stimulates the contraction of uterine muscle cells; in fact, it is usually prescribed for treating dysfunctional labor or preventing postpartum hemorrhage [35]. A prospective clinical trial was conducted to evaluate if oxytocin (20 u/ml/amp) was able to reduce operative blood loss during laparoscopic myomectomy; among patients receiving it, a significant reduction of blood loss and transfusion rate was observed (36). Another study conducted by the same authors group has provided overlapping results among patients undergoing laparoscopic-assisted vaginal myomectomy [37]. Interestingly, these results were contradicted in another study conducted by Agostini et al. on 94 patients undergoing vaginal or laparotomic myomectomy [38].

The hemostatic action of gelatin-trombin matrix was studies only with positive results during abdominal myomectomy [39]. More importantly, the use of a fibrin sealant applied on uterine suture during laparoscopic myomectomy demonstrated a significant reduction in intraoperative and postoperative bleeding and hemoglobin decrease. In addition, it showed a rapid healing of the suture by limiting the traumas of electrocoagulation [40].

The intraoperative injection of bupivacaine plus epinephrine during laparoscopy myomectomy was evaluated on 60 premenopausal patients in a double-blind randomized controlled trial (RCT). This double injection showed to be effective in reducing blood loss, operative time, surgical difficulty and postoperative pain [41].

Some surgical methods can be implemented to reduce the estimated blood loss: the preservation of the pseudocapsule during myoma excision has shown to be effective in minimizing blood loss. These results emerged from a prospective observational study by Tinelli et al. on 235 patients who underwent laparoscopic myomectomy for symptomatic fibroids. In this trial, the median blood loss was about 118 ± 27.9 ml; moreover, after surgery, 86.3% of patients did not present major post operative complications [42].

The use of unidirectional and bidirectional barbed sutures during laparoscopic myomectomy appears another interesting option: the action of small barbs can maintain the tension of the suture during the surgical procedure and eliminate the need of laparoscopic knots. In a randomized clinical study by Alessandri et al. 44 patients with similar preoperative hemoglobin concentration at baseline were enrolled and underwent laparoscopic myomectomy. The suture of uterine wall defect was performed by unidirectional knotless barbed suture or continuous suture with intracorporal knots. It was demonstrated that the use of unidirectional knotless barbed suture reduced the surgical times required for doing the suture ($p < .001$), the intraoperative bleeding ($p = .004$) and the degree of surgical difficulty ($p < .001$). However, a significant difference in the operative time between the two groups was not shown [43]. Confirmatory data on these findings emerged from a meta-analysis conducted by Tulandi et al. which demonstrated that barbed suture can definitively facilitate laparoscopic reparation of uterine wall after myomectomy incision. Furthermore, the use of barbed sutures seems to be characterized by a significant reduction of total operative time, suturing time and estimated blood loss [44].

Laparoscopic bilateral uterine artery ligation during myomectomy is a radical approach to minimize blood loss. In a comparative observational study, 84 patients underwent transient uterine artery ligation plus myomectomy and 83 patients underwent direct laparoscopic myomectomy. The transient uterine artery ligation group showed lower intraoperative blood loss, lower recurrence rates and no significant adverse effect on fertility [45]. Overlapping results were observed in another prospective controlled clinical trial by Alborzi et al. on 152 patients with symptomatic fibroids. In this study, women who underwent uterine artery occlusion before laparoscopic myomectomy showed a lower blood loss and lower request of blood transfusions; overall, no impact on fertility ($p = .966$) and live birth rates ($p = 63$) was reported for this procedure [46]. In a RCT by Zhao et al. the loop ligation of the myoma pseudocapsule combined with vasopressin demonstrated to significantly reduce blood loss ($p < .001$), length of hospital stay ($p < .001$), transfusion request ($p = .024$) and conversion to abdominal surgery ($p < .001$) during laparoscopic myomectomy for the presence of large uterine fibroids (>6 cm) [47]. Another RCT conducted by Vercellino et al. evaluated the efficacy of the temporary occlusion of the uterine arteries by vascular clips during laparoscopic myomectomy. During this procedure, a statistically reduction of hemoglobin loss ($p < .05$) was demonstrated; moreover, no patients required blood transfusion and no patient experienced conspicuous side effects [48]. Confirmatory data were observed in another RCT with a similar patients' population, in which a reduction of estimated blood loss was demonstrated [49].

According to a Cochrane review, a cervical tourniquet during surgical procedures for myomectomy can significantly decrease blood loss, transfusion rates, nevertheless not increasing the global surgical time or causing relevant postoperative side effects [50]; however, when compared with other hemostatic techniques (such as vasopressin and uterine artery ligation), the pericervical tourniquet obtains significant greater blood loss [51, 52]. Thus, the use of pericervical tourniquet tends to be associated with other hemostatic procedures.

Numerous medical or surgical strategies can be intraoperatively or preoperatively used to reduce blood loss, rate of transfusions and complications [53–57]. Anyway, the association of these techniques should be taken into consideration only in patients with preoperative anemia or those with higher risk of intraoperative or postoperative complications.

4. Enucleation Procedure and Tissue Extraction

The number of incisions on the uterine wall during myomectomy should be limited. Overall, it is preferable to perform a single incision in the presence of adjacent multiple myomas [15].

Transverse and longitudinal incisions (Figure 1) do not lead to significant differences regarding to intraoperative blood loss; however, the transverse incision can facility the closure of the uterine breach [58], moreover, the uterine incision should be not done too laterally in order to limit injury in critical nearby structures such as adnexa and uterine artery [15].

Electrosurgical methods like monopolar needle, bipolar forceps and laparoscopic scissors are usually employed aiming to reduce intraoperative bleeding. A RCT by Litta et al. investigated the use of an ultrasonically activated scalpel (Harmonic™, Ethicon, Cincinnati, OH) in comparison with that of electrosurgical pencil and dilute epinephrine (50 mL of saline solution and 0.5 mL of epinephrine). The harmonic scalpel proved a significant improvement on global intraoperative time (71.8 ± 26.7 vs 88.8 ± 35.5), blood loss (135.2 ± 89.1 vs 182.8 ± 116.8), recovery time and lower immediate (24h) postoperative pain at VAS (visual analogue scale, 5.6 ± 0.8 vs 4.4 ± 1.1) without an increased surgical difficulty [59]. It has been supposed that the differences between the two techniques may be linked to the capacity of the harmonic scalpel to seal and divide blood vessels <2 mm as well as to simultaneously cut and coagulate.

Overall, the enucleation of an intramural myoma should be performed by pushing away the tissue adjacent to the dissection plane; it should avoid a strong traction on the fibroid due to the risk of avulsion and subsequent injury of the endometrial wall (Figures 2a-2b, Figure 3).

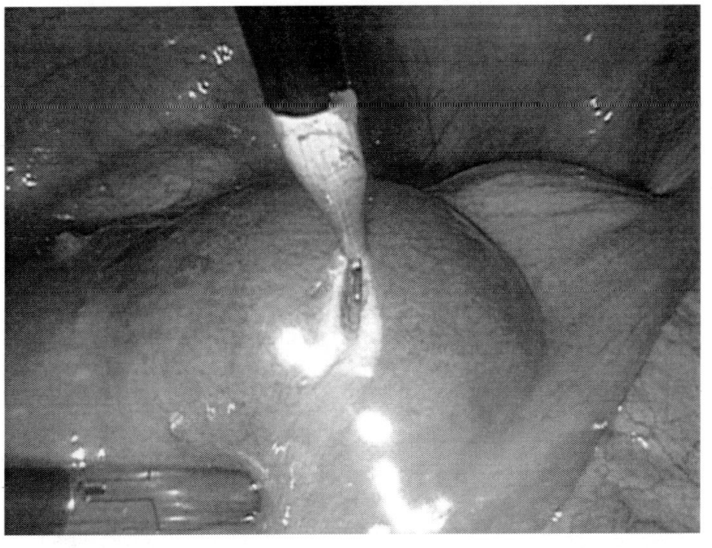

Figure 1. Incision of the uterine wall.

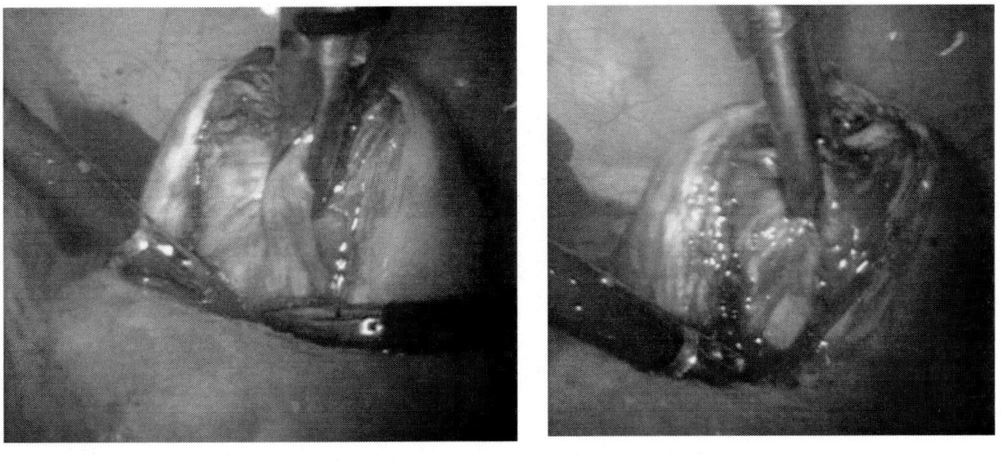

(a) (b)

Figure 2a-2b. Visualization and demarcation of the myoma.

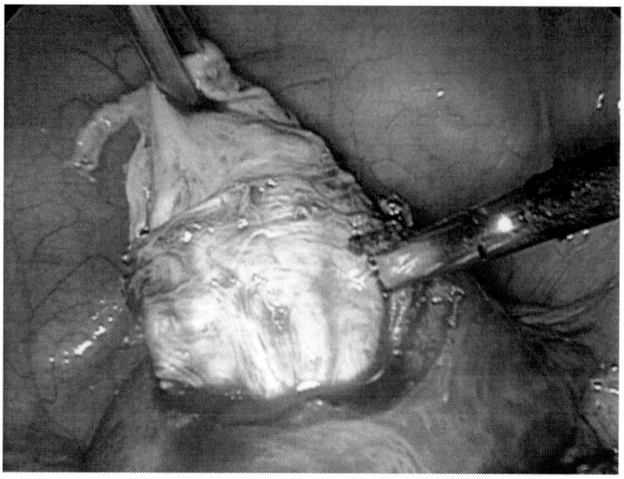

Figure 3. Extraction of the myoma.

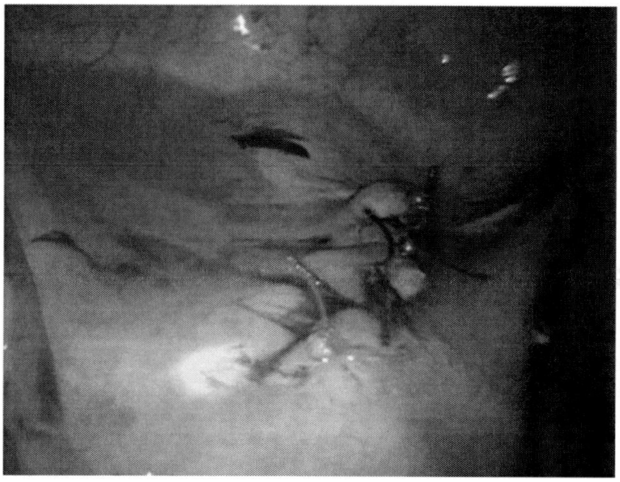

Figure 4. Suture of the myometrial bed after the myoma removal.

5. Closure of the Uterine Breach

After the myoma enucleation and extraction, the uterine breach should immediately be repaired by a resorbable fine suture (Figure 4). In order to facilitate the recognition of possible perforations, infusion of methylene blue solution into the endometrial cavity during the procedure can be considered [15].

The suture should be performed by 2 layers for the rapprochement of the myometrium; an additional third layer can be considered for reproaching the serosa [60, 61]. The aim of an accurate closure of the uterine breach is to reduce the risk of uterine rupture in future pregnancies.

Emerging evidence support the use of barbed knotless suture (Quill™ SRS, Angiotech Pharmaceuticals, Inc. Vancouver, Canada; V-Loc™, Covidien, USA) for closing myometrium as it seems to reduce operating times as well as intraoperative bleeding.

The efficacy of the barbed suture compared with the traditional one was observed in a meta-analysis in which a significant reduction in operative time and overall degree of suturing difficulty was shown [44]. A prospective control study on 60 patients by Song et al. compared the surgical outcomes between the two groups of suture during laparoscopic single-site myomectomy. Interestingly, the use of barbed suture led to a significant reduction in both suturing ($p = .014$) and total operative times ($p = .027$). Moreover, patients undergoing uterine closure by barbed suture had also lower intraoperative blood loss ($p = .040$); at least, the surgeons experienced less technical difficulty ($p = .001$) compared with performing traditional suture [62].

In general, depending on the surgeon's laparoscopic experience or whenever difficult hemostasis occurs, uterine closure can be performed through minilaparotomic approach [15].

6. Adhesion Prevention Barriers

The incidence of new adhesions with laparotomic and laparoscopic myomectomies of 98% and 41.3%, respectively [63]. It is currently known that the most important factor for preventing post-surgical adhesion is an optimal surgical procedure including meticulous hemostasis. Subsequently, the use of adhesion prevention barriers has been evaluated in the literature.

The use of Interceed™ (Johnson & Johnson Patient Care Inc., New Brunswick, NJ), an oxidized cellulose, during pelvic surgery has been associated with a reduction of adhesion after a second-look laparoscopy, even if the quality of this evidence is low [64].

A RCT evaluates the efficacy of this oxidized cellulose for the prevention of new adhesions after laparoscopic myomectomy. The study, performed by Mais et al. demonstrated a significant reduction in their incidence following the application (OR, 0.45; CI 95%, 0.28-0.75) [10]. Similar results emerged from another prospective blinded observational study conducted by Tinelli et al. on the use of oxidized regenerated absorbable adhesion barriers. In this study a total of 694 patients undergoing laparoscopic or abdominal myomectomy was enrolled. It was demonstrated a higher rate of adhesion after laparotomic and laparoscopic surgery without using any barrier (28.1% and 22.6% versus 22% and 15.9%). In particular, the incidence of cohesive adhesions were higher in women without the application of barriers [65].

Overall, the use of adhesion barriers may be particularly indicated in patients with desire of pregnancy and presence of posterior myoma, as they tend to have a higher risk of tubo-ovarian adhesions after myomectomy, needing a posterior uterine incision [66].

7. Surgical Outcomes

It has demonstrated that laparoscopic myomectomy has a low rate of intraoperative conversion to laparotomy. A retrospective cohort study performed by Sanberg et al. evaluated the risk of conversion among 731 patients undergoing laparoscopic myomectomy. The conversion was required in 8 women (1.1%); all conversions were associated with longer hospital stay ($p \leq .001$) and greater blood loss ($p \leq .001$) [67].

A Cochrane review summarized the results from 6 studies evaluating the operative times of laparoscopic myomectomy compared with open myomectomy. Operating time was demonstrate to be significantly higher for the minimally invasive procedure with a mean difference of 13 minutes (95% CI; 9.61-16.56 min) [5]. Moreover, a reduction of median length of hospital stay (hours) was observed in patients undergoing laparoscopic myomectomy [11, 68, 69]. Another study comparing laparoscopic myomectomy to laparoscopically assisted mini-laparotomy showed no clear evidence for reduction of mean operative time between the two study groups (mean difference 5.52 hours; 95% CI, 0.13-2.52 hours) [70].

Regarding the complication rate of laparoscopic myomectomy, a single-center retrospective review on 514 women was conducted by Bean et al. Overall, 18 patients had complications, among which the most frequent was blood loss >1000 ml ($n = 15$); the others were bowel ($n = 1$) and bladder ($n = 1$) injury, small bowel obstruction secondary to port site hernia ($n = 1$) [12]. Another trial including 148 women evaluated the performance of laparoscopic myomectomy in comparison with mini-laparotomy. The authors demonstrated the onset of surgical complications only in one case (bowel perforation) in the laparoscopic group; anyway, this difference was not judged significant [11]. In another trial, Alessandri et al. compared the postoperative pain (by VAS scale) among 148 patients after 6 hours from laparoscopic or mini-laparotomic myomectomies; patients in the laparoscopic group had lower intensity of pain at 6 hours from the procedure ($p < .001$); moreover, in this group the request for post-operative analgesics was significantly lower in the 48 hours following the intervention ($p < .001$). Moreover, women who undergoing laparoscopic myomectomy demonstrated a more frequent full recuperation at day 15 from the intervention [11]. Two other studies comparing postoperative pain after laparoscopic myomectomy with open myomectomy provided similar results. From a global analysis, it was shown that postoperative pain (at VAS) after 48 hours was significantly lower for patients undergoing the laparoscopic approach (mean difference, −1.90; 95% CI, −2.80 to −1.00) [10, 71].

A review on six studies including 635 women demonstrated that the onset of postoperative fever was significantly lower in patients undergoing laparoscopic myomectomy compared with open myomectomy (OR 0.44, 95% CI 0.26 to 0.77) [5]. The same review analyzed other six studies enrolling 549 patients for evaluating the hemoglobin drop during laparoscopic myomectomy in comparison with mini-laparotomy, unmodified open myomectomy and laparoscopically assisted mini-laparotomy. These studies reported a significant reduction in blood loss for laparoscopic myomectomy [5]. Only one study provided a statistically more reduced hemoglobin drop for laparoscopically assisted mini-laparotomy in comparison to laparoscopic myomectomy [70].

8. EFFECTS ON FERTILITY

The presence of uterine fibroids as sole causal factor is observed only in 3% of infertile patients. Most of them tend to be affected by submucosal myomas that can be easily approached by hysteroscopy [72].

The correlation between infertility and myomas is linked to several factors including their type and position or general physical alterations of the uterus, cervix, ovaries and fallopian tubes. Globally, these alterations can influence the myometrial contractile activity, thus causing a reduction in vascular perfusion and in blastocysts implantation [14, 73–76]. In addition, fibroids can negatively affect fertility causing multiple pro-inflammatory reactions; overall, uterine fibroids have been associated with pre-term birth (<37 w), reduced birth weight, breech presentation and higher incidence of primary cesarean section [15].

Some studies showed that myomectomy leads to a reduction in the number of miscarriage in patients with myomas worsening the profile of uterine cavity [18, 77, 78]. On the other hand, results obtained from two RCTs did not demonstrate an improvement of fertility after the performance of myomectomy by any route [79, 80].

Other data suggested the utility of doing myomectomy in patients affected by submucosal fibroids aiming to increase pregnancy and live birth rates [80]. No differences have been demonstrated for fertility outcomes of patients with subserosal myomas in comparison with healthy patients; for this reason, myomectomy should not be recommended in this setting. No significant improvement in pregnancy and live-birth rates were equally found after the removal of intramural myomas [80].

A systematic review with meta-analysis was conducted in order to evaluate the influence on fertility of intramural fibroids not distorting the endometrial cavity in patients undergoing IVF. The analysis of 6087 cases showed a significant reduction in pregnancy (RR = 0.85, 95% CI: 0.77-0.94, P = .002) and live-birth (RR = 0.79, 95% CI: 0.70-0.88, P < .0001) [81].

A retrospective design study collecting the data of 265 women undergoing laparotomic or laparoscopic surgery for symptomatic fibroids demonstrated an increase of live-birth (up to 86%) and pregnancy rates (up to 70%) without significant differences between the two surgical routes. In particular, size of the largest myoma and the number of extracted fibroids were judged as negative factors for obtaining pregnancy ($p = .02$ and $p < .010$, respectively); a higher number of complication was shown in patients who received the extraction of more than three myomas ($p = .0471$) [82].

One prospective RCT showed an improvement in pregnancy rate after the surgical removal of submucosal, intramural and submucosal-intramural myomas. This result was especially achieved in patients who had been trying to conceive for at least one year without success. Notably, no significant results were obtained for the removal of intramural and submucosal-intramural myomas. This study under lighted how the position of the fibroid can affect the chances of fertilization and pregnancy maintenance [83].

CONCLUSION

Laparoscopic myomectomy can provide many advantages compared with traditional laparotomic myomectomy. Currently, it is considered a gold-standard treatment for treating patients with symptomatic myomas with desire to preserve the fertility.

After the failure or the non-feasibility of hysteroscopic resection, laparoscopic myomectomy should be considered for myomas with a submucous component.

The literature demonstrates that postoperative pain measured by VAS score is significant lower in women who undergo laparoscopic surgery than laparotomic one. With regard to the reduction of global blood-loss, the laparoscopic approach demonstrates to be most effective; in particular, it tends to reduce intraoperative blood-loss, consequently ameliorating postoperative hemoglobin; in general, the eventual performance of several hemostatic options can be consider for this purpose. At the moment, the use of adhesion prevention barriers requires more study in order to assume their real effectiveness. Moreover, laparoscopic approach has showed lower incidence of postoperative fever and reduced recovery time compared with laparotomic myomectomy.

The practice of unconfined morcellation for myoma extraction should not be currently recommended for the risk of eventually disseminating tumor cells; instead, the performance of an endo-bag morcellation is considered a safer way to prevent cell dissemination.

Overall, surgical removal of submucosal myomas demonstrates to improve patients' fertility outcomes; however, it is still not clear the role of myomectomy for improving fertility of women affected by intramural and subserous myomas. Better-designed and larger RCTs with longer follow-up need to be conducted to establish the definitive effectiveness of laparoscopic myomectomy for this purpose.

REFERENCES

[1] Donnez J, Dolmans MM. Uterine fibroid management: From the present to the future. *Hum Reprod Update*. 2016; 22(6):665-686.

[2] Ferrero S, Abbamonte LH, Giordano M, Parisi M, Ragni N, Remorgida V. Uterine myomas, dyspareunia, and sexual function. *Fertil Steril*. 2006 Nov;86(5):1504-10.

[3] Donnez J, Donnez O, Dolmans MM. With the advent of selective progesterone receptor modulators, what is the place of myoma surgery in current practice? *Fertil Steril*. 2014; 102(3):640-8.

[4] Segars JH, Parrott EC, Nagel JD, Guo XC, Gao X, Birnbaum LS, et al. Proceedings from the third national institutes of health international congress on advances in uterine leiomyoma research: Comprehensive review, conference summary and future recommendations. *Hum Reprod Update*. 2014; 20(3):309-33.

[5] Bhave Chittawar P, Franik S, Pouwer AW, Farquhar C. Minimally invasive surgical techniques versus open myomectomy for uterine fibroids. *Cochrane Database of Systematic Reviews*. 2014;(10):CD004638

[6] Gobern JM, Rosemeyer CJ, Barter JF, Steren AJ. Comparison of Robotic, Laparoscopic, and Abdominal Myomectomy in a Community Hospital. *JSLS J Soc Laparoendosc Surg*. 2013; 17(1): 116–120.

[7] Shen Q, Chen M, Wang Y, Zhou Q, Tao X, Zhang W, et al. Effects of Laparoscopic Versus Minilaparotomic Myomectomy on Uterine Leiomyoma: A Meta-analysis. *Journal of Minimally Invasive Gynecology*. 2015; 22(2):177-84.

[8] Takeuchi H, Kitade M, Kikuchi I, Shimanuki H, Kumakiri J, Takeda S. Influencing factors of adhesion development and the efficacy of adhesion-preventing agents in patients undergoing laparoscopic myomectomy as evaluated by a second-look laparoscopy. *Fertil Steril*. 2008;89(5):1247-53.

[9] Dubuisson JB, Fauconnier a, Fourchotte V, Babaki-Fard K, Coste J, Chapron C. Laparoscopic myomectomy: predicting the risk of conversion to an open procedure. *Hum Reprod*. 2001; 16(8):1726-31.

[10] Mais V, Ajossa S, Piras B, Guerriero S, Marongiu D, Melis GB. Prevention of de-novo adhesion formation after laparoscopic myomectomy: A randomized trial to evaluate the effectiveness of an oxidized regenerated cellulose absorbable barrier. *Hum Reprod*. 1995; 10(12):3133-5.

[11] Alessandri F, Lijoi D, Mistrangelo E, Ferrero S, Ragni N. Randomized study of laparoscopic versus minilaparotomic myomectomy for uterine myomas. *J Minim Invasive Gynecol*. 2006; 13(2):92-7.

[12] Bean EMR, Cutner A, Holland T, Vashisht A, Jurkovic D, Saridogan E. Laparoscopic Myomectomy: A Single-center Retrospective Review of 514 Patients. *J Minim Invasive Gynecol*. 2017; 24(3):485-493.

[13] Halaska MJ, Haidopoulos D, Guyon F, Morice P, Zapardiel I, Kesic V, et al. European Society of Gynecological Oncology Statement on Fibroid and Uterine Morcellation. *Int J Gynecol Cancer*. 2017; 27(1):189-192.

[14] Donnez J, Jadoul P. What are the implications of myomas on fertility? A need for a debate? *Human Reproduction*. 2002;17(6):1424-30.

[15] Flyckt R, Coyne K, Falcone T. Minimally Invasive Myomectomy. *Clinical Obstetrics and Gynecology*. 2017; 60(2):252-272.

[16] Nezhat C, Lavie O, Hsu S, Watson J, Barnett O, Lemyre M. Robotic-assisted laparoscopic myomectomy compared with standard laparoscopic myomectomy-a retrospective matched control study. *Fertil Steril.* 2009; 91(2):556-9.

[17] Malzoni M, Tinelli R, Cosentino F, Iuzzolino D, Surico D, Reich H. Laparoscopy versus minilaparotomy in women with symptomatic uterine myomas: Short-term and fertility results. *Fertil Steril.* 2010; 93(7):2368-73.

[18] Parazzini F, Tozzi L, Bianchi S. Pregnancy outcome and uterine fibroids. *Best Pract Res Clin Obstet Gynaecol*. 2016; 34:74-84.

[19] Sinha R, Hegde A, Mahajan C, Dubey N, Sundaram M. Laparoscopic Myomectomy: Do Size, Number, and Location of the Myomas Form Limiting Factors for Laparoscopic Myomectomy? *J Minim Invasive Gynecol.* 2008; 15(3):292-300.

[20] Granata M, Tsimpanakos I, Moeity F, Magos A. Are we underutilizing Palmer's point entry in gynecologic laparoscopy? *Fertil Steril.* 2010; 94(7):2716-9

[21] Choi CH, Kim TH, Kim SH, Choi JK, Park JY, Yoon A, et al. Surgical Outcomes of a New Approach to Laparoscopic Myomectomy: Single-Port and Modified Suture Technique. *J Minim Invasive Gynecol*. 2014; 21(4):580-5.

[22] Lewis EI, Srouji SS, Gargiulo AR. Robotic single-site myomectomy: Initial report and technique. *Fertil Steril.* 2015; 103(5):1370-7.e1.

[23] Nezhat C, Nezhat F, Bess O, Nezhat CH, Mashiach R. Laparoscopically assisted myomectomy: a report of a new technique in 57 cases. *Int J Fertil Menopausal Stud.* 1994; 39(1):39-44.

[24] Kalogiannidis I, Prapas N, Xiromeritis P, Prapas Y. Laparoscopically assisted myomectomy versus abdominal myomectomy in short-term outcomes: A prospective study. *Arch Gynecol Obstet.* 2010; 281(5):865-70.

[25] Advincula AP, Xu X, Goudeau IV S, Ransom SB. Robot-assisted laparoscopic myomectomy versus abdominal myomectomy: A comparison of short-term surgical outcomes and immediate costs. *J Minim Invasive Gynecol*. 2007; 14(6):698-705.

[26] Abbott JA, Munro MG, Singh SS, Scheib S, Jackson TR, Jansen F, et al. AAGL practice report: practice guidelines on intrauterine adhesions developed in collaboration with the European Society of Gynaecological Endoscopy (ESGE). *Gynecol Surg.* 2017; 24(5):695-705.

[27] Tal R, Segars JH. The role of angiogenic factors in fibroid pathogenesis: Potential implications for future therapy. *Hum Reprod Update.* 2014; 20(2):194-216.

[28] Frederick S, Frederick J, Fletcher H, Reid M, Hardie M, Gardner W. A trial comparing the use of rectal misoprostol plus perivascular vasopressin with perivascular vasopressin alone to decrease myometrial bleeding at the time of abdominal myomectomy. *Fertil Steril.* 2013; 100(4):1044-9.

[29] Lin X-N, Zhang S-Y, Fang S-H, Wang M-Z, Lou H-Y. [Assessment of different homeostatic methods used in laparoscopic intramural myomectomy]. *Zhonghua Yi Xue Za Zhi*. 2008; 88(13):905-8.

[30] Tulandi T, Beique F, Kimia M. Pulmonary edema: A complication of local injection of vasopressin at laparoscopy. *Fertil Steril.* 1996; 66(3):478-80.

[31] Hobo R, Netsu S, Koyasu Y, Tsutsumi O. Bradycardia and cardiac arrest caused by intramyometrial injection of vasopressin during a laparoscopically assisted myomectomy. *Obstet Gynecol*. 2009; 113(2 Pt 2):484-6.

[32] Nezhat F, Admon D, Nezhat CH, Dicorpo JE, Nezhat C. Life-threatening hypotension after vasopressin injection during operative laparoscopy, followed by uneventful repeat laparoscopy. *Am Assoc Gynecol Laparosc.* 1994; 2(1):83-6.

[33] Shokeir T, Shalaby H, Nabil H, Barakat R. Reducing blood loss at abdominal myomectomy with preoperative use of dinoprostone intravaginal suppository: A randomized placebo-controlled pilot study. *Eur J Obstet Gynecol Reprod Biol.* 2013; 166(1):61-4.

[34] Kalogiannidis I, Xiromeritis P, Prapas N, Prapas Y. Intravaginal misoprostol reduces intraoperative blood loss in minimally invasive myomectomy: A randomized clinical trial. *Clin Exp Obstet Gynecol.* 2011; 38(1):46-9.

[35] Arrowsmith S, Wray S. Oxytocin: Its mechanism of action and receptor signalling in the myometrium. *Journal of Neuroendocrinology*. 2014; 26(6):356-69.

[36] Wang CJ, Lee CL, Yuen LT, Kay N, Han CM, Soong YK. Oxytocin infusion in laparoscopic myomectomy may decrease operative blood loss. *J Minim Invasive Gynecol.* 2007;14(2):184-8.

[37] Wang CJ, Yuen LT, Yen CF, Lee CL, Soong YK. A simplified method to decrease operative blood loss in laparoscopic-assisted vaginal hysterectomy for the large uterus. *J Am Assoc Gynecol Laparosc*. 2004; 14(2):184-8.

[38] Agostini A, Ronda I, Franchi F, Bretelle F, Roger V, Cravello L, et al. Oxytocin during myomectomy: A randomized study. *Eur J Obstet Gynecol Reprod Biol.* 2005; 118(2):235-8.

[39] Raga F, Sanz-Cortes M, Bonilla F, Casañ EM, Bonilla-Musoles F. Reducing blood loss at myomectomy with use of a gelatin-thrombin matrix hemostatic sealant. *Fertil Steril.* 2009; 92(1):356-60.

[40] Angioli R, Plotti F, Ricciardi R, Terranova C, Zullo MA, Damiani P, et al. The use of novel hemostatic sealant (Tisseel??) in laparoscopic myomectomy: A case-control study. *Surg Endosc Other Interv Tech.* 2012; 26(7):2046-53.

[41] Zullo F, Palomba S, Corea D, Pellicano M, Russo T, Falbo A, et al. Bupivacaine plus epinephrine for laparoscopic myomectomy: A randomized placebo-controlled trial. *Obstet Gynecol*. 2004; 104(2):243-9.

[42] Tinelli A, Hurst BS, Hudelist G, Tsin DA, Stark M, Mettler L, et al. Laparoscopic myomectomy focusing on the myoma pseudocapsule: Technical and outcome reports. *Hum Reprod*. 2012; 27(2):427-35.

[43] Alessandri F, Remorgida V, Venturini PL, Ferrero S. Unidirectional barbed suture versus continuous suture with intracorporeal knots in laparoscopic myomectomy: A randomized study. *J Minim Invasive Gynecol.* 2010; 17(6):725-9

[44] Tulandi T, Einarsson JI. The use of barbed suture for laparoscopic hysterectomy and myomectomy: A systematic review and meta-analysis. *Journal of Minimally Invasive Gynecology*. 2014; 21(2):210-6

[45] Liu L, Li Y, Xu H, Chen Y, Zhang G, Liang Z. Laparoscopic transient uterine artery occlusion and myomectomy for symptomatic uterine myoma. *Fertil Steril.* 2011; 95(1):254-8.

[46] Dunghav VA. A comparison of combined laparoscopic uterine artery ligation and myomectomy vs laparoscopic myomectomy in treatment of symptomatic myoma. *World Journal of Laparoscopic Surgery*. 2015; 8(2):52-56.

[47] Zhao F, Jiao Y, Guo Z, Hou R, Wang M. Evaluation of loop ligation of larger myoma pseudocapsule combined with vasopressin on laparoscopic myomectomy. *Fertil Steril*. 2011; 95(2):762-6.

[48] Vercellino G, Erdemoglu E, Joe A, Hopfenmueller W, Holthaus B, Köhler C, et al. Laparoscopic temporary clipping of uterine artery during laparoscopic myomectomy. *Arch Gynecol Obstet*. 2012; 286(5):1181-6.

[49] Kwon Y-S, Jung D-Y, Lee S-H, Ahn JW, Roh HJ, Im KS. Transient occlusion of uterine arteries with endoscopic vascular clip preceding laparoscopic myomectomy. *J Laparoendosc Adv Surg Tech A*. 2013; 23(8):679-83.

[50] Neilson JP. Interventions to reduce haemorrhage during myomectomy for fibroids. *Obstetrics and Gynecology*. 2007; 109(5):1197-8.

[51] Helal AS, Abdel-Hady ES, Refaie E, El Shamy M, El Fattah RA, Mashaly AEM. Preliminary uterine artery ligation versus pericervical mechanical tourniquet in reducing hemorrhage during abdominal myomectomy. *Int J Gynecol Obstet.* 2010; 108(3):233-5.

[52] Fletcher H, Frederick J, Hardie M, Simeon D. A randomized comparison of vasopressin and tourniquet as hemostatic agents during myomectomy. *Obstet Gynecol.* 1996; 87(6):1014-8.

[53] Ferrero S, Alessandri F, Vellone VG, Venturini PL, Leone Roberti Maggiore U. Three-month treatment with ulipristal acetate prior to laparoscopic myomectomy of large uterine myomas: a retrospective study. *Eur J Obstet Gynecol Reprod Biol.* 2016; 205:43-7.

[54] Bizzarri N, Ghirardi V, Remorgida V, Venturini PL, Ferrero S. Three-month treatment with triptorelin, letrozole and ulipristal acetate before hysteroscopic resection of uterine myomas: prospective comparative pilot study. *Eur J Obstet Gynecol Reprod Biol.* 2015; 192:22-6.

[55] Leone Roberti Maggiore U, Scala C, Venturini PL, Ferrero S. Preoperative treatment with letrozole in patients undergoing laparoscopic myomectomy of large uterine myomas: A prospective non-randomized study. *Eur J Obstet Gynecol Reprod Biol.* 2014; 181:157-62.

[56] Ferrero S, Vellone VG, Barra F. Pharmacokinetic drug evaluation of ulipristal acetate for the treatment of uterine fibroids. *Expert Opin Drug Metab Toxicol.* 2018;14(1):107-16.

[57] Ferrero S, Vellone VG, Barra F, Scala C. Ulipristal Acetate before Hysteroscopic and Laparoscopic Surgery for Uterine Myomas: Help or Hindrance? *Gynecol Obstet Invest.* 2018:1-13.

[58] Falcone T, Parker WH. Surgical management of leiomyomas for fertility or uterine preservation. *Obstetrics and Gynecology.* 2013; 121(4):856-68.

[59] Litta P, Fantinato S, Calonaci F, Cosmi E, Filippeschi M, Zerbetto I, et al. A randomized controlled study comparing harmonic versus electrosurgery in laparoscopic myomectomy. *Fertil Steril.* 2010; 94(5):1882-6.

[60] Paul PG, Paul G, Radhika KT, Bulusu S, Shintre H. Laparoscopic Myomectomy for a Plethora of Submucous Myomas. *J Minim Invasive Gynecol.* 2017; 24(6):893-894.

[61] Glasser MH. Minilaparotomy myomectomy: A minimally invasive alternative for the large fibroid uterus. *J Minim Invasive Gynecol.* 2005; 12(3):275-83.

[62] Song T, Kim TJ, Kim WY, Lee SH. Comparison of barbed suture versus traditional suture in laparoendoscopic single-site myomectomy. *Eur J Obstet Gynecol Reprod Biol.* 2015; 185:99-102.

[63] Dubuisson JB, Fauconnier A, Chapron C, Kreiker G, Nörgaard C. Second look after laparoscopic myomectomy. *Hum Reprod.* 1998; 13(8):2102-6.

[64] Ahmad G, O'Flynn H, Hindocha A, Watson A. Barrier agents for adhesion prevention after gynaecological surgery. *Cochrane Database of Systematic Reviews.* 2015; (2):CD000475.

[65] Tinelli A, Malvasi A, Guido M, Tsin DA, Hudelist G, Hurst B, et al. Adhesion formation after intracapsular myomectomy with or without adhesion barrier. *Fertil Steril.* 2011; 95(5):1780-5.

[66] Tulandi T, Murray C, Guralnick M. Adhesion formation and reproductive outcome after myomectomy and second-look laparoscopy. *Obs Gynecol.* 1993; 82(2):213-5.

[67] Sandberg EM, Cohen SL, Jansen FW, Einarsson JI. Analysis of Risk Factors for Intraoperative Conversion of Laparoscopic Myomectomy. *J Minim Invasive Gynecol.* 2016; 23(3):352-7.

[68] Cicinelli E, Tinelli R, Colafiglio G, Saliani N. Laparoscopy vs Minilaparotomy in Women with Symptomatic Uterine Myomas: A Prospective Randomized Study. *J Minim Invasive Gynecol.* 2009; 16(4):422-6.

[69] Seracchioli R, Rossi S, Govoni F, Rossi E, Venturoli S, Bulletti C, et al. Fertility and obstetric outcome after laparoscopic myomectomy of large myomata: A randomized comparison with abdominal myomectomy. *Hum Reprod.* 2000; 15(12):2663-8.

[70] Tan J, Sun Y, Dai H, Zhong B, Wang D. A Randomized Trial of Laparoscopic Versus Laparoscopic-Assisted Minilaparotomy Myomectomy for Removal of Large Uterine Myoma: Short-Term Outcomes. *J Minim Invasive Gynecol.* 2008; 15(4):402-9.

[71] Holzer A, Jirecek ST, Illievich UM, Huber J, Wenzl RJ. Laparoscopic versus open myomectomy: A double-blind study to evaluate postoperative pain. *Anesth Analg.* 2006; 102(5):1480-4.

[72] Farquhar C. Do uterine fibroids cause infertility and should they be removed to increase fertility? *BMJ.* 2009; 338:b126.

[73] Inagaki N, Ung L, Otani T, Wilkinson D, Lopata A. Uterine cavity matrix metalloproteinases and cytokines in patients with leiomyoma, adenomyosis or endometrial polyp. *Eur J Obstet Gynecol Reprod Biol.* 2003; 111(2):197-203.

[74] Kroon B, Johnson N, Chapman M, Yazdani A, Hart R. Fibroids in infertility - Consensus statement from ACCEPT (Australasian CREI Consensus Expert Panel on Trial evidence). *Australian and New Zealand Journal of Obstetrics and Gynaecology.* 2011; 51(4):289-95.

[75] Yoshino O, Nishii O, Osuga Y, Asada H, Okuda S, Orisaka M, et al. Myomectomy decreases abnormal uterine peristalsis and increases pregnancy rate. *J Minim Invasive Gynecol.* 2012; 19(1):63-7.

[76] Galliano D, Bellver J, Díaz-García C, Simón C, Pellicer A. Art and uterine pathology: How relevant is the maternal side for implantation? *Hum Reprod Update.* 2015; 21(1):13-38.

[77] Bernardi TS, Radosa MP, Weisheit A, Diebolder H, Schneider U, Schleussner E, et al. Laparoscopic myomectomy: A 6-year follow-up single-center cohort analysis of fertility and obstetric outcome measures. *Arch Gynecol Obstet.* 2014; 290(1):87-91.

[78] Saravelos SH, Yan J, Rehmani H, Li TC. The prevalence and impact of fibroids and their treatment on the outcome of pregnancy in women with recurrent miscarriage. *Hum Reprod.* 2011; 26(12):3274-9.

[79] Metwally M, Cheong YC, Horne AW. Surgical treatment of fibroids for subfertility. In: *Cochrane Database of Systematic Reviews.* 2012; 11:CD003857.

[80] Pritts EA, Parker WH, Olive DL. Fibroids and infertility: an updated systematic review of the evidence. *Fertil Steril.* 2009; 91(4):1215-23.

[81] Sunkara SK, Khairy M, El-Toukhy T, Khalaf Y, Coomarasamy A. The effect of intramural fibroids without uterine cavity involvement on the outcome of IVF

treatment: A systematic review and meta-analysis. *Human Reproduction.* 2010; 25(2):418-29.

[82] Kundu S, Iwanuk C, Staboulidou I, Garcia-Rocha GJ, Soergel P, Hertel H, et al. Morbidity, fertility and pregnancy outcomes after myoma enucleation by laparoscopy versus laparotomy. *Arch Gynecol Obstet.* 2018;297(4):969–976.

[83] Casini ML, Rossi F, Agostini R, Unfer V. Effects of the position of fibroids on fertility. *Gynecol Endocrinol. 2006*; 22(2):106-9.

In: Uterine Fibroids
Editors: S. Ferrero and F. Barra

ISBN: 978-1-53615-046-9

Chapter 8

HYSTEROSCOPIC MYOMECTOMY

Gloria D'Alessandro, MD, Fabio Barra, MD, Federico Casabona, MD and Simone Ferrero*, MD, PhD

Obstetrics and Gynecology, Department of Neurosciences, Rehabilitation, Ophthalmology, Genetics, Maternal and Child Health (DiNOGMI), University of Genoa, Italy

Academic Unit of Obstetrics and Gynecology, Ospedale San Martino, Genoa, Italy

ABSTRACT

Nowadays the standard minimally invasive surgery for the removal of submucous fibroids is represented by the hysteroscopic myomectomy, which may be performed in operating or office-based setting by using a smaller resectoscope. The most common indications for this endoscopic operation are abnormal uterine bleeding and infertility; in fact, it has been demonstrated to be an effective technique to treat menstrual disorders as well as to achieve a pregnancy rate ranging between 29.7% and 58.9% among infertile patients. The preoperative evaluation of these patients may be done by previous office hysteroscopy, transvaginal ultrasonography and sonohysterography; it aims to give accurate information regarding the "myometrial free margin," the volume of fibroids and their protrusion into the uterine cavity. According to these myomas features, several operative techniques may be performed (such as Mazzon, Litta or OPPIuM techniques). Moreover, during them, it is possible to employ electrosurgical (thermal loops and vaporizing electrodes) and mechanical (cold loops) or alternative (laser fibers and intrauterine morcellator devices) instruments. The main complications during hysteroscopic myomectomy are represented by uterine perforation, cervical injury, bleeding, fluid deficit and air embolism. In order to permit an easier procedure, to shrink the nodule size or to correct anemia before surgery, different drugs have been proposed, such as GnRH-as and SPRMs.

---

* Corresponding Author's E-mail: simoneferrero@me.com.

Keywords: submucous fibroids, resectoscopic myomectomy, hysteroscopic procedure, thermal loops, cold loops

1. Introduction

The incidence of myomas ranges from 20% to 25% in women of reproductive age and submucous myomas account for 5.5% to 16.6% of all uterine myomas [1]. Thanks to the development of endoscopy and the introduction of operative hysteroscopy, a new conservative and effective procedure has been offered to the treatment of submucous fibroids that a resectable from the inner of uterus; thus, resectoscopic myomectomy has become, over the years, the standard minimally invasive surgery for their removal [2, 3].

Approximately 540.000 hysterectomies are performed annually in the United States, of which the most common indication is the myomas [4, 5]. Symptoms, such as menorrhagia, metrorrhagia, pelvic pain, colicky dysmenorrhea (due to the attempt of the uterus to expel fibroids through contractions) and sub fertility, constitute the general indications to perform this surgical procedure [6].

The first hysteroscopic myomectomy was performed by Neuwirth and Amin [7] in 1976 using a urologic resectoscope with monopolar current. In 1987, Hallez [8] performed the procedure with a new gynecological resectoscope by a continuous-flow device with a 0° optic, cutting current and 1.5% glycine as distension medium. At the beginning, fibroids were removed by rugged methods using ovum forceps to twist pedunculated lesions and scissors outside the hysteroscopic sheath in order to cut the fibroid pedicle. During the last 2 decades, better instruments have been employed and the development of pioneering techniques has made hysteroscopic myomectomy a *fully-fledged* surgical operation, becoming successfully the treatment of choice in the management of patients with symptomatic submucous myomas [1].

This endoscopic operation, being feasible and effective, is associated with little postoperative pain, short hospital stays, and rapid recovery time [9].

2. Indication to Hysteroscopic Myomectomy

The most common indications for operative hysteroscopy are abnormal uterine bleeding (AUB), ranging from 60% to 84.1% of cases, and infertility [3, 10–12]. Uterine bleeding has been more associated with the presence of submucous myomas rather than subserous and intramural ones, probably due to the uterine cavity distortion and to the increase of the endometrial bleeding surface [13].

The myomectomy is more frequently performed for the relief of patients' symptoms, such as abnormal bleeding, iron deficiency, dysmenorrhea, not specific pelvic pain or bulk pain; in cases of asymptomatic patients with reproductive problems or recurrent pregnancy loss, the existing literature is controversial, being the impact of the procedure on fertility and pregnancy outcomes less clear [1, 14].

There is insufficient evidence regarding the effect of myomas on the reduction of chance of achieving pregnancy with or without performing assisted reproductive technology (ART). Moreover, it is controversial which nodule characteristics (excluding submucosal or intramural myomas impacting the endometrial cavity contour) influence pregnancy rates and early pregnancy loss and if hysteroscopic myomectomy reduces the likelihood of early pregnancy loss in infertile women with a submucous fibroid (Grade C recommendation) (14); instead, there is clear evidence of improving pregnancy outcomes after the removal of fibroids that distorts uterine cavity whereas there is insufficient evidence regarding this effect on early pregnancy loss or live birth. Contrary to submucosal myomas, it is established that subserosal myomas do not provide a negative impact on fertility [15, 16]. For all these reasons, myomectomy is generally not suggested or increasing fertility in asymptomatic infertile women with non-cavity-distorting myomas [14], whereas it is recommended in asymptomatic infertile women with submucous fibroid, as claimed by the latest French guidelines (Grade A); moreover, it is suggest using bipolar energy and anti-adhesion gel during the procedure (Grade C) [17]. Therefore, in current clinical practice infertile patients with submucosal myomas should be counseled to remove hysteroscopically them in order to maximize their chances of spontaneous conception or subsequent ART.

The reason of the negative impact on fertility of fibroids distorting the endometrial cavity can be attributed to multiple reasons, such as endometrium alteration, abnormal myometrial contractility and vascularization, eventual physical obstruction of the uterine cornua [18] as well as interference with sperm migration, ovum transport or embryo implantation [1].

Finally, an asymptomatic woman starting a hormone replacement therapy can represent another uncommon indication to perform the operative hysteroscopy [8].

Given all these indications, it is important to know which patients should not undergo hysteroscopic removal of fibroids. A prophylactic myomectomy should not be systematically performed with the aim of reducing the risk of malignant transformation of the fibroid due to leiomyosarcoma rarity in childbearing age (0.1% [19]). Moreover, a rapid increase in size of the fibroid in premenopausal patients is generally not associated with this development. Whenever a suspicion of malignant transformation is high, it is appropriate to get necessary oncologic investigations. Additionally, a prophylactic myomectomy should not even be performed to prevent obstetric complications (such as miscarriage, cesarean section, premature delivery, malpresentation and placental abruption), because pregnancy in most of cases of women affected by fibroids tend to evolve without complications. Moreover, it is impossible to predict during future pregnancy a relevant myoma increase or its potential of becoming symptomatic; moreover, 70% of women with fibroids of >10cm of diameter can achieve vaginal delivery [20].

General contraindications to hysteroscopy in pregnancy include cervicitis, acute pelvic inflammatory disease and the concomitant presence of cervical or endometrial cancer.

3. Preoperative Evaluation

The most widespread pre-surgical diagnostic techniques to detect number, size and invasion of the myometrium of myomas are office hysteroscopy, the transvaginal ultrasound scanning (TVS) and sonohysterography (SHG) [1].

Office hysteroscopy provides for view of cavity, exact fibroids location, its relationship with uterine structures, characteristics of the endometrium and eventual intracavitary pathologies which may require other surgical approaches. Moreover, it can give some indirect details regarding the depth of myometrium [1].

TSV allows to measure the dimensions of the uterus [9] and to evaluate two important factors: the "myometrial free margin" (FMM), which is the myometrial thickness between the myoma and the uterine serosa, and other potential uterine affections. Furthermore, it allows to evaluate the exact volume of the fibroid [21–23].

It is possible to know more accurate details about the myoma protrusion by using SHG than TVS [1].

The preoperative diagnosis of myomas may become complicated in some situations like in case of a large uterus, multiple fibroids or in obese patients; in these cases, the recurs to magnetic resonance imaging (MRI) may give further details for correctly detecting the presence of myomas. Moreover, in particular situations, MRI may help to accurately distinguish fibroids from adenomyosis. Overall, due to high costs, it is not routinely employed for the pre-operative work-up for myomas [6].

The virtual hysteroscopy has also been proposed for the evaluation of submucosal nodules. This radiologic method is less invasive compared to a hysteroscopic exam because the acquisition of the image of uterine cavity is processed by a multislice helical computed tomography (CT) scanner, using 3D computer graphics (3DCG) software [24].

3.1. Classification of Submucous Fibroids

The European Society for Gynecological Endoscopy (ESGE) adopted the classification system developed by Wamsteker et al. [25] in 1993, which takes account of the degree of penetration of the submucous nodule in the myometrium. In accordance also with their size and the proportion of the myoma protruding into the uterine cavity, submucous myomas are divided into three grades (Table 1). This classification is efficient for discriminating the complexity of hysteroscopic myomectomies [26].

Table 1. Classification of the European Society of Hysteroscopy depending on the degree of intramural involvement. Although type 0 myomas are usually removed completely in a 1-step procedure, complete removal of myomas with intramural development (particularly G2) in a 1-step procedure is often difficult. The resection of G2 fibroids should be undertaken by experienced hysteroscopic surgeons [52]

Classification of the European Society of Hysteroscopy(106)	
Type 0 (G0)	Myoma is completely in the endometrial cavity without intramural extension
Type I (G1)	Myoma has its larger portion (>50%) in the endometrial cavity with intramural extension <50%
Type II (G2)	Myoma has its smaller portion (<50%) in the endometrial cavity with intramural extension >50%

Table 2. Presurgical Lasmar score classification.
Score 0-4 (Group I): low complexity hysteroscopic myomectomy.
Score 5-6 (Group II): complex hysteroscopic myomectomy, consider preparing with gonadotropin-releasing hormone agonists (GnRHa) and/or two step surgery.
Score 7-9 (Group III): recommend an alternative non hysteroscopic technique

Lasmar's pre-surgical classification of submucous myomas					
Score	Extention of base	Size (cm)	Location within uterus	Penetration into myometrium	Lateral wall involvement
0	≤1/3	≤2	Lower third	0	Absent
1	>1/3 to ≤2/3	>2-5	Middle third	≤50%	Present
2	>2/3	>5	Upper third	>50%	

Lasmar et al. [21] proposed a further preoperative classification of submucous fibroids (Table 2). The authors include five aspects to be evaluated in the preoperative setting for myomas: extension of myomas in relation to the uterine wall, their size and topography into the uterine cavity, their penetration into the myometrium and lateral wall involvement. Each parameter gives a score by which it is possible to allocate patients into one of three levels of surgical difficulty.

Lasmar score >7 and myoma size >5 cm are considered significant predictors for performing a 2-step hysteroscopical procedure [27]. Overall, several studies [28] suggest that a large myoma (>3-5 cm) is the main factor associated with an incomplete removal and operative complications.

Finally, it appears essential to consider the FMM because it prevents the uterine perforation during hysteroscopic operation, if it results appropriate. Most authors consider a thickness between 5 and 10mm as ideal to proceed safely with resectoscopic surgery [29]. A further attention should be taken when submucous fibroids are near the cornual region in order to avoid injury to the tubal ostia [1].

4. Operative Hysteroscopic Procedure

The endoscopic operation is usually performed under general anesthesia (spinal or local anesthesia represents valid alternatives [30]) that takes place in operating room or in an outpatient setting.

The traditional procedure requires the use of a resection loop introduced into the resectoscope channel and connected to an energy source. A continuous and constant irrigation through a liquid medium is adopted to distend uterine cavity and allows a good visual. In case of the use of monopolar energy, the liquid is constituted by glycine 1.5% or sorbitol 3% as these fluids do not disperse current, whereas in case of the use bipolar energy, a safer isotonic saline is employed. The intrauterine cavity pressure is set between 90 and 110 mmHg, depending on the type of intervention. The liquid balance needs a careful monitoring to avoid complications such as the intravasation syndrome and other electrolyte disorders.

The surgical procedure usually starts with the "slicing technique" using the thermal loop, mentioned before, set in "pure cutting" mode; it carries on with a cold loop for the intramural portion of the myoma. The monopolar energy, employed at the beginning for the submucous part, acts only where the loop comes into contact with the myomas (in fact, the bipolar loop does not need tissue contact for activation). This minimizes the danger coming from the passage through the uterine structures and it has a direct cutting action on the tissue.

The procedure may be executed in one or two surgical steps. Finally, samples of myomas collected are sent to histological evaluation.

Some authors [31, 32] described the use of transrectal ultrasound for the intraoperative monitoring of myomas in order to reduce the risk of uterine perforation and to perform a complete removal in one surgical step.

4.1. Hysteroscopic Equipment and Surgical Techniques

Several improvements in instrumentation and in operative techniques have been made for endoscopic resection of submucous myoma in order to make the procedure easier, more effective and tolerated. Different methodologies have been proposed; currently, the choice of the best surgical technique and instrumentation depends on the surgeon preference and experience and on the myoma characteristics [3]. One of these discoveries is the use of the bipolar energy with normal saline as distending medium. However, despite of this innovation, it is still needed and essential the continuous and careful monitoring of patient and fluid status [4].

The classical technique is performed under anesthetic by a surgical hysteroscope with a diameter of 10 mm; the introduction requires cervical dilatation. The nodule is removed by a cutting loop performing repeated and progressive passages on fibroid surface until the nodule is chopped into slices (slicing technique) (Figure 1a-b-c-d) [26]. The cut usually starts from the top of the nodule and carries on towards its base; when the myoma is pedunculated, the pedicle may be cut also from the basis [6, 22].

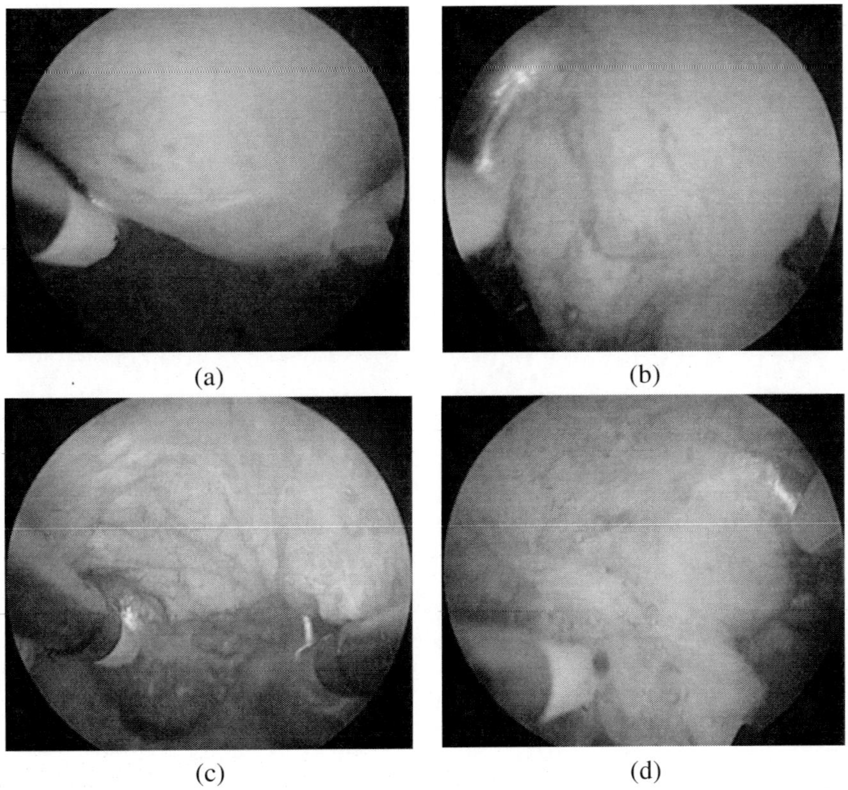

Figure 1. a-b-c-d. Resection of a submucous myomas by Thermal loop.

Further hysteroscopic innovations have been introduced over the last years, such as myoma morcellation, its ablation by different kind of lasers and the developing of hysteroscopes with smaller diameter, more suitable for the office myomectomy. In fact, hysteroscopy may allow simultaneous diagnostic and operative procedures ("see and treat") without cervical dilatation and anesthesia [33, 34].

Despite several improvements, myomectomy is performed up to 40% in the operating room [26] and slicing technique still represents the "gold standard" for treating myomas

[3]. Furthermore, no technique is proven to be better for the treatment of G1 and G2 fibroids. It is important to remove only the intramural portion of myomas avoiding a uterine perforation during the passage of the loop. The use of cold loop currently represents the best option to save healthy myometrium and to remove completely the myoma in one step procedure [1].

4.1.1. Hysteroscopic Resectoscope

The hysteroscopic resectoscope allows the removal of submucous myomas under a constant visual control. Several components need to be assembled before this procedure (Figure 2).

The resectoscope has been modified from the urologic one, including a straight-forward telescope (0°) or a slightly fore-oblique 12–30° telescope with an outer diameter of 3-4 mm and as heath of 24-27 Fr. This latter contains channels providing a constant inflow and outflow of distension fluid in which it is possible to introduce operating instruments and to move them through a spring handle [35].

The operating instruments are divided into electrosurgical (thermal loops and vaporizing electrodes) and mechanical (cold loops). Moreover, there is the possibility to employ laser fibers or intrauterine morcellator (IUM) device [1].

Several thermal loops with different shapes and sizes have been developed (Figure 3a): the smaller ones are usually used for bipolar instruments (rather than monopolar resectoscopes with the same outer diameter) that need more time for resection [6].

The vaporizing electrodes need a power of 150-300 W of pure cut current (coming from an electrosurgical generator) in order to vaporize tissue [36]. This tool can be used also in a mechanical way to dissect the fibroid from myometrium [1].

The cold loops are structurally stronger than the thermal loops due to their mechanical action during intramural enucleation without needing electrical energy (Figure 3b) [1].

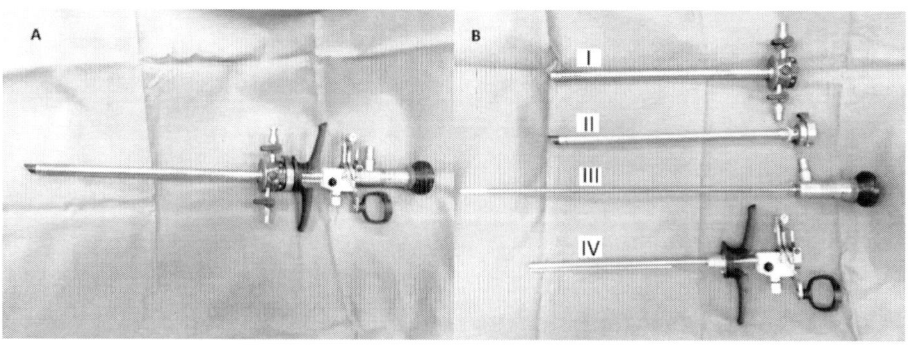

Figure 2. a. Hysteroscopic resectoscope with continuous flow double-sheath system, rotatable; b. It consists of a set of I outer sheaths, II inner sheaths, III optics, IV working element.

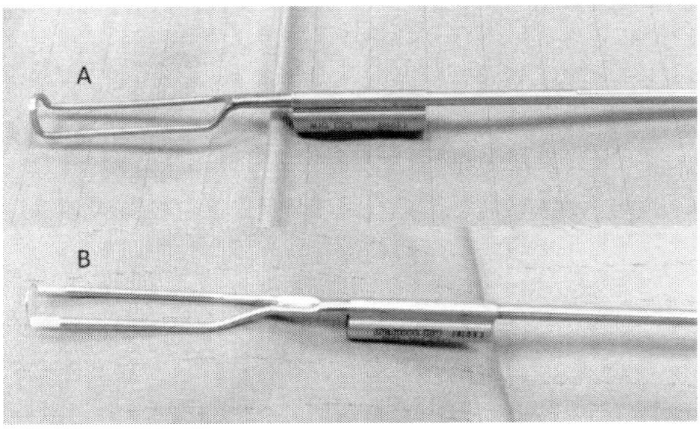

Figure 3. a. Cold loop 90° for resectoscopic myomectomy; b. Thermal loop (bipolar), 90° for resectoscopic myomectomy.

4.1.2. Hysteroscopic Miniresectoscope

A smaller resectoscope, developed from the pediatric one, has been recently introduced in the medical practice. It has been elaborated by Karl Storz and its clinical application has been described for the first time by Papalampros et al. [37].

This miniresectoscope permits to enucleate small myomas in a office-based setting: this technique can be performed without anesthesia and cervical dilatation; the device can be inserted using either a speculum and a tenaculum applied to the anterior lip of the cervix or through vaginoscopic approach without speculum.

The complete nodule excision and the slides extraction are not always achieved by using this instrument. Thus, the procedure can be longer, especially if myoma is deep into the myometrium with an increase in the perforation risk [3].

4.1.3. Hysteroscopic Morcellator

The introduction of IUM allowed shorter operating time and less fluid overload complications compared to the traditional hysteroscopic methods [4, 38].

IUM consists of two disposable tubes to fit into each other and to insert inside the hysteroscope channel. The surgeon has the control, by a foot pedal, of the inner tube, which rotates as result of an electrically powered control unit activation connected to a handheld motor drive. This mechanical technique combines cutting and aspiration: the tissue is cut when the inner tube is rotated and sucked into a window-opening located at the end of this tube [1]. These two simultaneous actions may explain the reduction in operating time during myomectomy [39]. Lastly, the aspirated specimen tissues are sent for pathologic evaluation. IUM can be used also as a hook for the removal of a G2 myoma, as reported by Pakrashi et al. [40]. Currently, the procedure may be potentially performed in outpatient rooms since a smaller device can be inserted through a 5 mm endoscope [4].

Hysteroscopic morcellation presents some advantages compared with bipolar resectoscopy: firstly, it does not provoke electrical damage of surrounding myometrium because the tissue is mechanically cut; secondly, no gas bubbles are formed, permitting a better view together with a reduction of gas embolism risk [22]; thirdly, the continuous aspiration of myoma fragments ensures again a good vision. Among the disadvantages, IUM procedure does not allow to coagulate bleeding vessels [36]; moreover, it results more expensive compared with the reusable instruments for resectoscopy [39].

4.1.4. Laser Technology

CO_2 laser and argon and krypton and neodymium-doped yttrium aluminum garnet (Nd:yAG) lasers have been successfully used in the hysteroscopy field. In particular, Nd:yAG lasers became particularly widespread between 1980s and 1990s [41]. These two techniques have been developed by using the laser technology, and they can be type "touch" and type "non-touch." The first one maintains contact between the endoscopic tool and the tissue, while few millimeters divide the laser from the myoma in the "non-touch" technique [41]. Laser methodology presents some disadvantages, such as lack of possibility of sending specimens for histological analysis, longer time to reduce the nodule size [42] and high cost; therefore, its utilization is not widely diffuse in clinical practice [1]. Recently, a Spanish group [3] has re-adopted the technique and published its experience with office hysteroscopic laser enucleation of submucous myomas without anesthesia. The group always tried to perform a biopsy of a little myoma sample for histological analysis despite of the laser use. Moreover, it left inside the cavity the remnant portion of the nodule whenever the mass extraction was not possible. During the 2-3-monthfollow-up, the authors did not find patients presenting residual myoma inside the uterine cavity, probably because a subsequent expulsion occurred during the menstruation or in a spontaneous way. They demonstrated that leaving free tissue inside the uterus after a laser treatment may be a feasible and safe therapeutic option.

4.1.5. Treatment of Myomas Completely within the Uterine Cavity (G0)

Intracavitary fibroids (GO) are easier to remove in one-step procedure than G1 and G2 myomas. The size is the main factor to consider during excision of G0 myomas. A pedunculated fibroid may be cut by resectoscopic loop by performing standard technique [22], or by using Nd:yAG laser or vaporizing electrode [43].

After the cut obtained by endoscopic loop, the free chips into the cavity may meddle in the visual. It is possible to catch them by the loop electrode taking out the resectoscope. This process, which is supervised by resectoscopic view, may require several steps. In general, there are further methods to withdraw free fragments: for example, it is possible to collect them by forceps or through the use of a resectoscope with automatic chip aspiration, by which the tissue is immediately sucked after been cut. At the end of the excision, the base of the implant should be smooth and regular; the fasciculate structure of the myometrium should be always showed [1].

Nd:yAG laser is a suitable option in case of small fibroids (≤2cm). This technique allows to coagulate vessel and to flatten the nodule by repeated touches with laser fibers (touch technique) [1].

It is also possible to "vaporize" the fibroid using spherical or cylindrical electrodes. The operation needs a slow movement across the surface of the nodule done by electrodes. The depth of vaporization depends on duration of contact, resistance and wattage of the generator. The power should be activated only when moving in the direction towards the operator. Moreover, it should avoid a long pressure with high current on tissue, considering the perforation risk [43]. Compared to the classical resectoscopic myomectomy, fibroid vaporization turns out to be faster and it does not present visual interference due to fragments [36]; anyway, the lack of tissue sample for histological analysis makes it necessary to obtain a myoma sample by another technique prior to perform vaporization [43]. Another disadvantage is that gas bubbles, produced by the high power, could enter into the vascular system [1].

Lastly, for the treatment of this type of fibroids, the morcellation technique has been described; it offers the advantage of obtaining tissue for pathology. Moreover, it is effective and faster than conventional resectoscope [44].

4.2. Treatment of Myomas with Intramural Extension (G1-G2)

Several techniques have been proposed for the resection of the intramural portion of submucous myomas. This part is often considered a challenge for the operators; the aim of all these approaches is to extrude the intramural portion inside the uterine cavity in a safe and effective way [45].

Even if some surgeons succeed to treat G2 myomas in 1-step, others recommend a 2-step procedure. On opposite, others surgeons prefer to avoid the hysteroscopic surgery for excising myomas larger than 5 cm [42].

The following techniques represent the most widely used procedures for treating myomas with intramural component.

4.2.1. Mazzon Technique

The intramural portion of the myoma is enucleated by a cold loop ("cold loop myomectomy") by using a mechanical traction and a system of leverage. The aim of this procedure is to avoid a thermal myometrial lesion and to maintain untouched myometrial fibers, nevertheless ensuring a complete myoma enucleation. The surgeon cuts the connective bridges of the pseudocapsule of the myoma without using any energy source on the myometrium. The pseudocapsule anchors the myoma to the myometrium; its preservation ensures less complications rate, avoids thermal damage and reduces the postoperative intracavitary adherences [2]. Moreover, it allows to preserve myometrial integrity providing a better healing and also a potential improvement of infertility outcomes after endoscopic myomectomy [45–49].

At the beginning of the intervention, the surgeon usually performs an excision of the endometrial portion of the myoma by the traditional slicing technique, in particular by using an electric loop. When it is visible the cleavage plane between the nodule and myometrium, the thermal loop (never used under the endometrial lining) is replaced by the cold loop; the fibers anchoring the myoma are mechanically detached from the myometrium through a blunt dissection and the intramural portion is thus enucleated without the use of the electrical cutting.

The free endocavitary tissue can be removed by using the thermal loop again through a cutting action that starts from the nodule and is directed toward the uterine cavity. It necessary to prevent the opposite direction where the uterine wall is thinner, avoiding the perforation risk.

In a retrospective study [50] recruiting 1215 patients, published by Mazzon, originator of the technique, it has been concluded that this procedure is effective and safe (Table 3).

Table 3. Main published studies illustrating the principal techniques used for the hysteroscopic removal of intramural portion of the myoma

Authors	Technique	Study Design, Number of Casesand Inclusion Criteria	Results	Comments
Mazzon et al., (2018) [50]	Mazzon technique: enucleation of the intramural portion by cold loops	Retrospective cohort study: - 1215 patients; -1434 myomectomies; - G1 and G2 myomas; - FMM $\leq$ 2 mm	1252 (87.3%) one-step procedure 182 (12.7%) multiple-step procedure (p= 0.028)	Size, number of myomas and the age of patients were significantly correlated with a multiple-step procedure
Litta et al., (2003) [51]	Litta technique: enucleation in toto	Prospective study (Canadian Task Force classification II-1): - 41 patients; - single myoma (G2); - FMM >4mm; - absence of associated intracavitary lesions	38 (92.6%); one-step procedure 3 (7.4%) second-step procedure (p= 0.028)	3 patients who underwent second step procedure presented myomas > 4 cm (n = 2), myoma = 3 cm (n = 1)
Bettocchi et al., (2009) [52]	OPPIuM technique: office preparation of partially intramural myomas	Prospective pilot study: - 59 patients; - G1- G2 myomas.	The conversion of G1 and G2 myomas into G0 or G1 was observed in 93.2% (55/59) of cases: G1 (n = 27) were converted into G0 in all cases (100%). G2 (n = 32) were converted in 29/32 (90.6%) cases. The conversion into G1 was achieved in 22 (75.9%) cases and into G0 in 7 (24.1%) cases	In 3 cases of failure, the myomas, originally classified as G2, were still graded as G2 at follow-up hysteroscopy. In 2 of these cases, the myoma size was 4 cm. One case excluded for total spontaneous expulsion of the myoma at the subsequent menstrual cycle

Authors	Technique	Study Design, Number of Casesand Inclusion Criteria	Results	Comments
Haimovich et al., (2013) [26]	Two-step myomectomy technique, Bertocchi technique modified, using laser	Prospective pilot study: - 43 women; - G1- G2 myomas; - myomas ≤ 4cm.	Successfully performed in 34 (79.1%) patients: complete enucleation was achieved in 80.9% (17/21) of G1 myomas and in 77.3% (17/22) of G2 myomas ($p = 1.000$). Enucleation based on: -Size ($p < 0.001$): 100% ≤ 18 mm, 85% 19-30 mm, - Location ($p = 0.020$): 87.9% anterior/posterior 50% fundus/lateral - Parity ($p = 0.009$): 95.5% nulliparous 61.9% parous	In 9 patients in whom large masses were left free in the uterine cavity, ultrasound follow-up two months later showed a total disappearance of myoma in all of them. Enucleation was not achieved in: 4 patients with G1, 5 patients with G2. Success of surgery was associated with size, location, and women's parity.
Zayed et al., (2015) [9]	Combination of techniques: manual massage, hydro massage and applying traction on the myoma by a resectoscope loop	Prospective study (Canadian Task Force classification II-3): - 49 patients; - G1- G2 myomas; - myomas ≥4cm.	91.84% (45/49) one-step complete resection. Resection based on: - Size ($p = .002$): 97.73% <6 cm 40% >6 cm - Number ($p = 0.016$): 97.5% single 66.67% multiple - Lasmar score ($p = 0.011$): 100% <7 76.47% >7 - Type of myomas ($p = 0.042$): 100% G0-G1 82.61% G2 The rate of 1-step complete removal of myomas was 95% for G2 < 6 cm	Follow up after 2-months with office hysteroscopy revealed residual myomas in 4 patients. 100% incompletely removed myomas were G2, Lasmar score ≥7. One-step complete resection of myomas was more frequent in patients with myomas <6 cm, single myomas, principle myomas with a Lasmar score <7, myomas G1
Indaman, (2004) [53]	Pharmacological -aided techniques: intracervical carboprost administered to facilitate resection	Review of 10 cases: 13 myomas that otherwise could not be resected completely.	8/10 complete resection 2/10 incomplete resection	In the two cases with incomplete resection approximately 10% of each myoma remained
Murakami et al., (2003, 2006) [54]	Transabdominal injection of prostaglandin F (PGF)-2a under laparoscopic monitoring	Case report: a 38-year-old patient with sessile submucous leiomyoma of 3 cm.	The intramural remnant portion of the myoma is squeezed into the cavity during the contraction of the uterus provoked by the drug.	Local injection is superior to systematic administration because a local and short-term effect is desired to induce uterine contractions.

4.2.2. Litta Technique

Litta et al. [51] described an enucleation *in toto* of the myomas, which consists in making an elliptical incision on the mucosa covering the myoma, seeking its reflection over the uterine wall until the cleavage plane by using the resectoscope and Collins electrode. The handling should lead to a disconnection of the connective fibers that anchor the nodule to the myometrium and promote its enucleation into the uterine cavity. Lastly, the detached piece can be removed using the traditional slicing technique.

The logical explanation of the extrusion into the cavity can be found in the dynamic structure of the myometrium: during the growing of the nodule, the myometrial fibers are pressed and stretched without rupturing and preserving a normal contractility. Overall, it is considerable that greater is the intramural myoma portion, higher are the muscular elastic forces; therefore, a G2 myomas are thought to have a higher expulsion force than a G1 or G0 myomas. Once the shallow elliptic incision is performed, the myoma expulsion towards cavity starts, decreasing the diving force until zero when there is no more intramural myoma tissue. At the same time of the expulsion process, the uterine wall returns to its normal thickness.

4.2.3. OPPIuM Technique

Bettocchi et al. [52] described the office preparation of partially intramural myomas (OPPIuM) technique which consists of two-step procedure for deep myomas. The first step is performed in office setting without anesthesia using a Versapoint Bipolar Electrosurgical System (Gynecare ™; Ethicon Inc., Somerville, NJ) to incise the mucosa covering the myoma at the level of its reflection on the uterus. It has the purpose to disconnect the fibroid from its pseudocapsule and to facilitate the expulsion. The second step takes place in surgery room during the proliferative phase of the patient's menstrual cycle after 2 menstrual cycles from the first procedure. It is performed by resectoscopy and bipolar electrode by which the submucous fibroid is divided into two halves and then it is sliced into segments. The reason of these two step procedures is to wait a spontaneous extrusion of the intramural portion of the nodule during the subsequent menstrual cycles following the first step preparation.

4.2.4. Haimovich: OPPIuM Technique Modified

Haimovich et al. [26] reported a modification of the technique described by Bertocchi et al.: the first step preparation of the intramural portion of myoma may be done by using the laser diode rather than by the standard bipolar energy. Moreover, after the second step, the free nodule is left inside the cavity also when it is large enough to be entirely extracted. During the first step, it is possible to collect a tissue sample for histological diagnosis by means of high-power diode laser 1000 micron and diamond probe. In the second step, done after four weeks from the first one, the excision of the myoma may be finalized by the laser diode again or by a mechanical technique. If the size of myoma does not allow to completely remove it at the end of the enucleation, it is left free into the cavity, under the assumption that it will be spontaneously expelled. These authors performed an ultrasound follow-up 2 months later to verify the complete expulsion, which was achieved in all cases.

4.2.5. Combination of Techniques

Zayed et al. [9] proposed a combination of techniques, which includes: bimanual massage, hydromassage and application of traction on the myoma by the resectoscope loop inserted in a cleavage plane between myoma and myometrium.

All of these techniques aim to facilitate the expulsion of the intramural portion of the myoma into the uterine cavity. After the removal of the submucous myoma portion by traditional slicing technique, the surgeon applies a traction towards the cleavage plane between the myoma and the myometrium by a resectoscope loop in order to promote its extrusion. In each maneuver, saline infusion is stopped and is restarted to establish rapid changes in the intrauterine pressure, performing a uterine hydromassage that provokes contractions. It is also possible to massage the uterus holding the right hand in the posterior fornix of the vagina and the left hand on the anterior abdominal wall. This induces the extrusion of intramural portion of the nodule. Lastly, the myoma fragments may be removed from the cavity by an ovum forceps.

5. Pharmacological-Aided Techniques

Drugs inducing uterine contractions have been proposed to facilitate the expulsion of the intramural part of the fibroid into the cavity. Uterine contraction scan provokes a further extrusion of partially resected and extrudes myomas, which are frequent problem (especially for type II) after myomectomy. In this regard, Indman [53] proposed the use of intracervical carboprost, a methyl analogue of prostaglandin F (PGF-2a), and Murakami et al. [54] described a transabdominal injection of PGF-2a under laparoscopic monitoring. These techniques are safe, respecting the surrounding health myometrium. Anyway, they present some disadvantages such as the side effects drug-related (nausea, vomiting, diarrhea, fever, bronchospasm in patients with bronchial asthma), the interference with hysteroscopic visual and a high operator ability to maneuver the resectoscope in case of vigorous contractions. Moreover, using them it is unpredictable the entity of following contractile myometrial reaction and, in the Murakami's technique, it is necessary a laparoscopic monitoring. Indman proposed an off-label use of carboprost, since this compound has been approved by the U.S. Food and Drug Administration (FDA) for the treatment of refractory postpartum hemorrhage and for complications of second-trimester abortion; therefore, the literature rarely reports its use in non-pregnant uterus.

6. Effects of Hysteroscopic Myomectomy on Menstrual Pattern and Infertility

6.1. Success Rate in Controlling Abnormal Uterine Bleeding

Hysteroscopic myomectomy is safe and effective to treat menstrual disorders, with high success rate (70-97%) [43, 55] and low symptoms recurrence (4-20%). A discrete rate of patients (16-21%) may benefit from a reoperation at 4 years [12, 56–58].

Several studies report a recurrence of abnormal bleeding as the follow-up period after myomectomy increases [1], probably it is due to a re-growth of the submucous portion of the myoma left inside the uterus or the development of further nodules. Moreover, it is necessary to consider different causes such as dysfunctional bleeding or coexistent presence of adenomyosis.

The technique employed for myomectomy does not seem to have any influence on the recurrence of myomas. Therefore, a long-term follow-up does not accurately evaluate the efficacy of the surgical approach, considering that a future return of symptoms may be caused by other factors; on opposite, an immediate success may be associated to the specific surgical technique used, the operator experience and the myoma characteristics (size and type) [9]. With special regard to the size, some authors [59] published a success rate of 78% after the treatment of myoma less than 3 cm of diameter and a 14% rate of success for myomas more than 5 cm; others [27] reported a94.4% of bleeding control in case of submucous myomas measured 5 cm or more.

Another important factor to consider in the recurrence of patients' symptomatology is represented by the eventual incomplete resection of intramural portion of the fibroid [25, 60].

6.2. Pregnancy Rates after Hysteroscopic Myomectomy

Most studies report a pregnancy rates after hysteroscopic myomectomy ranging between 29.7% and 58.9% [9]. This wide percentages may be explained for the heterogeneity of the studies, which include different myomas characteristics, surgical approaches, patients' characteristics (age, primary or secondary infertility) and infertility etiology as well as discrepancies in follow-up [61].

Pritts et al. [15] first declared that the endoscopic myomectomy may increase only the ART success, nevertheless not influencing implantation, miscarriage, preterm delivery and live birth rates.

Overall, myomas represent a very rare cause of infertility as isolated factor, ranging from 1% to 2.4% [62, 63]. Particularly, some authors [59] showed a pregnancy rate of

41.6% in patients whose fibroids appeared the only infertility cause, compared to 26.3% of success among patients that presented another apparent infertility cause and to 6.3% when the infertility factors were multiple.

Referring to myoma characteristics, it is important to evaluate type, number and size. Multiple and intramural myomas are generally related to negative impact on postoperative pregnancy rates. However, intramural myomas do not distort the cavity, as showed during an hysteroscopic follow-up performed after their resection; therefore, it is reasonable to assume other causes to explain eventual infertility due to their presence [1].

Stamatellos et al. [64] corroborated the importance of intramural extension of the myoma, reporting an increase of fertility success after resection of G0 and G1 myomas and a decrease after resection of G2 myomas.

Some authors [65] indicated better outcomes after myomectomy by recurring to ART in case of intramural myomas measured more than 5 cm of diameter; others suggested the same results also for spontaneous pregnancy rates. Fernandez et al. [59] reported a 57% of success after the removal of fibroids more than 5 cm compared to 23% in case of fibroids measuring less; Jayakrishnan et al. [66] published a 50% of success for myomas greater or equal to 3 cm versus a pregnancy rate of 24.3% for those of less than 3 cm.

7. Complications of Hysteroscopic Myomectomy

The most frequent intraoperative complications described in literature include uterine perforation, cervical injury, bleeding, fluid deficit (in case of loss more than 2000 mL) and air embolism [9]. Among them, uterine perforation represents the most common complication [48]. About half of these events occurs during hysteroscopic entrance into the uterus [48], despite of the current utilization of dilators for the cervix and the common custom of giving locally prostaglandin analogs prior the procedure [67].

Table 4. Illustration of intraoperative, short-term and long-term complications related to hysteroscopic myomectomy

Intraoperative and short-term complications	Long-term complications
Uterine perforation	Intrauterine adhesions
Cervical injury	Abnormal placentation
Bleeding	Uterine rupture in subsequent pregnancies
Fluid deficit >2000 mL (intravasation syndrome)	
Air embolism	
Endometritis	

The long-term complications are intrauterine adhesions, abnormal placentation and uterine rupture in subsequent pregnancies [9]. Intrauterine adhesions represent the greater tardive problem and it has a rate between 1 to 13% (Table 4) [8, 25].

7.1. Intraoperative and Short-Term Complications

Cervical lacerations range from 1% to 11% of hysteroscopic myomectomy and they occur more frequently during cervix dilatation [48, 68]. If the patient has previously taken a gonadotropin-releasing hormone agonist (GnRH-a), the risk increases due to the induced hypoestrogenic state, which has a negative impact on tissue tropism [1].

The rate of uterine perforation is about 1.3% [48, 68]. This adverse event can occur in several procedures: not only during the dilatation of the cervix but also over the course of hysteroscope entrance into the uterus or the excision of the submucous portion of the myoma by slicing or while the operator tries to enucleate the intramural portion by cold loop [1]. With respect to the late maneuver, the risk becomes particularly high if the intramural spreading is enough to imply an aggressive resection into the myometrium [22] and if the FMM is low (it is generally considered safe an FMM of 10 mm) [45].

If a uterine perforation occurs, the hysteroscopy should be stopped and, even if there is not any bowel lesion, the patient should be undergone to a period of observation and then be discharged; otherwise, in case of suspicion of bowel damage, it is needed to perform an exploratory laparoscopy [6]. Jansen et al. [48], during the performance of 2515 hysteroscopic myomectomy, reported 19 cases of uterine perforations among which 4 patients had an important bleeding. One of these underwent to hysterectomy and one presented a bowel injury treated with laparotomic approach.

Less frequent but the most dangerous reported complication during the procedure is the intravasation of the fluid used to distend the cavity. If the fluid absorption is elevated, it may occur severe complications: pulmonary and cerebral edema, hypoosmolarity and electrolyte imbalance (such as hyponatremia and hyperammonemia) and heart failure [69].

The intravasation can occur through damaged vessels of fibroid during myomectomy or through the fallopian tubes as a result of a retrograde flow of fluid used to distend the cavity. In case of threshold of fluid above, it is required to stop the procedure. There are several methods to assess the difference between inflow and outflow fluid that operating room personnel should monitor by accurate electronic balances. An amount of 750 ml is considered enough to plan a term of the procedure [70]; a fluid intravasation over 1000 ml requires the imminent end of it [71]. Together with the fluid monitoring, another parameter to consider is the intraoperative measure of sodium, whose limit is set at 125 mm Eq/L for performing a safe myomectomy [2].

The main risk factors for intravasation complication include the depth of intramural portion and size of myoma (due to the possibility to provoke veins injury), the length of the procedure and the volume of fluid inflow [69, 72]. The risk of hyponatremia is associated to low-viscosity distending media and to accumulation of free water. Regarding to this, the more recent bipolar technology is considered safer as it allows to use isotonic saline [73], however, an excessive intravasation (like 1500 ml) can still be correctly considered dangerous [22].

An infusion pressure of saline less than 100 mmHg, a suction pressure from 30 to 40mmHg during the whole procedure and several actions aiming to occlude myoma vessels (hydro massage or bimanual massage of the uterus and preoperative use of misoprostol to stimulate uterus contractions) may be performed as preventive measures to avoid this complication [9].

Some authors [74] have reported the phenomenon of gas embolism related to both monopolar and bipolar energy source and whose severity corresponded to the severity of intravasation; however, any case of cardiovascular instability has been never demonstrated.

Finally, the transfusion rate after endoscopic myomectomy using electric energy is widely variable in the literature [75–77]. Agostini et al. [78] found a 0.38% of hemorrhagic complication, whereas only 1 case of important uterine bleeding (0.07%) has been described in another study [45], without did not have necessity of blood transfusion.

7.2. Long-Term Complications

The most common complication after myomectomy is the development of synechiae inside the uterine cavity related to the postoperative healing process or to an eventual perforation of the uterine wall [79]. These adverse events may have a negative impact on future fertility and lead to recurrent pregnancy loss, placenta accrete, and intrauterine growth restriction (IUGR) in subsequent pregnancies [2]. The incidence of intrauterine adhesions widely ranges in the literature and depend on the presurgical characteristics fibroids, the electrosurgical system adopted and the use of anti-adhesive material during the operative procedure [18].

Thermal damage of myometrium and of endometrium surrounding the myoma induced by the resection seems to be the main risk factor for developing fibrotic reactions in the tissue [8, 25]. The number and the position of fibroids, such as in case of multiple nodules "in face-to face" position, may similarly cause the adhesions growth, as reported by several authors [79, 80]. Another studied risk factor for fibrotic reactions is represented by the type of electrical energy adopted during myomectomy [81]. Taskin et al. [79] reported a 31% rate of postoperative synechiae after the use of monopolar energy for the treatment of solitary fibroids and a 45% rate in case of multiple nodules, whereas others authors [81] showed a rate of 7.5% using bipolar diathermy. The bipolar source of energy was judged by them safer and characterized by fewer risks (such as accidental electric fluxes on healthy myometrium), in comparison with the monopolar energy.

Several authors [6, 46] proposed various methods to reduce the risk of uterine synechiae; they under lighted for example the necessity to avoid an excessive manipulation of the cervix and trauma on tissue surrounding the fibroid as well as to minimize the electrical energy use, particularly during the removal of intramural portion of the nodule or in case of multiple fibroids "in face-to face" position. Some authors [82] performed an early second-look hysteroscopy after endoscopic myomectomy to prevent and treat precocious adherences detected. Lastly, it has been suggested the use of uterine anti-adhesive barriers based on hyaluronic acid gel ("auto-cross-linked hyaluronic acid gel" and "polyethylene oxide-sodium carboxymethylcellulose gel"), which showed promising results [83, 84]. A randomized controlled trial [84] found a significant reduction of postoperative synechiae when hyaluronic gel was applied after myomas resection (16% in the group when gel was used versus 33.3% when it was not used, $p < .005$).

Abnormal placentation is considered another long-term complication of hysteroscopic myomectomy, although the available literature reports that its risk is low. Gyamfi-Bannerman et al. [85] did not find any cases of placenta accrete analyzing 176 pregnancy of women previously undergone myomectomy. Anyway, the incidence of abnormal placentation is unknown because of the small number of reported cases [86].

The uterine rupture during pregnancy after hysteroscopic myomectomy represents another adverse event reported by several authors [87–90]. Regarding to its prevention, common opinion is to wait at least one year between the uterine operation and a future pregnancy; however, some surgeons prefer to perform a caesarian if the previously removed fibroid had an intramural component [91, 92]. The current evidence concerning the mode of delivery after uterine operation are weak [1].

8. Preoperative and Intraoperative Medical Therapy Role

Several drugs have been proposed for treating symptoms related to fibroids (such as the excessive bleeding). Some of these compounds have been commonly used in their preoperative setting to shrink the nodule size or to correct anemia. The most adopted treatments include tranexamic acid, non-steroidal anti-inflammatory drugs, progestins, oral contraceptives, GnRH-as and selective progesterone-receptor modulators (SPRMs), Among them, only GnRH-a and SPRMs have been demonstrated to obtain a real reduction on myoma volume [93].

Gutmann et al. [94] claimed that the treatment of patients with submucous fibroids is most clinically relevant indication for the use of preoperative GnRH-a. In fact, GnRH-as induce a status of amenorrhea and a subsequent reduction of endometrial thickness, myoma size and vascularization, which improve preoperative anemia of patients affected [95]; therefore, they have been generally used to minimize the risks related to hysteroscopic myomectomy [96, 97]. Some authors [82] prefer to not pre-operatively treat patients with a fibroid diameter <2 cm by the use of GnRH-as. They consider a 3 weeks preparation with a progestogen or danazol for myomas ranging between 2 to 4 cm and reserve GnRH-as for fibroids >4 cm. The main disadvantages regarding the preoperative use of GnRH-as are menopausal side effects, which can make more difficult the cervical dilatation during the procedure, determining the "sinking" phenomenon (as the consequence of a reduced estrogenic level and the decreased elasticity of myometrial tissue). Moreover, they increase the uterine perforation risk due to a reduced myometrial thickness [96, 98, 99]. On the other hand, evidences show that ulipristal acetate (UPA) is not inferior to leuprolide acetate in improving patients' bleeding and it does not present the hypoestrogenic effects typically experienced by the use of GnRH-as. Thus, UPA is better tolerated, despite some cases of liver dysfunction have been reported after its assumption [100-102]. The preoperative use of UPA before performing hysteroscopic removal of submucosal myomas has been evaluated in several studies with positive outcomes [103, 104].

A different use is reserved for prostaglandin analogues and vasopressin, whose up-take has been closely described in the surgery setting. As said before, Indman [53] and Murakami [54] proposed the intracervical or laparoscopic use of prostaglandin (PG)F-2a, with the aim of inducing uterine contractions and facilitating extrusion of the intramural part of myoma during the procedure. Misoprostol, a synthetic PGE1 analogue, may be administered vaginally 3 hours before surgery to facilitate dilatation of the cervix. Cooper et al. [105] published a systematic review in which they demonstrated a reduction of pain when dilating the cervix >5mm by the use of misoprostol, especially in postmenopausal patients. On the contrary, others authors [106] did not notice significant difference about time for dilation and the decrease of intra- and post-operative complications related to the hysteroscope entrance into the cavity. On the other hand, they reported misoprostol-associated side-effects (preoperative vaginal bleeding, nausea and diarrhea). Therefore, the preoperative use of misoprostol is chosen by each operator [4].

The use of vasopressin has been more described during abdominal and laparoscopic myomectomy [107] rather than in hysteroscopic surgery. Some studies [72, 108, 109] report the intracervical injection of vasopressin during the endoscopic procedure with the purpose of obtaining a local vasoconstrictive effect, thus reducing blood loss and improving surgical visual. This system allows to use less fluid for distend cavity with the result of a reduction of intravasation syndrome risk.

REFERENCES

[1] Di Spiezio Sardo A, Mazzon I, Bramante S, Bettocchi S, Bifulco G, Guida M, et al. *Hysteroscopic myomectomy: A comprehensive review of surgical techniques. Human Reproduction Update*. 2008; 14(2):101-19.

[2] Mazzon I, Favilli A, Cocco P, Grasso M, Horvath S, Bini V, et al. Does cold loop hysteroscopic myomectomy reduce intrauterine adhesions? A retrospective study. *Fertil Steril*. 2014;101(1):294-298.e3.

[3] Haimovich S, López-Yarto M, Urresta Ávila J, Saavedra Tascón A, Hernández JL, Carreras Collado R. Office hysteroscopic laser enucleation of submucous myomas without mass extraction: A case series study. *Biomed Res Int*. 2015.

[4] Pakrashi T. New hysteroscopic techniques for submucosal uterine fibroids. *Current Opinion in Obstetrics and Gynecology*. 2014;26(4):308-13

[5] Falcone T, Parker WH. Surgical management of leiomyomas for fertility or uterine preservation. *Obstetrics and Gynecology*. 2013;121(4):856-68.

[6] Indman PD. Hysteroscopic treatment of submucous myomas. *Clinical Obstetrics and Gynecology*. 2006;121(4):856-68

[7] Neuwirth RS, Amin HK. Excision of submucus fibroids with hysteroscopic control. *Am J Obstet Gynecol*. 1976;126:95-99.

[8] Hallez JP. Single-stage total hysteroscopic myomectomies: indications, techniques, and results. Fertil Steril. 1995;63(4):703-8.

[9] Zayed M, Fouda UM, Zayed SM, Elsetohy KA, Hashem AT. Hysteroscopic myomectomy of large submucous myomas in a 1-step procedure using multiple slicing sessions technique. *J Minim Invasive Gynecol*. 2015;22(7):1196–202.

[10] Campo S, Campo V, Gambadauro P. Short-term and long-term results of resectoscopic myomectomy with and without pretreatment with GnRH analogs in premenopausal women. *Acta Obstet Gynecol* Scand. 2005;84(8):756-60.

[11] Marziani R, Mossa B, Ebano V, Perniola G, Melluso J, Napolitano C. Transcervical hysteroscopic myomectomy: Long-term effects on abnormal uterine bleeding. *Clin Exp Obstet Gynecol*. 2005; 32(1):23-6.

[12] Polena V, Mergui JL, Perrot N, Poncelet C, Barranger E, Uzan S. Long-term results of hysteroscopic myomectomy in 235 patients. *Eur J Obstet Gynecol Reprod Biol*. 2007;130(2):232-7.

[13] Maher PJ. Endoscopic management of fibromyomata. *Reviews in Gynaecological Practice*. 2003.

[14] Penzias A, Bendikson K, Butts S, Coutifaris C, Falcone T, Fossum G, et al. Removal of myomas in asymptomatic patients to improve fertility and/or reduce miscarriage rate: a guideline. *Fertil Steril*. 2017;108(3):416–25.

[15] Pritts EA, Parker WH, Olive DL. Fibroids and infertility: an updated systematic review of the evidence. *Fertil Steril*. 2009; 91(4):1215-23..

[16] Klatsky PC, Tran ND, Caughey AB, Fujimoto VY. Fibroids and reproductive outcomes: a systematic literature review from conception to delivery. *American Journal of Obstetrics and Gynecology*. 2008;198(4):357-66.

[17] Marret H, Fritel X, Ouldamer L, Bendifallah S, Brun JL, De Jesus I, et al. Therapeutic management of uterine fibroid tumors: Updated French guidelines. *European Journal of Obstetrics Gynecology and Reproductive Biology*. 2012;165(2):156–164.

[18] Legendre G, Brun JL, Fernandez H. [The place of myomectomy in woman of reproductive age]. *J Gynecol Obs Biol Reprod*. 2011; 40(8):875-84.

[19] Wallach EE, Vlahos NF. Uterine myomas: An overview of development, clinical features, and management. *Obstetrics and Gynecology*. 2004;104(2):393-406.

[20] Qidway GI, Caughey AB JA. Obstetric outcomes in women with sonographically identified uterine leiomyomata. *Obs Gynecol.* 2006;107:376-82.

[21] Lasmar RB, Barrozo PRM, Dias R, De Oliveira MAP. Submucous myomas: A new presurgical classification to evaluate the viability of hysteroscopic surgical treatment - Preliminary report. *J Minim Invasive Gynecol.* 2005;12(4):308-11.

[22] Murakami T, Tamura M, Ozawa Y, Suzuki H, Terada Y, Okamura K. Safe techniques in surgery for hysteroscopic myomectomy. *Journal of Obstetrics and Gynaecology Research.* 2005;31(3):216–223.

[23] Sutton C. Hysteroscopic surgery. Best Practice and Research: *Clinical Obstetrics and Gynaecology.* 2006.

[24] Takeda A, Manabe S, Hosono S, Nakamura H. Preoperative evaluation of submucosal myoma by virtual hysteroscopy. *J Am Assoc Gynecol Laparosc.* 2004;11(3):404-9.

[25] Wamsteker K, Emanuel MH, de Kruif JH. Transcervical hysteroscopic resection of submucous fibroids for abnormal uterine bleeding: results regarding the degree of intramural extension. *Obstet Gynecol.* 1993;82(5):736-40.

[26] Haimovich S, Mancebo G, Alameda F, Agramunt S, Solé-Sedeno JM, Hernández JL, et al. Feasibility of a new two-step procedure for office hysteroscopic resection of submucous myomas: Results of a pilot study. *Eur J Obstet Gynecol Reprod Biol.* 2013;168(2):191–4.

[27] Camanni M, Bonino L, Delpiano EM, Ferrero B, Migliaretti G, Deltetto F. Hysteroscopic Management of Large Symptomatic Submucous Uterine Myomas. *J Minim Invasive Gynecol.* 2010;17(1):59-65.

[28] Saccardi C, Conte L, Fabris A, De Marchi F, Borghero A, Gizzo S, et al. Hysteroscopic enucleation in toto of submucous type 2 myomas: Long-term follow-up in women affected by menorrhagia. *J Minim Invasive Gynecol.* 2014;21(3):426-30.

[29] Rakotomahenina H, Rajaonarison J, Wong L, Brun JL. Myomectomy: Technique and current indications. *Minerva Ginecologica.* 2017;69(4):357-369.

[30] Florio P, Puzzutiello R, Filippeschi M, D'Onofrio P, Mereu L, Morelli R, et al. Low-dose spinal anesthesia with hyperbaric bupivacaine with intrathecal fentanyl for operative hysteroscopy: A case series study. *J Minim Invasive Gynecol.* 2012; 19(1): 107-112.

[31] Ludwin A, Ludwin I, Pityński K, Basta P, Basta A, Banas T, et al. Transrectal Ultrasound-Guided Hysteroscopic Myomectomy of Submucosal Myomas With a Varying Degree of Myometrial Penetration. *J Minim Invasive Gynecol.* 2013;20(5):672-85.

[32] Ghirardi V, Bizzarri N, Venturini PL, Remorgida V, Ferrero S. Intraoperative bidimensional and 4-D transrectal ultrasonography for hysteroscopic metroplasty. *J Minim Invasive Gynecol.* 2014;21(6):S61.

[33] Hamerlynck TWO, Dietz V, Schoot BC. Clinical implementation of the hysteroscopic morcellator for removal of intrauterine myomas and polyps. A retrospective descriptive study. *Gynecol Surg*. 2011; 8(2):193-196.

[34] Serden SP. Diagnostic hysteroscopy to evaluate the cause of abnormal uterine bleeding. *Obstetrics and Gynecology Clinics of North America*. 2000; 27(2): 277-286.

[35] Emanuel MH. New developments in hysteroscopy. *Best Pract Res Clin Obstet Gynaecol*. 2013; 27(3):421-9..

[36] Vilos GA, Abu-Rafea B. New developments in ambulatory hysteroscopic surgery. *Best Practice and Research: Clinical Obstetrics and Gynaecology*. 2005; 19(5) 727-42.

[37] Papalampros P, Gambadauro P, Papadopoulos N, Polyzos D, Chapman L, Magos A. The mini-resectoscope: A new instrument for office hysteroscopic surgery. *Acta Obstet Gynecol Scand*. 2009; 88(2):227-30.

[38] van Dongen H, Emanuel MH, Wolterbeek R, Trimbos JB, Jansen FW. Hysteroscopic Morcellator for Removal of Intrauterine Polyps and Myomas: A Randomized Controlled Pilot Study among Residents in Training. *J Minim Invasive Gynecol*. 2008;15(4):466-71.

[39] Hamerlynck TWO, Schoot BC, Van Vliet HAAM, Weyers S. Removal of endometrial polyps: Hysteroscopic morcellation versus bipolar resectoscopy, a randomized trial. *J Minim Invasive Gynecol*. 2015;22(7):1237-43.

[40] Pakrashi T, Ressler IB, Sroga JM, Dipaola KB, Thomas M a, Lindheim SR. Hysteroscopic Enucleation of Type II Submucosal Uterine Leiomyomas Using a TRUCLEAR Hysteroscopic Morcellator: Case Report and Review of the Literature. *J Laparoendosc Adv Surg Tech A*. 2013; 23(4):378-82.

[41] Ubaldi F, Tournaye H, Camus M, Van der Pas H, Gepts E, Devroey P. Fertility after hysteroscopic myomectomy. *Hum Reprod Update*. 1995;1(1):81-90.

[42] Donnez J, Gillerot S, Bourgonjon D, Clerckx F, Nisolle M. Neodymium: YAG laser hysteroscopy in large submucous fibroids. *Fertil Steril*. 1990;54(6):999-1003.

[43] Glasser MH. Endometrial ablation and hysteroscopic myomectomy by electrosurgical vaporization. *J Am Assoc Gynecol Laparosc*. 1997;4(3):369-74.

[44] Emanuel MH, Wamsteker K. The Intra Uterine Morcellator: A new hysteroscopic operating technique to remove intrauterine polyps and myomas. *J Minim Invasive Gynecol*. 2005;12(1):62-6.

[45] Mazzon I, Favilli A, Grasso M, Horvath S, Di Renzo GC, Gerli S. Is cold loop hysteroscopic myomectomy a safe and effective technique for the treatment of submucous myomas with intramural development? A series of 1434 surgical procedures. *J Minim Invasive Gynecol*. 2015;22(5):792-8.

[46] Mazzon I. Nuova tecnica per la miomectomia isteroscopica: enucleazione con ansa fredda. In: Cittadini E, Perino A, Angiolillo M ML, editor. *Atlante di Chirurgia Endoscopica Ginecologica*. COFESE. Palermo, Italy; 1995.

[47] Leone FPG, Calabrese S, Marciante C, Cetin I, Ferrazzi E. Feasibility and long-term efficacy of hysteroscopic myomectomy for myomas with intramural development by the use of non-electrical "cold" loops. *Gynecol Surg*. 2012; 9(2):155-161.

[48] Jansen FW, Vredevoogd CB, Van Ulzen K, Hermans J, Trimbos JB, Trimbos-Kemper TCM. Complications of hysteroscopy: a prospective, multicenter study. *Obstet Gynecol*. 2000;96(2):266-70.

[49] Tinelli A, Hurst BS, Hudelist G, Tsin DA, Stark M, Mettler L, et al. Laparoscopic myomectomy focusing on the myoma pseudocapsule: Technical and outcome reports. *Hum Reprod*. 2012;27(2):427-35.

[50] Mazzon I, Favilli A, Grasso M, Horvath S, Bini V, Carlo G, et al. *Risk Factors for the Completion of the Cold Loop Hysteroscopic Myomectomy in a One-Step Procedure: A Post Hoc Analysis*. 2018; 8429047.

[51] Litta P, Vasile C, Merlin F, Pozzan C, Sacco G, Gravila P, et al. A new technique of hysteroscopic myomectomy with enucleation in toto. *J Am Assoc Gynecol Laparosc*. 2003;10(2):263-70.

[52] Bettocchi S, Di Spiezio Sardo A, Ceci O, Nappi L, Guida M, Greco E, et al. A New Hysteroscopic Technique for the Preparation of Partially Intramural Myomas in Office Setting (OPPIuM technique): A Pilot Study. *J Minim Invasive Gynecol*. 2009;16(6):748-54.

[53] Indman PD. Use of Carboprost to Facilitate Hysteroscopic Resection of Submucous Myomas. *J Am Assoc Gynecol Laparosc*. 2004: 11(1):68-72.

[54] Murakami T, Shimizu T, Katahira A, Terada Y, Yokomizo R, Sawada R. Intraoperative injection of prostaglandin F2αin a patient undergoing hysteroscopic myomectomy. *Fertil Steril*. 2003;79;1439–41.

[55] Vercellini P, Zàina B, Yaylayan L, Pisacreta A, De Giorgi O, Crosignani PG. Hysteroscopic myomectomy: Long-term effects on menstrual pattern and fertility. *Obstet Gynecol*. 1999;94(3):341-7.

[56] Emanuel MH, Wamsteker K, Hart AAM, Metz G, Lammes FB. Long-term results of hysteroscopic myomectomy for abnormal uterine bleeding. *Obstet Gynecol*. 1999;93(5 Pt 1):743-8.

[57] Fernandez H, Kadoch O, Capella-Allouc S, Gervaise A, Taylor S, Frydman R. Transcervical hysteroscopic resection of submucous leiomyomas: Long-term results. *Ann Chir*. 2001;16(7):1489-92.

[58] Hart R, Molnár BG, Magos A. Long term follow up of hysteroscopic myomectomy assessed by survival analysis. *BJOG An Int J Obstet Gynaecol*. 1999;106(7):700-5.

[59] Fernandez H, Sefrioui O, Virelizier C, Gervaise a, Gomel V, Frydman R. Hysteroscopic resection of submucosal myomas in patients with infertility. *Hum Reprod.* 2001;16(7):1489-92.

[60] Van Dongen H, Hans Emanuel M, Smeets MJ, Trimbos B, Willem Jansen F. Follow-up after incomplete hysteroscopic removal of uterine fibroids. *Acta Obstet Gynecol Scand.* 2006;85(12):1463-7.

[61] Somigliana E, Vercellini P, Daguati R, Pasin R, De Giorgi O, Crosignani PG. Fibroids and female reproduction: a critical analysis of the evidence. *Hum Reprod Update.* 2007;13(5):465-76.

[62] Wallach EE, Verkauf BS. Myomectomy for fertility enhancement and preservation. *Fertil Steril.* 1992;58(1): 1–15.

[63] Wallach EE, Buttram VC, Reiter RC. Uterine leiomyomata: etiology, symptomatology, and management. *Fertil Steril.* 1981;36(4):433-45.

[64] Ioannis S, Aristotelis A, Antonios T, Panagiotis S, John B. Fertility rates after hysteroscopic treatment of submucous myomas depending on their type. *Gynecol Surg.* 2006; 3(3):206-210 .

[65] Bulletti C, De Ziegler D, Setti PL, Cicinelli E, Polli V, Stefanetti M. Myomas, pregnancy outcome, and in vitro fertilization. *Annals of the New York Academy of Sciences.* 2004;1034:84-92.

[66] Jayakrishnan K, Menon V, Nambiar D. Submucous fibroids and infertility: Effect of hysteroscopic myomectomy and factors influencing outcome. *J Hum Reprod Sci.* 2013; 6(1): 35–39.

[67] Polyzos NP, Zavos A, Valachis A, Dragamestianos C, Blockeel C, Stoop D, et al. Misoprostol prior to hysteroscopy in premenopausal and post-menopausal women. A systematic review and meta-analysis. *Human Reproduction Update.* 2012; 18(4), 393–404.

[68] Capmas P, Levaillant JM, Fernandez H. Surgical techniques and outcome in the management of submucous fibroids. Current Opinion in *Obstetrics and Gynecology.* 2013;25(4):332-8.

[69] Emanuel MH, Hart A, Wamsteker K, Lammes F. An analysis of fluid loss during transcervical resection of submucous myomas. *Fertil Steril.* 1997;68:881–886.

[70] Loffer FD. Preliminary experience with the VersaPoint bipolar resectoscope using a vaporizing electrode in a saline distending medium. *J Am Assoc Gynecol Laparosc.* 2000; 7(4) 498-502.

[71] Muñoz JL, Jiménez JS, Hernández C, Vaquero G, Pérez Sagaseta C, Noguero R, et al. Hysteroscopic myomectomy: our experience and review. *JSLS.* 2003; 7(1): 39–48.

[72] Corson SL, Brooks PG, Serden SP, Batzer FR, Gocial B. Effects of vasopressin administration during hysteroscopic surgery. *J Reprod Med.* 1994;39(6):419-23.

[73] Munro MG, Christianson LA. Complications of hysteroscopic and uterine resectoscopic surgery. *Clin Obstet Gynecol*. 2015;58(4):765-97.

[74] Dyrbye BA, Overdijk LE, Van Kesteren PJ, De Haan P, Riezebos RK, Bakkum EA, et al. Gas embolism during hysteroscopic surgery using bipolar or monopolar diathermia: A randomized controlled trial. *Am J Obstet Gynecol*. 2012;207(4):271.e1-6.

[75] Corson SL, Brooks PG. Resectoscopic myomectomy. In: *Fertility and Sterility*. 1991;55(6):1041–1044.

[76] Derman SG, Rehnstrom J, Neuwirth RS. The long-term effectiveness of hysteroscopic treatment of menorrhagia and leiomyomas. *Obstet Gynecol*. 1991;77(4):591-4.

[77] Aydeniz B, Gruber I V, Schauf B, Kurek R, Meyer a, Wallwiener D. A multicenter survey of complications associated with 21,676 operative hysteroscopies. *Eur J Obstet Gynecol Reprod Biol*. 2002;104(2):160-4.

[78] Agostini A, Cravello L, Desbrière R, Maisonneuve AS, Roger V, Blanc B. Hemorrhage risk during operative hysteroscopy. *Acta Obstet Gynecol Scand*. 2002;81(9):878-81.

[79] Taskin O, Sadik S, Onoglu A, Gokdeniz R, Erturan E, Burak F, et al. Role of endometrial suppression on the frequency of intrauterine adhesions after resectoscopic surgery. *J Am Assoc Gynecol Laparosc*. 2000;7(3):351-4.

[80] Yang JH, Chen MJ, Wu MY, Chao KH, Ho HN, Yang YS. Office hysteroscopic early lysis of intrauterine adhesion after transcervical resection of multiple apposing submucous myomas. *Fertil Steril*. 2008;89(5):1254-9.

[81] Touboul C, Fernandez H, Deffieux X, Berry R, Frydman R, Gervaise A. Uterine synechiae after bipolar hysteroscopic resection of submucosal myomas in patients with infertility. *Fertil Steril*. 2009;92(5):1690-3.

[82] Wheeler JM TO. Second-look office hysteroscopy following resectoscopy: the frequency and management of intrauterine adhesions. *Fertil Steril*. 1993.

[83] Di Spiezio Sardo A, Spinelli M, Bramante S, Scognamiglio M, Greco E, Guida M, et al. Efficacy of a Polyethylene Oxide-Sodium Carboxymethylcellulose Gel in Prevention of Intrauterine Adhesions after Hysteroscopic Surgery. *J Minim Invasive Gynecol*. 2011;18(4):462-9.

[84] Guida M, Acunzo G, Di Spiezio Sardo A, Bifulco G, Piccoli R, Pellicano M, et al. Effectiveness of auto-crosslinked hyaluronic acid gel in the prevention of intrauterine adhesions after hysteroscopic surgery: A prospective, randomized, controlled study. *Hum Reprod*. 2004;19(6):1461-4.

[85] Gyamfi-Bannerman C, Gilbert S, Landon MB, Spong CY, Rouse DJ, Varner MW, et al. Risk of uterine rupture and placenta accreta with prior uterine surgery outside of the lower segment. *Obstet Gynecol*. 2012;120(6):1332-7.

[86] Tanaka M, Matsuzaki S, Matsuzaki S, Kakigano A, Kumasawa K, Ueda Y. Placenta accreta following hysteroscopic myomectomy. *Clin Case Reports.* 2016; 4(6): 541–544.

[87] Cooper JM, Brady RM. Late complications of operative hysteroscopy. *Obstetrics and Gynecology Clinics of North America.* 2000;27(2):367-74.

[88] Sentilhes L, Sergent F, Roman H, Verspyck E, Marpeau L. Late complications of operative hysteroscopy: Predicting patients at risk of uterine rupture during subsequent pregnancy. *European Journal of Obstetrics Gynecology and Reproductive Biology.* 2005;120(2):134-8.

[89] Gerli S, Baiocchi G, Favilli A, Di Renzo GC. New treatment option for early spontaneous rupture of a postmyomectomy gravid uterus. *Fertil Steril.* 2011;96:e97–8.

[90] Howe RS. Third-trimester uterine rupture following hysteroscopic uterine perforation. *Obstet Gynecol.* 1993;81(5 (Pt 2)):827-9.

[91] Cravello L, Agostini a, Beerli M, Roger V, Bretelle F, Blanc B. [Results of hysteroscopic myomectomy]. *Gynécologie, Obs Fertil.* 2004;32(9):825-8.

[92] Keltz, Varasteh, Levin, Neuwirth. Pregnancy rates following hysteroscopic polypectomy, myomectomy, and a normal cavity in infertile patients. *Prim Care Update Ob Gyns.* 1998;5(4):168.

[93] Stewart EA. Uterine fibroids. *Lancet.* 2001;357(9252):293-8.

[94] Gutmann JN, Corson SL. GnRH agonist therapy before myomectomy or hysterectomy. *Journal of Minimally Invasive Gynecology.* 2005;12(6):529-37.

[95] Donnez J, Schrurs B, Gillerot S, Sandow J, Clerckx F. Treatment of uterine fibroids with implants of gonadotropin-releasing hormone agonist: Assessment by hysterography. *Fertil Steril.* 1989;51(6):947-50.

[96] Wong ASW, Cheung CW, Yeung SW, Fan HL, Leung TY, Sahota DS. Transcervical intralesional vasopressin injection compared with placebo in hysteroscopic myomectomy: A randomized controlled trial. *Obstet Gynecol.* 2014;124(5):897–903.

[97] Lethaby A, Vollenhoven B, Sowter MC. Pre-operative GnRH analogue therapy before hysterectomy or myomectomy for uterine fibroids. In: *Cochrane Database of Systematic Reviews.* 2001;(2):CD000547.

[98] Lin BL, Akiba Y, Iwata Y. One-step hysteroscopic removal of sinking submucous myoma in two infertile patients. *Fertil Steril.* 2000;74(5):1035–8.

[99] Bradley LD. Complications in hysteroscopy: Prevention, treatment and legal risk. *Current Opinion in Obstetrics and Gynecology.* 2002;14(4):409-15.

[100] Donnez J, Tomaszewski J, Vàzquez F, Bouchard P, Lemieszczuk B, Barò F, et al. Ulipristal acetate versus leuprolide acetate for uterine fibroids. *N Engl J Med* 2012; 366:421-432

[101] Ferrero S, Vellone VG, Barra F. Pharmacokinetic drug evaluation of ulipristal acetate for the treatment of uterine fibroids. *Expert Opin Drug Metab Toxicol.* 2018;14(1):107-16.

[102] Tafi E, Scala C, Leone Roberti Maggiore U, Bizzarri N, Candiani M, Venturini PL, et al. Drug safety evaluation of ulipristal acetate in the treatment of uterine fibroids. *Expert Opin Drug Saf.* 2015;14(6):965-77.

[103] Ferrero S, Racca A, Tafi E, Alessandri F, Venturini PL, Leone Roberti Maggiore U. Ulipristal Acetate Before High Complexity Hysteroscopic Myomectomy: A Retrospective Comparative Study. *J Minim Invasive Gynecol.* 2016;23(3):390-5.

[104] Ferrero S, Vellone VG, Barra F, Scala C. Ulipristal Acetate before Hysteroscopic and Laparoscopic Surgery for Uterine Myomas: Help or Hindrance? *Gynecol Obstet Invest.* 2018:1-13.

[105] Cooper NAM, Smith P, Khan KS, Clark TJ. Does cervical preparation before outpatient hysteroscopy reduce women's pain experience? A systematic review. *BJOG: An International Journal of Obstetrics and Gynaecology*. 2011;118(11): 1292-301.

[106] Selk A, Kroft J. Misoprostol in operative hysteroscopy: A systematic review and meta-analysis. *Obstetrics and Gynecology*. 2011;118(4):941-9.

[107] Kongnyuy EJ, van den Broek N, Wiysonge CS. A systematic review of randomized controlled trials to reduce hemorrhage during myomectomy for uterine fibroids. *Int J Gynaecol Obstet*. 2008; 100(1):4-9.

[108] Wong ASW, Cheung ECW, Leung K-T, Yeung S-W, Leung T-Y, Fung T-Y. Transcervical intralesional vasopressin injection in hysteroscopic myomectomy--description of a new technique. *J Laparoendosc Adv Surg Tech A*. 2013; 23(3):258-62.

[109] Phillips DR, Nathanson HG, Milim SJ, Haselkorn JS, Khapra A, Ross PL. The effect of dilute vasopressin solution on blood loss during operative hysteroscopy: A randomized controlled trial. *Obstet Gynecol*. 1996;88(5):761-6.

In: Uterine Fibroids
Editors: S. Ferrero and F. Barra
ISBN: 978-1-53615-046-9

Chapter 9

LEVONORGESTREL-RELEASING INTRAUTERINE DEVICE FOR THE TREATMENT OF HEAVY MENSTRUAL BLEEDING CAUSED BY UTERINE MYOMAS

Barbara Gardella**, MD, Giulia Muscettola, MD, Anna Orlandini, MD, Mattia Dominoni, MD and Arsenio Spinillo, MD
Department of Obstetrics and Gynecology,
IRCCS Policlinico San Matteo, University of Pavia, Italy

ABSTRACT

Abnormal uterine bleeding (AUB) is a very common condition with a high prevalence in women and consists in excessive menstrual bleeding related or not to pelvic pain which can affect the quality of women life.

For now, the etiology of heavy menstrual bleeding (HMB) is not yet fully understood but different mechanisms have been hypothesized.

Epidemiological studies suggested that approximately 10% to 30% of reproductive-aged women were affected by menorrhagia. HMB are currently treated both with medical or surgical interventions and both methods can be considered safe, acceptable and effective.

Uterine fibromatosis is a problem affecting almost the 70% of women in their reproductive age. Among these only approximately the 25% of reproductive-age women with uterine fibromatosis show symptoms related to this condition. Symptom presentation usually depends on myoma position in the uterus. Regarding the symptoms caused by

* Corresponding Author's E-mail: Barbara.gardella@gmail.com.

Uterine fibromatosis, the most common ones associated with uterine leiomyomas are irregular and excessive bleeding that can often be a cause of anemia. It is important to evaluate each individual patient and to make an adequate and personal counselling before starting any therapeutic choices. Medical therapy must be considered as a first choice and only secondarily we should consider the surgical approach.

Before choosing the right medical or surgical treatment for the HMB associated with uterine fibromatosis, it is important to perform a complete gynecological examination, with ultrasound scan and may be a hysteroscopy.

The levonorgestrel intrauterine device (LNG-IUD) is a T-shaped device that releases levonorgestrel into endometrium that can possible stay in the uterus for 5 years. In 2009, LNG intrauterine device, Mirena, has been approved as a treatment for HMB by FDA. The LNG-IUD has become the leading choice as the most effective first-line medical therapy for the treatment of HMB. It can be used by a large variety of patients, particularly patients who need a long-term therapy, which have major or relative contra-indications for surgical intervention, who do not seek a pregnancy in the short term, or who have contraindications to oral contraceptive therapy or POP. As a result of this treatment is shown an atrophic involution of the endometrium, and this is precisely the mechanism that greatly reduces menorrhagia over time.

Several literature reviews evaluated the outcomes in term of reduction of menstrual bleeding treated with LNG-IUD. Almost the 85% of patients with menorrhagia saw a normal menstrual flow re-established, after a six months therapy with LNG-IUDs.

Keywords: uterine myomas, abnormal uterine bleeding, heavy menstrual bleeding, levonorgestrel-releasing intrauterine device

1. Introduction

1.1. Definition of HMB

HMB is a highly prevalent condition, characterized by excessive menstrual blood loss and cramping, that interferes with activities of daily life.

The National Institute for Health and Care Excellence in the United Kingdom proposed a definition of HMB as an excessive menstrual blood loss that interferes with the woman's physical, emotional, social and material quality of life itself or a menstrual blood loss that occurs in combination without her symptoms.

This is certainly a useful definition for women that don't meet the standard blood loss criteria for HMB but the menstrual blood loss has in any case a significant impact on their quality of life.

A normal menstrual cycle has an average duration of menstrual bleeding of 4.5–8 days an interval of 24–38 days between the onsets of menses with 2–20 days of cycle to cycle variation over 12 months.

The most blood loss occurs during the first 2 days of menstruation.

The average blood loss with menstruation for normal women is ≤30 ml and menstrual blood loss more than 80 ml is considered abnormal.

Therefore, menorrhagia is to be considered as an excessively heavy flow during the menstrual period, and is one of the abnormalities that can be included in the category ofirregular and excessive bleeding [1].

The definition of menorrhagia comprehends multiple conditions, such as:

- More than 7 days of uterine bleeding.
- Needing to wear more than one pad at a time to control menstrual flow.
- Needing to change several pads or tampons during the night.
- Bleeding that soaks through one or more tampons or pads every hour for several hours in a row.
- Abundant menstrual flow with blood clots

But summarizing, we can say that menorrhagia is defined as total menstrual flow >80ml per cycle, or that soak a pad or a tampon every 2 hours or less.

1.2. Etiology of Menorrhagia

The pathogenetic mechanisms of HMB is not yet fully understoodand different mechanisms have been hypothesized [2].

There are multiple pathways as leading cause of menorrhagia including the fibrinolytic system particularly the plasminogen activator and its inhibitor, the increasing levels of prostaglandin E2, local cytokines, and the increase number of leukocytes into the endometrial stroma.

Women with HMB seems to have an increased level of tPA, and on the other hand a reduction of PAI-1 levels [3].

The result of this process is the increasing collagenase and fibrinolytic activity.

Progesterone also increases endometrial cyclooxygenase 2 (COX-2) enzyme, that lead to an increase synthesis and secretion of prostaglandin E2 (PGE2), and prostaglandin F2 alpha (PGF2a). Women with HMB have been demonstrated to have increased prostaglandin synthesis and COX-2 enzymes associated with HMB [4].

Endometrial cytokines and metalloproteinases (MMPs) have been reported to be involved in HMB causing the dissolution of endometrial collagen.

But not a single pathway explains the cause of HMB.

1.3. Social Aspects and Costs

A large American cohort study evaluated the healthcare resources and the direct and indirect costs related with HMB in the US.

Epidemiological studies suggested that approximately 10% to 30% of reproductive-aged women were affected by menorrhagia.

Using some parameters such as: lost work productivity and medical costs for HMB treatment [5].

Based on the reported prevalence, utilization rate, and unit costs, current estimated annual direct cost associated with HMB in the US is approximately 1 billion dollars while the estimated indirect costs is definitely higher and can be considered approximately 12 billion dollars because of the impact on work, considering days lost at work, and quality of life for the woman.

This included the costs of physician visits, drug therapy, and treatment with hysterectomy and ablation.

Cost for hysterectomy alone may have accounted for approximately half of the total treatment cost.

The costs and productivity loss due to absenteeism are caused essentially by the iron deficiency anemia with its symptoms of fatigue, weakness, pallor, and dizziness that is to be considered a major medical problem related to menorrhagia.

Or this reason the costs related to HMB and anemia is higher than for menorrhagia alone [5].

The AUB has a broad impact on the women quality of life.

Menorrhagia is the most common cause of iron-deficiency anemia in the developed world.

Excessive menstrual bleeding considering monthly blood loss more than 60 ml itself can deplete iron stores, which leads to iron-deficiency anemia.

HMB is currently treated both with medical or surgical interventions and both methods can be considered safe, acceptable and effective.

Studies have suggested that medical treatment with LNG-IUD and surgical treatment with endometrial ablation or hysterectomy can all significantly improve women's quality of life [6].

Although hysterectomy is a definitive treatment for HMB related or not to other uterine anomaly, a medical treatment is the preferred primary intervention in most cases.

In fact, surgery is associated with higher of internal organ injury particularly the ones located in the pelvis: but also hemorrhage, infection and mortality.

The main goal is to control the episode of heavy bleeding and to reduce menstrual blood loss in subsequent cycles. The American College of Obstetricians and gynecologists suggested that the selection of treatment for each woman depends on clinical stability, overall acuity, etiology of the bleeding, desire for future pregnancy and comorbidities.

2. Alternative Methods to Quantify the Intensity of the Menstrual Cycle and Establish the Causes of HMB

2.1. PBAC

An alternative method to quantify the menstrual blood loss is the pictorial blood loss assessment chart (PBAC) that visually estimates the extent of blood on sanitary pad and tampons (Figure 1).

The Royal College of Obstetricians and Gynecologists in 2016 established a pictorial chart to diagnose HMB the PBAC [7].

The PBAC is a semi-quantitative measurement tool. Women are instructed to count their number of used towels or tampons each day and then divide them by level of soiling. The chart is scored using the scoring system revised by Higham et al.

This measurement method has a specificity and sensitivity of 80–90% when compared with the gold standard, alkaline hematin method.

To define HMB most studies use a score of more than 150 points in the PBAC chart.

A PBAC score of 150 is related to more than 80 ml of blood loss.

However, at the momentis not that certainwhether the PBAC score is also useful as a toolfor the evaluation of theoutcome ofa specific treatment [7].

	DATE							
	TOWEL	1	2	3	4	5	6	7
1		II	I			I		
5			I	II				
20			I		IIII			
	TAMPON	1	2	3	4	5	6	7
1			I			I		
5			II	II		I		
10			I	II	I			
	DAILY SCORE	**2**	**47**	**40**	**90**	**7**		

Figure 1. PBAC chart: PBAC-menorrhagia, is a simple and non laboratoristic method for semi-objective diagnosis of heavy menstrual bleeding. It has a sensitivity of 86%(doesn not miss the Dx) and a specificity of 89% (does not overcall the Dx). The FDA studies established a PBACmore than 250 to diagnose menorrhagia, and for normal menses the PBAC score is less or equal to 75.

This is true because even with a score below of 150 the quality of life of patients could not be improved.

2.2. PALM –COEIN

The PALM-COEIN classification (Figure 2) is a method designed to simplify and easily remember what are the main causes of AUB [8].

The categories were developed based on the group of AUB in acute, chronic, and intermenstrual.

Each is designed to facilitate the development of subclassification systems. It was hypothesized that the first part of the system would be used in primary care and that the subclassification would be most relevant at specialist and research levels. The system has been approved by the FIGO Executive Board as a FIGO classification system.

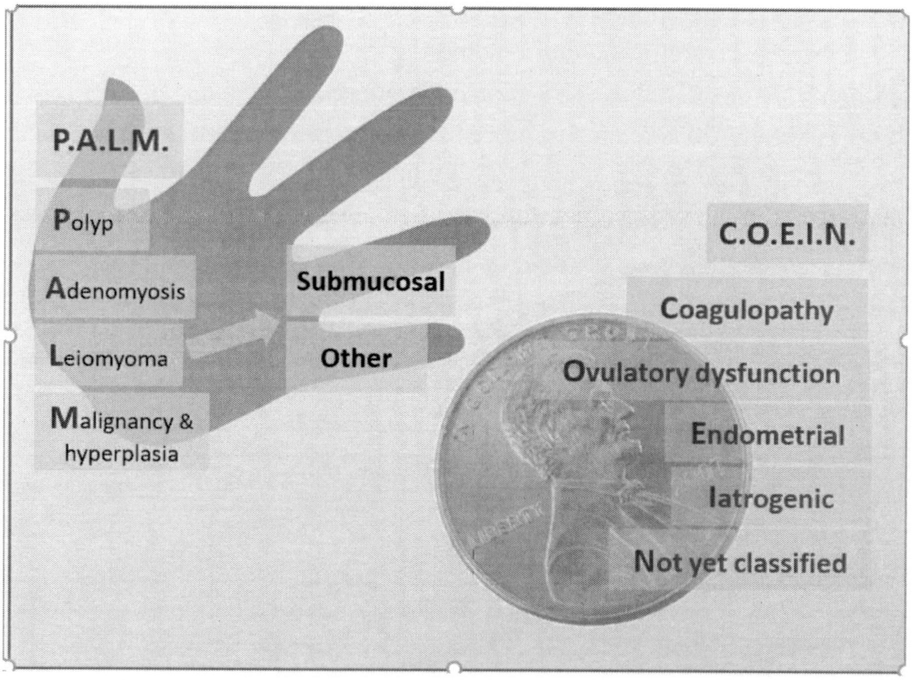

Figure 2. The FIGO classification system (PALM-COEIN) for causes of abnormal uterine bleeding in nongravid women of reproductive age, Malcolm G. Munro et al. The PALM COEINsystem includes 4 structural categories that can defined by objective structural criteria with ultrasound scan or hystopatology (PALM: polyp; adenomyosis; leiomyoma; andmalignancy and hyperplasia), the second part of the system includes 4 entities that are unrelated to structural anomalies (COEI: coagulopathy; ovulatory dysfunction; endometrial; iatrogenic), and 1 reserved for entities that are not yet classified (N). Furthermore, the leiomyoma category (L) is subdivided into submucosal myoma (LSM) andmyomas that do not impact the endometrial cavity (LO).

There are 9 main categories, which are arranged according to the acronym PALM-COEIN.

Thecategories are: polyp; adenomyosis; leiomyoma; malignancy and hyperplasia; coagulopathy; ovulatory dysfunction; endometrial; iatrogenic; and not yet classified. The characteristics of the PALM group can be measured visually with ultrasound scan or other imaging techniques and/or histopathology examination, on the other hand the COEIN group is related tonon-structuralentities, so for this reason those can't be defined by ultrasound scan or histopathologic examination [9].

Among the causes of menorrhagia, the main ones have to be considered:

2.2.1. Polyps

It has long been controversial whether or not to include cervical or endometrial polyps in this classification.

These epithelial lesions are due to endometrial proliferation with a variable increase of the vascular, glandular, fibromuscular components andof the connective tissue.

Polyps are often asymptomatic, but it is generally accepted that in some cases they contribute to the genesis of AUB.

These lesions are usually benign but a small minority may have atypical or malignant features.

The diagnosis is made with the imaging and confirmed with the histologic examination.

2.2.2. Adenomyosis

The correlation between adenomyosis and the HMB is still unclear.

The prevalence in the female population of adenomyosis varies from 5% to 70% [10].

Generally, the diagnostic criteria of adenomyosis have been based on the histopathologic evaluation of the depth of endometrial tissue beneath the endometrial–myometrial interface.

However, because there are diagnostic criteria by using sonographic images and magnetic resonance imaging (MRI), adenomyosis has been included in this classification system.

The ultrasound scan image of adenomyosis is partly related to the presence of heterotopic endometrial tissue in the thickness of the myometrium but it's also partly due at the same time to a related myometrial hypertrophy.

Issues that must be addressed in such an imaging-based system include the minimum sonographic criteria for diagnosis, the distinctions between diffuse and focal (or multifocal) adenomyosis, and whether a metric indicating volume or extent of the disease should or can be included at this time [11].

2.2.3. Malignancy and Others

Although relatively uncommon, atypical hyperplasia and malignancy are important potential causes of AUB and must be considered as differential diagnosis in nearly all women of reproductive age.

During the diagnostic procedure in women with HMB malignancy must be considered and if a premalignant hyperplastic or malignant process is identified during the clinical investigation in a woman with menorrhagia, it has to be classified using the appropriate WHO or FIGO system.

2.2.4. Ovulatory Dysfunction

Anovulatory cycles due may lead to a decrease in progesterone levels compared to a normal menstrual cycle in which ovulation occurs. In conclusion this leads to a hormonal imbalance that determines menorrhagia.

During a normal menstrual cycle, it must exist a balance between the estrogen and progesterone. Those hormones cyclically regulate the thickness of the endometrium. Therefore, the hormone's activity causes the endometrial flaking during menstruation.

A hormone imbalance can cause a thickening of the endometrium, so the increased thickness of the endometrium can eventually shed by way of HMB. A number of conditions can cause hormone imbalances, including polycystic ovary syndrome (PCOS), obesity, insulin resistance and thyroid problems.

2.2.5. Disorders of Hemostasis and Coagulopathy

Coagulopathy can be a cause of HMB including systemic disorders of hemostasis or coagulopathies.

The VonWillebrand disease is reported to be the most common coagulopathy related to HMB with the highest prevalence [12].

Is it possible to use some screening criteria to identify a coagulopathy:

- HMB since menarche
- Postpartum hemorrhage or bleeding elated to a surgical procedure or bleeding associated with dental work
- Epistaxis 1 or 2 times/month, or a family history of bleeding symptoms.

2.2.6. Endometrial

When no other definable causes are identified and AUB occurs in a normal ovulary menstrual period, the mechanism is probably a primary disorder of the endometrium.

Is it possible that may exist a primary disorder of the mechanisms that locally regulate hemostasis in the endometrium itself.

Such disorders may be secondary to: endometrial inflammation or infection; abnormalities in the local inflammatory response; or aberrations in endometrial angiogenesis.

For this reason, considering the PALM-COEIN classification system, the diagnosis of endometrial disorders should probably be determined excluding some other identifiable abnormalities in the patients, typically in women of reproductive age who seem to have normal ovulatory function.

2.2.7. The Uterine Fibromatosis

The mechanism of leiomyoma-associated to menorrhagia is still unknown. Possible explanations are the increased endometrial surface area, but also a condition of vascular dysregulation.

Another possible explanation could be the interference with endometrial hemostasis. Cause of menorrhagia are particularly the submucosal myomata which are located in the endometrium thickness. This kind of myoma represent about 5-10% of all fibroids [13].

Although this percentage may be underestimated due to the difficult diagnosis.

They tend to be responsible for most of the symptoms and therefore create particular discomfort to patients who present this condition.

Particularly they are responsible of menorrhagia ad infertility due to a distortion of the endometrium.

The main organic causes determining menometrorrhagia in women of age between 20 and 50 years are leiomyomas (36% -68%), especially the submucous type, secondly the endometrial polyps (6% -20%) and diffuse adenomyosis (20%-25%) [14].

Uterine leiomyomas (fibroids or myomas) are the most common benign tumors of fertile women, originating from myometrial smooth muscle cells of the uterus.

This pathology, which is able to alter significantly the quality of life of the woman, is proper to the fertile age: the myomas rarely appear before the menarche, the incidence increases with the age of the woman, and often regress after the menopause.

3. HMB Caused by Leyomioma

Uterine fibromatosis is a problem affecting almost the 70% of women in their reproductive age. Among these only approximately the 25% of reproductive- age women with uterine fibromatosis show symptoms related to this condition [15].

The incidence and severity of symptoms typically depend on size, number, and also location of the fibroid.

Several risk factors have been identified such as ethnicity, genetics factors, nulliparity, but certainly the sex hormones effect in the etiology and biology of uterine fibroids.

We should also remind that uterine leiomyomas are classified as subserosal, intramural, and submucosal based on the location that they have in the uterus.

So, we can define as follow: intramural if they are found in the thickness of the myometrium, submucosal if they protrude into cavities of the uterus and subserosal if they modify the external profile of the uterus.

These three classes are not so well distinguished in clinical practice, it is not rare to observe myomas in intermediate positions, the recent FIGO's classification system takes into consideration any kind of localization by dividing fibroids in as many as 10 different categories [16].

But we should notice that uterine leiomyoma can be also classified by different histological types.

At the moment the exact molecular and cellular changes that led to the development and growth of uterine leiomyoma are not well understood.

However, a major and common characteristic of uterine leiomyoma is the excessive accumulation of extracellular matrix (ECM) components including: collagens, laminins proteoglycans and fibronectin.

A large number of studies indicate that ECM accumulation and function is regulated by growth factors cytokines and steroid hormones.

And it is precisely the ECM's accumulation the critical event that lead to the production of the rigid structure of leiomyoma.

As a result of this, the ECM stiffness is thought to be one of the causes of abnormal bleeding and pelvic pain or pressure caused by uterine fibromatosis [17].

Therefore, regarding the etiology of uterine fibromatosis, it has been widely demonstrated that sex hormones both estrogen and progesterone regulate and induct the myoma's growth.

In fact, several studies have shown that the cells of the fibroids express a higher concentration both of estrogen and progesterone receptors compared to normal myometrium.

Symptom presentation usually depends on myoma position in the uterus.

Regarding the symptoms caused by uterine fibromatosis, the most common ones associated with uterine leiomyomas are irregular and excessive bleeding that can often be a cause of anemia.

This symptom is almost every time caused by intramural and submucosal myoma.

Another common condition related to uterine fibromatosis is pain in the back or on the legs, pelvic pain or sensation of pelvic pressure, bowel and bladder dysfunctions [18].

It can also lead to sensation of pressure in the lower abdomen, pain during sexual intercourse, infertility, and recurrent abortion. Generally, these conditions are caused by intramural and subserosal myomata.

Those symptoms are not exclusive to uterine fibromatosis. Whenever a patient complains about these symptoms in important to make a differential diagnosis.

Differential diagnosis may include plural conditions such as endometriosis, infection, pelvic inflammatory disease adhesions form prior surgeries but also malignancies.

In this chapter we will focus on the irregular and excessive bleeding caused by myomata.

So far for these and many other reasons uterine leiomyomas are to be considered at the moment the most common indication for hysterectomy in the world.

3.1. Counselling

It is important to evaluate each individual patient and to make an adequate and personal counselling before starting any therapeutic choices.

First of all, we can divide patients with AUB into three categories:

- the adolescents
- the woman in her reproductive age
- the woman in her post-reproductive age.

Each category of patients has specific needs and therefore is important to settle different therapeutic approaches.

The importance of a right therapeutic choice is evident also according to national and international guidelines (Figure 3).

The indications for the surgical treatment in women with AUB are:

- inability to utilize medical therapies (i.e., side effects, contraindications);
- anomalous uterine bleeding not controlled with another clinical therapeutic approach and so failure to respond to medical therapy;
- compressive symptoms such as pain or pelvic pressure, incontinence, hydronephrosis or constipation;
- fibroids greater than 8 centimeters;
- fibroids with a rapid growth;
- infertility,
- prevention of obstetric complications(19).

The surgical approach is the main therapeutic strategy for fertile patients looking for a pregnancy.

Several studies show a significant increase in the rate of pregnancy after myomectomy [20].

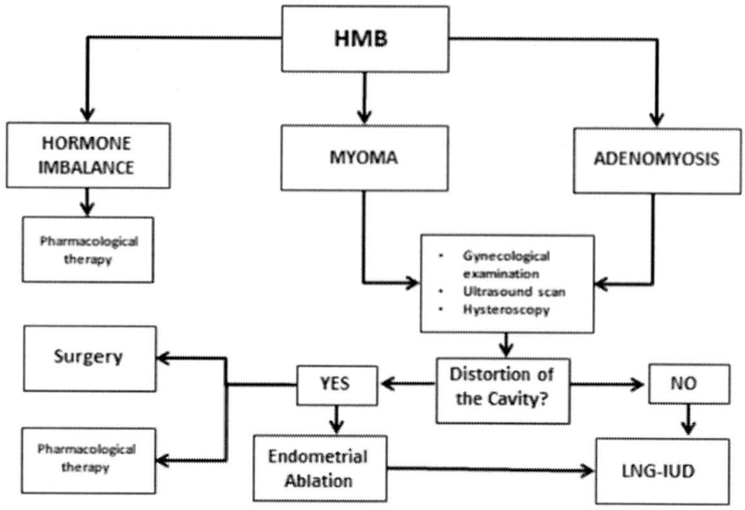

Figure 3. Management of uterine fibromatosis: after a clinical examination, considering if symptomatic or asymptomatic. It is possible to have a waiting behaviour, if asymptomatic. Is necessary discuss with the symptomatic patients the possible clinical options considering the age, the willing to maintain the fertility and the presence of comorbidities. Considering the size of the myomata and the uterus it is possible to choose between a surgical or a pharmacological treatment.
Mym = myomectomy.

A rate of pregnancy after surgery increase from about 20 to 40% in patient with submucosal myomas and from 15 to 40% in patient with submucosal-intramural myomas respectively was demonstrated.

However also for menopause patients a surgical approach should be evaluated.

A positive family history of gynecological cancers should always be investigated.

And can determine the choice of a type of demolition surgery, such as hysterectomy, instead of the use of a medical treatment.

Women with both intramural and submucosal fibroids, who are not eligible for a demolition surgery, are candidates for laparoscopy and hysteroscopy in the same intervention.

Medical therapy must be considered as a first choice and only secondarily we should consider the surgical approach [21]. Pharmacological treatment is the best option for some patients.

Some pharmacological therapies can also be use aiming to reduce the size of the fibroid and consequently decrease the menstrual bleeding and so far improve the hemoglobin levels before surgery.

Regarding Adolescents, we should notice that they frequently have irregular and/or painful cycles but rarely they experienceunpredictable and prolonged uterine bleeding or excessive menstrual bleeding that could suddenly become a medical emergency [22].

Even if HMB, in adolescents is most often the result of an immature hypothalamic-pituitary ovarian axis, we should notice that the menorrhagia is often multifactorial.

At the moment multiple non-hormonal and hormonal treatment modalities have been described for the treatment of HMB in adolescents [12, 22].

Anyhow there aren't official guidelines for an optimal management of HMB in adolescents and specific recommendations cannot be made presently regarding the superiority of one intervention compared with the other.

Oral contraceptives are at the moment the most commonly used method of hormonal contraception in the adolescent population of patients, are useful for regulation of menstrual flow, also allow for regular shedding of endometrium and reduce the menstrual flow,

Oral contraceptives also improve the menstrual pain and can be used for the prevention of ovulation bleeding.

The progesterone-only contraceptives (POP and progestin implant) in adolescent may also reduce menstrual flow and are another alternative to oral contraceptives in adolescents with HMB but they aren't commonly used because of the greater frequency of adverse effects such as weight gain.

Another possible treatment is the LNG-IUD that steadily releases 20 mcg of levonorgestrel every 24 h for a maximum of 5 years, locally and directly into the endometrial cavity.

The use is increasing in the United States and in Europe, particularly among older adolescents.

Recent studies on acceptability and use of IUDs in adolescents suggest that using a LNG IUD for one year in continuous shows an improvement of dysmenorrhea and HMB among the 75% of the patients.

In any case the main goal for all the possible therapies, surgical and pharmaceutical, is to stop the AUB [23].

Considering the pharmacological therapies for the HMB at the moment the main possibilities are:

- Ulipristal Acetate
- Analogues of Gonadotropin-Releasing Hormone (GnRH analogues)
- Combined oral contraceptives or only progestins contraceptives
- Medicated LNG IUD.

Ulipristal acetate is a synthetic steroid derived from 19-norprogesterone. The molecule belongs to the Modulator class Progesterone Receptor Selective (SPRM) and is the first of this class of compounds to have obtained the indication for the treatment of symptomatic uterine fibroids [14]. The effectiveness of ulipristal acetate on reducing the volume of the myoma is the main reason why this therapy is frequent used before surgery. Another possible treatment is the administration of the GnRH analogues. It is a treatment that works by reducing the level of estrogen and progesterone through the induction of a pseudo-menopausal hormonal state. As a result of this treatment the menstrual bleeding are blocked, and so the AUB. This therapy also caused a reduction of the size of the fibroma and consequently to the less blood loss an improvement of the hemoglobin levels solving the anemia condition. The treatment can be taken by injection every month or every three months. However, the main limits of the use of GnRH analogues is that they must be administrated for a maximum of six months, because a major side effect is the loss of bone mass and therefore the risk of fractures.

Add-back therapy with low-dose estrogen and progestins will minimize adverse effects, and should be administered if therapy is to extend beyond 6 months [24].

Other side effects complained by the patients are hot flashes, fatigue, headache and reduction of sexual desire, related to the pseudo-menopausal state. At the end of the treatment the growth of the fibroids begins again and the associated symptoms, such as pelvic pain or HMB, may recur. Even though effective the therapies with GnRH analogues or ulipristal acetate modify relationships between myoma and itspseudocapsula and the consistency of myoma. For this reason, the myomectomy can become technically more difficult and surgery can be complicated by more blood loss. For these reasons, surgery should be postponed after theend of the therapyand these treatments must therefore be reserved for symptomatic patients with severe anemia awaiting surgery [25].

3.2. Clinical Approach

Before evaluating the possibility of a medical therapy for heavy menstrual period, or menorrhagia related to uterine fibromatosis, using a LNG IUD it is necessary to perform a careful gynecological check in order to exclude other possible causes of AUB, but also to exclude or diagnose the presence of comorbidities.

3.2.1. Gynecological Examination

Standard gynecological examination includes the vaginal examination but also the speculum examination.

This last one is particularly important for women with AUB, such as irregular bleeding, intermenstrual bleeding or menorrhagia, because during the speculum examination is it possible to directly examine the cervix.

During a cervical examination we can exclude the presence of any clinical condition that may directly cause the AUB, such as a presence of an ectropion, cervical polyp or malignancy.

At the same time if necessary, the patient can receive additional treatment or additional diagnostic testing [26].

The vaginal examination on the other hand give us information about the vagina, cervix and uterus. It determines the size, shape and mobility of these structures and may suggest the presence of fibroids, adenomyosis or possible malignancy.

During this examination is possible to diagnose the presence of a fibroid of medium or large size because it is possible to appreciate a deformed uterus or mass located in the pelvis. It is also possible to evaluate the increased consistency of a fibroid, usually is not associated with pain during the examination and the mobility of the mass depends on the size of the myoma.

3.2.2. Transvaginal Ultrasonography

Cornerstone in the diagnosis of uterine fibromatosis the ultrasounds allows to distinguish myomas from pelvic masses of other origin particularly from the ovarian ones.

At the ultrasound the uterine myomas appear as neoformations round and capsulated, with well-defined margins.

The echogenicity typically can vary widely in relation to the amount of muscle cells and connective tissue that compose the fibroid.

The role of the ultrasound scan is important because with this examination it is possible to determine the location of the fibroids inside of the uterus.

However, sometimes with the ultrasound scan we can't easily distinguish between polyps, submucous fibroids and adenomyosis [26].

Of considerable importance in the ultrasound evaluation of uterine myomas is the color Doppler assessment. It provides the evaluation of the organ vascularity, which may be useful in distinguishing between solid and cystic uterine masses. Vascular assessment may also be useful in preparation for minimally invasive treatment but may also be used to evaluate vessel splaying around the fibroid, and also allow to differentiate the fibroid from myometrial, or endometrial thickness. Finally, a Doppler evaluation may be useful in the differential diagnosis of myomas from adenomyosis.

As regards the ultrasound study of uterine pathology we currently refer to the MUSA (Morphological Uterus Sonographic Assessment) indications. The MUSA is a consensus statement on terms, definitions and measurements that should be used to describe the ultrasound characteristic of the uterus and of the endometrium [27].

3.2.3. Hysteroscopy

Hysteroscopy provides direct visualization of the uterine cavity by endoscopy with access through the cervix.

Allows a direct visualization of the uterine cavity, and therefore allows the diagnosis of intracavitary abnormalities, such as polyps or fibroids, that can be directly visualized.

During this procedure, if required, it is possible to perform a target biopsy or remove intracavitary abnormality.

It has been shown that ambulatory hysteroscopy, in addition to ascertaining the presence of the fibroma submucosal, it also allows to evaluate important parameters that can be useful in order to decide which should be the best medical approach [28].

In particular, hysteroscopy can be demonstrated:

- The location of the myoma.
- The volume.
- The consistency that is assessed indirectly by exerting pressure on training with the distal end of the hysteroscope or with the tip of the operative instruments.
- Depth of myometrial invasion e valuated by studying the angle of insertion of myoma with the endometrium.

For these reasons, hysteroscopy is a highly sensitive and specific test, both around 93–98%.

Hysteroscopy is essential in order to be able to carry out a differential diagnosis between submucous fibroids or which support the cavity of the uterine and adenomyosis.

As a matter of fact, fibroids and adenomyosis have common symptoms such as dysmenorrhea, menometrorrhagia, dyspareunia, low back pain [29].

From an ultrasound point of view, it can be difficult to differentiate these two medical conditions. Even if a hysteroscopy cannot directly diagnose the presence of adenomyosis.

These hysteroscopic features generally indicates a pathological condition:

- Fibrous cystic appearance of the endometrium.
- Intramyometrial hemorrhage.
- Hemorrhagic cystis with a dark blue or chocolate brown appearance.
- Irregular appearance of the endometrium.
- Hypervascularization of the endometrium.
- A "strawberry" pattern of the endometrium.

In patients with adenomyosis, hysteroscopy reveals an irregular endometrial vascular distribution pattern, during all the phases of the menstrual period. Moreover, it allows obtaining biopsy samples from the endometrium and underlying myometrium [30].

4. Intrauterine Device

An intrauterine device is a small, often T-shaped device that is inserted into a woman's *uterus* and has as a major indication the prevention of pregnancy.

There can be find two main types of intrauterine device:

- *Nonhormonal: Copper-containing IUD*
- *Hormonal: Progestogen-releasing IUD*

Among the medicated LNG IUD there are four different type of IUD (brand names Mirena, Skyla, Kyleena, and Liletta) that works by releasing *levonorgestrel* locally in the endometrium. Each type is different in size, level of levonorgestrel released, and duration of efficacy.

The IUD must be applied and removed by a gynecologist after a gynecological examination that includes:

- a complete medical history:
- a pregnancy test, to exclude pregnancy:
- PAP-test if not recent:
- an ultrasound scan.

The intrauterine device is equipped with two wires that protrude into the vagina; these can be used to verify that it is always positioned correctly.

The Only one registered for the treatment of HMB is the one that releases 20μg/day of levonorgestrel (Mirena) [31]. Not all women can use an intrauterine device, sometimes the shape or size of the uterus may not be compatible. Women with abnormal results in a recent pap test or with other contraindications could not use an IUD [32].

However, the placement of an IUD is contraindicated in the case of:

- sexually transmitted disease in active phase;
- pelvic inflammatory disease or occurred for less than 3 months;
- presence of other abnormal uterine bleeding;
- pregnancy;
- abortion, puerperal sepsis or purulent cervicitis;
- AUB not yet diagnosed;
- malignancies of the uterus or malignant tumor of the breast or liver;
- uterine dysmorphism abnormalities of the uterine cavity;
- venous thrombosis.

4.1. Eligible Patients for Levonorgestrel-Releasing Intrauterine System

Patients who are eligible for a pharmacological treatment for HMB with levonogestrel-treated IUDs are essentially patients who need a long-term therapy, which have major or relative contra-indications for surgical intervention, who do not seek a pregnancy in the short term, or who have contraindications to oral contraceptive therapy or POP.

In particular as regards the latter category of patients, LNG- intrauterine device has no contraindications for women with coagulation problems and thrombophilia [33].

On the other hand, the use of this device is for obvious reasons reserved for patients with normal uterine volume or at least less than 10,5 cm and in patient with normal conformation of the uterine cavity.

4.2. Levonorgestrel-Releasing Intrauterine System (Mirena)

The LNG-IUD is a T-shaped device that releases levonorgestrel into the uterus that can be still for up to 5 years.

Is commonly used as a method of contraception for which was approved by FDA in 2000.

In 2009, LNG IUD has been approved as a treatment for HMB by FDA, and this was registered as an additional use [34].

The effectiveness of the IUD has been documented in several clinical trials, in particular a Chinese study has identified the effect of high concentrations of LNG on the rate of proliferation and apoptosis of myoma cells.

The results of the study show that the high concentrations of LNG that is released by the intrauterine system directly into the uterine cavity, suppressed the proliferation of uterine myoma cells and promoted cell apoptosis.

Several studies reported that medicated LNG IUD is effective for reducing menstrual blood loss in women with fibroid-related menorrhagia and increasing hemoglobin values, but not for fibroid regression.

We must not forget the ethical problem related to the use of IUDs as medical treatment. The intrauterine device is however always a contraceptive method and for this reason it can't be accepted by some types of patients for religious reasons. A recent study published in 2018 by the research team of the "La paz" hospital in Madrid and the pontifical university in Rome, evaluate the ethical aspects of the use of the medicated intrauterine device with levonorgestrel in patients with HMB. As a result, this study concludes that although the intrauterine device, Mirena®, is still a contraceptive method, the use of the IUD in the treatment of the HMB, from the ethical point of view, can be tolerated against the good of the benefit that contributes [35]. However, patients who profess religions other than Catholic may not want to be treated with this kind of medical approach.

4.3. Indications

The LNG-IUD is indicated in the therapy of:

- HMB;
- Iron deficiency anemia;
- Uterine fibromas;
- Endometrial hyperplasia;
- Adenomyosis;
- Endometriosis;
- Abnormal bleeding due to disorders of the coagulation system;
- Symptomatic patients who also need a contraception method.

The LNG-IUD is not recommended for patients currently desiring fertility and will not effectively treat significant fibroid bulk symptoms instead [36]. The LNG-IUD releases 20 mcg/day of progestin in the endometrial site and ensures 5 years of treatment. Local administration leads to a low systemic injection of the progestin that is released continuously and constantly and avoids a peak plasma concentration. The endometrial concentration of LNG is 808 +/-511pg/ml, while the circulating share is 0.1-0.2ng/ml, compared to 1.7 ng/ml of LNG taken orally. The indications for which the LNG-IUD has been registered are the contraception, protection from endometrial hyperplasia while using therapy with estrogen. Its effectiveness has been demonstrated by a huge number of clinical trials. Several studies demonstrate that the LNG-IUD is a valid therapeutic option for women with abundant menstrual flows, especially if the menorrhagia is related to uterine fibromatosis, but is also useful in patient with comorbidities such as disorders of the coagulation system, hormones dysfunctions or adenomyosis.

The mechanism by which LNG-IUD reduces menstrual blood loss is likely to result from its suppressive effect on endometrial replication, inducing atrophy, and amenorrhea induced by LGN-IUS is mediated by vascular changes at the endometrial level, such as the thickening of the arterial walls and the obliteration of the spiral arterioles by the thrombosis of the capillaries.

In patients treated with LNG-IUD for menometrorrhagia, an increase in the mean resistance index of the uterine artery has been demonstrated.

The effect of the intrauterine device on the uterine arteries and their branches could also explain the reduction in the average uterine volume that is sometimes observed in patients treated with IUDs.

4.4. LNG Intrauterine Device in Obese Patients

Obesity can be considered one of the biggest public health problems of the current century.

It is possible to estimate that obesity has more than doubled since 1980.

In Europe at the moment the estimated prevalence of overweight adults, defined as a BMI > 25 but <30, is nearly 30-70% and the prevalence of obesity, defined as a BMI > 30 in the adult population in Europe is nearly 10-30% [37].

Besides being a public health problem, obesity contributing to elevated costs in health, not only because of the comorbidities such as diabetes, high blood pressure, etc, but also it imposes new challenges in the treatment of this kind of patients.

Obesity has been associated with dysfunctional uterine bleeding, secondary amenorrhea and PCOS. Furthermore, few studies have shown that an increased BMI is related to an increased risk of developing uterine fibromatosis. Many papers concerning contraception mention that LNG-intrauterine device can be effective in obese women for that purpose.

However, few studies were performed in order to evaluate if LNG-intrauterine device is effective in HMB treatment in elected obese women. Few studies tried to evaluate if there are any differences in terms of effectiveness of the LNG intrauterine device used as a treatment of HMB between obese and non-obese women [38, 39]. But in any case, the efficacy of LNG IUD is comparable in obese women compared to normal-weight patients.

Comparable results were obtained both in terms of decreased uterine bleeding and the improvement of the hemoglobin blood levels, solving the related problem of anemia in the patients with AUB [37].

4.5. Effects of LNG IUD on Fibrinolytic Factors in the Endometrium Cells

At the moment the currently accepted proposed mechanisms for the initiation of menstruation include hypoxia-induced vasoconstriction of the endometrial blood vessels and at the same time the inflammatory changes that involve the immune cell recruitment in the endometrium.

Several researches have been determined the main role of the hemostasis in the mechanism, in particular the predominant role of the plasminogen activator system.

During the secretory phase of the menstrual cycle the increasing levels of progesterone stimulates the decidual cells so that they started to express procoagulant factors, plasminogen activator inhibitor 1 (PAI-1) and tissue factor (TF).

With the decrease of the progesterone values, these factors also decrease, while the fibrinolytic factors increase allowing fibrinolytic activity to predominate.

A recent study however suggests that the blood vessels' hemostatic systems are still active during the menstrual period. This had been demonstrated by the presence of intravascular thrombi in uterine endometrial blood vessels detected from hysterectomy specimens removed between 3.5 and 72 hours after the onset of menstruation.

In addition, the presence of aberrant blood vessels in the endometrium of women with AUB have been reported.

Therefore, pathways specific to the endothelium may be important in understanding the pathophysiology of HMB [40].

Hemostatic and fibrinolytic mechanisms to control bleeding blood vessels are well-established. In particular, the plasminogen activator system regulates clot dissolution through changes in the balance between procoagulant and fibrinolytic factors in the endothelial cells. The tissue plasminogen activator (tPA) is a fibrinolytic factor secreted by the endothelium that converts plasminogen to plasmin and then plasmin degrades the fibrin in order to break and dissolve the clot. This mechanism could lead to bleeding and so, to prevent excessive hemorrhage, the protease activity of tPA is kept under control through its link with PAI.

The levonorgestrel-releasing intrauterine system has become the leading choice as the most effective first-line medical therapy for the treatment of HMB.

The LNG released locally into the endometrial cavity results in well-documented histological changes.

For instance, it has been shown the decidualization of endometrial stromal cells, the glandular and surface epithelium atrophy, and changes in the vascular morphology.

Although successfully used as a pharmacological therapy for menorrhagia, the mechanism by which LNG decreases blood flow in the menstrual bleeding is still unknown [40].

Available clinical data suggesting that the changes in the hemostatic mechanisms after a LNG exposure are evident.

One year of LNG-IUD use by women with HMB showed improved hemostatic profiles.

It also shows an increased hemoglobin levels and improved visual bleeding scores. Increased PAI-1 and tPA messenger RNA mRNA were observed in endometrial samples obtained after 6 months of LNG-IUD use.

However, it still needs to be investigated how the LNG is mediating its hemostatic effects and which specific cells of this multicellular tissue are the target of this medical treatment.

The plasminogen activator system is an important system by which the vascular endothelium mediates hemostasis and clot lysis.

And for now, little is known about hemostatic responses by the endometrial endothelial cells during the menstrual cycle, even if a biological model for the roles of TF and PAI-1 in implantation and menstruation it has been hypothesized by studying perivascular decidualized endometrial stromal cells.

Since fibrin clots were reported in the endometrial vasculature during the first 24 to 72hours of menstruation, it may be possible that the endothelium-mediated hemostatic mechanisms are critical for controlling blood loss during the tissue destruction and vascular disruption associated with menstruation.

The LNG-IUD has been used successfully for treating HMB it acts altering tPA and PAI-1 levels in normal and HMB endometrium [41].

Since it is known that LNG can bind to androgen receptors a recent study investigated whether LNG decreased tPA through the androgen receptor in immortalized human endometrial endothelial cells. This data demonstrate that LNG decreases the fibrinolytic factor tPA in endometrial endothelial cells acting through an androgen receptor–mediated pathway.

This decrease results in a shift of the hemostatic balance in favor of maintenance of the clot within the blood vessels.

This could be one of the possible mechanisms through which LNG could decrease abnormal menstrual bleeding through a direct interaction with the endothelial cell.

4.6. Hystological Effects of Locally Released Progesterone on the Endometrium Cells

The IUD medicated with LNG releases high concentrations of progestins locally, so some authors have wondered if there are other therapeutic effects related more specifically to the action of LNG.

In a recent clinical trial, the effect of LNG on the growth and apoptosis of myoma cells were studied analyzing myoma's cells obtained from biopsies and samples collected during surgeries [42].

This study showed that in myoma cells treated with LNG morphological and cyto-structural changes are observed.

According to this trial the cells appear altered, with vacuoles and granular material at the level of the cytoplasm.

When viewed with an electron microscope, myoma cells, after treatment with LNG, present vacuolization in the cytoplasm, expansion of the endoplasmic reticulum, core exfoliation and chromatin thickening; all early signs of apoptosis.

At the concentration of 10 mcg/ml the LNG presents notable inhibitory effects on the proliferation of the cells of the uterine myoma and increases the rate of apoptosis.

This effect is both dose and time dependent.

Assuming that the uterine fibroid is a steroid-dependent fibro-muscular formation, it must be said that progesterone plays a key role in its development [43].

Numerous clinical studies show that the number of myoma cells in the replicative phase is substantially higher during the luteal phase than in the follicular phase, when the progesterone levels are higher.

Progesterone antagonist therapies can suppress the growth of uterine fibroids, since the myoma progesterone receptor is overexpressed relative to the surrounding healthy tissue.

It is a general opinion that progesterone stimulates the mitotic activity of myoma and promotes cell multiplication [44].

However, during pregnancy, when circulating progesterone concentrations are markedly elevated, in the majority of patients with uterine fibromatosis there is no exaggerated increase in the volume of myomas.

These data suggest that progesterone probably plays a double role in regulating the growth of myomas.

Several studies have shown how progesterone and estrogen act in a combined way to stimulate myoma growth.

They possibly induce the expression of the Epidermal Growth Factor (EGF) and its receptor (EGF-R), but they also lead to the expression of a selective modulator factor of the progesterone receptor which acts inhibiting proliferation, stimulating apoptosis and suppressing synthesis collagen of leiomyoma cells in vitro [45].

The effects of progesterone are first of all an up-regulation of the proliferative cell nuclear antigen expression, that is an indicator of cell's proliferation, in smooth muscle cells of uterine leiomyomas.

Secondly an up-regulation on the Bcl-2 protein, which inhibits cell death mediated by apoptosis.

Experimental data therefore show that, in patients with uterine fibromatosis, the use of LNG-IUD is more appropriate than the use of natural progesterone.

In fact, the LNG-IUD releases 20 mcg of LNG daily at the level of the uterine cavity, therefore the LNG reaches at local level concentrations 1000 times higher than in the blood circulation.

Thanks to the slow release of progesterone, IUD at LNG has been shown to be effective in reducing bleeding duration and the extent of menstrual blood loss, by inhibiting endometrial proliferation and increasing cell apoptosis.

Even if intrauterine device with LNG is therefore a valid therapeutic option for menorrhagia and anemia associated with uterine fibromatosis.

Its therapeutic effect, causing the reduction of menometrorrhagia, however is weighed down by side effects, such as increased volume of the uterine cavity and intermittent spotting.

It should also be noted that during the use of the IUD medicated with LNG there is not reported a reduction in the size of the fibroids and of the whole uterus.

Even after a prolonged use of the device the fibroids dimensions remain unchanged.

On the other hand, there is instead an atrophic involution of the endometrium, and this is precisely the mechanism that greatly reduces menorrhagia over time.

Several literature reviews evaluated the outcomes in term of reduction of menstrual bleeding treated with LNG-IUD.

The data suggests that after a treatment of three months almost the 85% of patients with menorrhagia saw a normal menstrual flow re-established.

After twelve months of therapy with LNG- intrauterine device almost the 40% of the patients reported amenorrhea, and according to that an increasing hemoglobin concentration.

It's also to be considered that according to systematic reviews of the literature in patients with uterine fibromatosis, with or without menometrorrhagia, the contraceptive efficacy of LNG-IUD is optimal but is also to be noticed that in patients with uterine fibromatosis the rates of expulsion of IUD are higher than in women without fibroids.

Finally, it is important to notice that LNG-IUD significantly reduces menstrual bleeding and dysmenorrhea associated with uterine fibromatosis, while not determining a reduction in the total size of the uterus or those of uterine fibroids.

4.7. The Role of Inflammatory Pathway and AUB Related

Several recent studies have shown the presence of aromatase expression in the endometrium of patients with adenomyosis, myomas, and endometrial polyps.

It is therefore important to suppress the aromatase expression in order to achieve an amenorrhea condition.

Several different progestins have been shown to inhibit aromatase and so far, vascular endothelial growth factor expression, and cyclooxygenase-2, COX2 expression in the endometrium.

This can be achieved also using a LNG IUD.

The insertion of LNG IUD in the uterus inhibited the expression of aromatase and p450, thus exerting a local anti-estrogenic effect on the endometrium, which is optimal in the treatment of adenomyosis and myomas.

A high concentration of COX-2 expression in the endometrium of women correlates with the presence of AUB even if treated with LNG intrauterine device, oral progestins ore oral contraceptives.

That is a demonstration of the important role of prostaglandins causing inflammation in the endometrium cells related to the pathogenesis of both menorrhagia and breakthrough bleeding [4].

5. Adenomyosis and Uterine Fibromatosis Different Aspects and Treatments

Considering the AUB, we must not forget the possibility of co-presence of adenomyosis and uterine fibromatosis.

Adenomyosis is a widespread disease usually affecting women at their late reproductive years, which has also a great impact in the women health also causing infertility [46].

The most common form is the diffuse adenomyosis, focal adenomyosis presenting as a cystic variant, is instead very rare, particularly in patients younger than 30 years old.

Adenomyosis can be defined as the presence of ectopic endometrial tissue within the uterine myometrium, surrounded by the presence of smooth muscle hypertrophy.

By definition, they consist of epithelial as well stromal elements and situated at least 2.5 mm below the endometrial–myometrial junction.

Sex hormone receptors in adenomyosis foci respond to sex hormones less than normal endometrium.

Adenomyosis is a frequent cause of AUB and pelvic pain in women of reproductive age.

Although hysterectomy has always been considered an effective treatment, less invasive procedures such as endometrial resection have been proposed as an alternative, though it's also associated with lower success rates.

The poor rates of amenorrhea after endometrial resection may be caused by the intrinsic capacity of the endometrium to regenerate [47].

Endo-myometrial resection is most suited to patients with disease limited to the endo-myometrial junction as menstrual symptoms may be reduced and the pathology may be removed. It may also be useful when adenomyosis is not only localized in the myometrial junction but it is also present in the outer myometrium.

This is true because performing a laparoscopic myometrial excision alone may not cure the symptom of abnormal menstrual bleeding, either because the excision could be incomplete or because the menstrual symptoms are not caused by the outer myometrial adenomyosis.

The desire for a future pregnancy contraindicates endometrial/myometrial resection, that's why the insertion of a LNG IUD alone could be consider as an option for women in their fertile age and desiring pregnancy soon [48].

The technique of endometrial ablation has been widely well described.

The whole thickness of the endometrium should be removed during the procedure as menorrhagia may be due to factors other than the adenomyosis.

Deeper myometrial removal or ablation carries the risk of causing increased bleeding. That's because significant arteries are situated about 5 mm deep under the myometrial surface [49].

If an MRI or ultrasound scan demonstrate that the adenomyosis is extended beyond the thickness of the endometrial/myometrial junction, the procedure can be modified to include 2-3 mm of myometrium in the affected areas [50].

The Histological examination of the excised myometrial fragments can confirm or refute the diagnosis of adenomyosis.

After performing an endometrial/myometrial ablation as a single operative procedure, the symptom of abnormal menstrual bleeding usually remains controlled in 55% of women for at least 2 years.

A Brazilian clinical trial of 2012 shows that the use of LNG-IUD following endometrial resection in patients with adenomyosis is associated with higher rates of amenorrhea and lower rates of dysmenorrhea compared to women who use LNG IUD but who were not submitted to endometrial resection [41]. Another study shows that in women with adenomyosis treated only with the LNG IUD insertion or undergoing to endometrial resection alone the success rates for the treatment of menorrhagia are lower than when both methods are used together.

The most common histological pattern reported for the endometrium of patient with LNG IUD insertion consisted of an endometrium with atrophic glands and the presence in the stroma of a decidual reaction and/or atrophic changes.

In the aforementioned study those chances in the endometrium are always shown in the patients using a LNG IUD.

But in patient who had not previously been submitted to endometrial resection, even if the thickness of the endometrium is lower, however, the presence of dilated blood vessels has been detected. This finding that was not present in women who had an endometrial resection before the insertion of a LNG IUD.

In conclusion LNG IUD is an effective option for the suppression of aromatase and Cox-2 expression in the endometrium of patients with adenomyosis; however, inhibition appears to be greater when this device is inserted immediately following endometrial resection [51].

Nevertheless, it should be noted that endometrial resection is an alternative to hysterectomy that obviously is not an option for women who still want to preserve their fertility. In this case, particularly when used to treat adenomyosis-related menorrhagia, the insertion of LNG IUD alone is a viable option, since fertility returns promptly after removal of the device.

The combination of LNG IUD insertion and the endometrial resection represent an excellent and effective alternative therapy instead of hysterectomy for the management of menorrhagia and dysmenorrhea in patients with AUB caused by adenomyosis.

6. Target of the Medical Therapy

The pharmacological therapies currently used are mostly for the control of irregular bleeding symptoms, such as oral contraceptives (estro-progestogens or progestins only) and intrauterine devices (LNG IUD) medicated with progesterone.

Analogs (agonists/antagonists) of GnRH are used for many years, particularly in the preoperative phase in patients with anemia, in order to reduce the size of the fibroid and block the bleeding by solving the anemia, causing a temporary menopause [43].

The fundamental benefit of pharmacological therapies is not to be invasive.

On the other hand, we have to consider that they are not free from disadvantages.

The main disadvantages are:

- The symptoms related to uterine fibroma at the end of therapy can reappear.
- The pharmacological therapies are not to be considered as a long-term therapy, so is important to discuss with the patient the duration of the therapies.
- The possible appearance of the side effects.

For example, some patients are not suitable for surgery for severe comorbidities, on the other hand there also could be women of reproductive age who doesn't allow hysterectomy

Medical treatment is indicated in symptomatic subjects to resolve symptoms or in preparation for surgery for the purpose of:

- Some pharmacological therapies are indicated to reduce the size of the myoma before the surgery.
- It is proved that pharmacological therapies and LNG IUD particularly can reduce the AUB related to the uterine fibromatosis and so far improve the correlated anemia condition.
- to allow a less invasive surgery in relation to the reduction of myoma and blood loss [15].

As sad before the medical therapy most of all is temporary and the duration of the pharmacological therapy is to be settled at the beginning of the treatment and it should be discussed with the patients.

A chronic medical treatment can be contemplated in relation to the requests of the woman and it is also to be considered in the presence of non-acute deriving symptoms from the presence of the myoma.

Based on the known stimulus factors of the proliferation of myomas, medical therapy is based on the use of all compounds capable of reducing or abolishing stimulation hormone level in the myoma or to act directly with proliferative mechanism and apoptotic ones.

The clinical-therapeutic choice of the use of the intrauterine device is conditioned by a careful diagnostic evaluation that excludes the presence of possible contraindications that may influence the displacement or spontaneous expulsion of the device.

Even if at the moment most of the pathogenetic mechanism for the growth of the myomas are still unknown. It is a common opinion that sex hormones are the basis of the growth of the fibroid cells. The hormones that promote proliferation of the myomas cells are estrogens (E) and progesterone. Receptors for estradiol (E2), and receptors for progesterone (P4) are more expressed in myoma myocytes than in normal myometrium [23]. Estrogen and Progesterone increase local growth factors and their receptors (EGF and Insulin-Like Growth Factor [IGF-I]), and reduce the inductors of apoptosis factors (Tumor Necrosis Factor a, [TNF a]; BCL-2) at the same time.

This result in proliferation of the myoma as a final effect, with consequent increase in size of the mass but also of the entire uterus. The cause of all this is that apoptosis in myoma cells is inhibited. Recent biochemical and clinical studies have suggested that progesterone may increase the proliferative activity of fibroids and that ovarian steroids can influence their growth [34].

These observations therefore have generated the hypothesis that anti-progestin drugs could be useful in the medical treatment of uterine fibroids.

Few reviews have been written comparing the pharmacological therapies that are available at the moment for the treatment of HMB related to uterine fibromatosis.

Considering the possible pharmacological treatment available at the moment we can't forget that Ulipristal Acetate have anti progestins effects not only locally in the uterus and must be considered as a limited treatment over time, and should be used before surgery.

POP therapy and Oral contraceptives could give a rebound effect and acting on the estroprogestinic receptors, overexpressed at the level of the fibroid cells, can lead to an increase in the size of the myoma itself.

LNG intrauterine device instead would have a minimal share of action at the myometrial and systemic level of progesterone because it exerts its mechanism of action mostly in the thickness of the endometrium.

6.1. Efficacy of Levonorgestrel-Releasing Intrauterine Device as Treatment of HMB Compared with Oral Progestins in Women with Uterine Leiomyoma

The medical treatment available as treatment for HMB related or not with uterine fibromatosis are NSAID progesterones, gestrinone, mifepristone, danazol, oral contraceptives and GnRH agonists.

At the moment patients with uterine fibromatosis are still treated by hysterectomy in about 35% of the cases.

Oral progesterone though used very frequently for the treatment of dysfunctional uterine bleeding for over 30 years has proved to have poor effects. Between fifth to 5th days of menstrual cycles 10 mg a day dosage for norethindrone acetate (NETA) has decreased bleeding to 80-85%.

In a large number of contrast studies LNG-IUD has proved to provide effective treatment for abnormal menstrual bleeding, endometrial hyperplasia, endometriosis, adenomyosis and guaranteed a strong contraception effectiveness [52].

The main problem related to the oral progesterone administration is poor patient compliance

After sixth months of treatment the ratio of attendance to the medical treatment is up to 77% in women with HMB treated with LNG intrauterine device, and almost the 22% in patients treated with oral progesterone administration instead [52].

Difference are found also in the reduction of menstrual blood loss, in patients treated with a medicated LNG intrauterine device the reduction of abnormal menstrual bleeding was up to 80%, on the other hand in women treated with oral progesterone the rate of success in the reduction of HMB is to be considered around the 56%.

The reduction of HMB have as a consequent that the hemoglobin values rises. So far, the hemoglobin values increase in the patients treated with LNG intrauterine device much more than in the patient treated with the administration of oral progesterone.

The long-term effects of using LNG-IUD are amenorrhea and oligomenorrhea.

In literature the ratios of amenorrhea and oligomenorrhea in patients treated with a LNG IUD are from 20 to 55%.

Fewer data are available in literature on the rate of amenorrhea in women treated with oral progesterone but summarizing the results of several studies those rates are lower compared with the LNG IUD treatment and are up to 5-10%.

Comparing the side effects reported by women using LNG IUD and NETA we can say that the main side effects complained by women treated with LNG-IUD are mostly mastalgia, weight gain and edema; rarely women complained hirsutisms, acne and headache

The most frequent adverse effect complained for LNG-IUD treatment is spotting for the first month of therapy.

On the other hand, the main side effects complained by women treated by NETA are weight gain, mastalgia, the difficulty in a regular drug usage and depression.

7. Follow up After LNG IUD Placement

After the placement of the LNG IUD in the uterine cavity, subsequently, the correct seat of the spiral is evaluated with an ultrasound scan with follow-up every six months.

The aim of this behavior is to promptly diagnose if there are any displacements of the device in the uterine cavity.

A close follow up of the patient is important, so we are able to evaluate the effectiveness of the therapy on the symptoms, particularly on the menstrual blood loss.

It's also important to report the appearance of possible side effects that could decrease the patient's compliance.

For these reasons it's important to inform and discuss, before starting the medical therapy, with the patients the rate of success of the treatment with LNG intrauterine device and which are the most common side effects [41].

References

[1] Sriprasert I, Pakrashi T, Kimble T, Archer DF. Heavy menstrual bleeding diagnosis and medical management. *Contracept Reprod Med.* 2017.

[2] Singh S, Best C, Dunn S, Leyland N, Wolfman WL. No. 292-Abnormal Uterine Bleeding in Pre-Menopausal Women. *J Obstet Gynaecol Canada.* 2018;40(5):e391–413.

[3] Report FA. Menstrual Bleeding. *Am J Obstet Gynecol.* 2011;217:574.e1-574.e9.

[4] Maia H, Haddad C, Casoy J, Maia R, Pinheiro N, Coutinho EM. Effect of a hormone-releasing intrauterine system (Mirena®) on aromatase and Cox-2 expression in patients with adenomyosis submitted or not, to endometrial resection. *Int J Womens Health.* 2012;4(1):175–83.

[5] Liu Z, Doan Q V., Blumenthal P, Dubois RW. A systematic review evaluating health-related quality of life, work impairment, and health-care costs and utilization in abnormal uterine bleeding. *Value Heal.* 2007;10(3):183–94.

[6] Food US. Evaluation and Management of Abnormal Uterine Bleeding in *Premenopausal Women.* 2012;35–43.

[7] Herman MC, Mak N, Geomini PM, Winkens B, Mol BW, Bongers MY. Is the Pictorial Blood Loss Assessment Chart (PBAC) score associated with treatment outcome after endometrial ablation for heavy menstrual bleeding? A cohort study. *BJOG An Int J Obstet Gynaecol.* 2017;12(1):15–20.

[8] Deneris A. PALM-COEIN Nomenclature for Abnormal Uterine Bleeding. *J Midwifery Women's Heal.* 2016;61(3):376–9.

[9] Munro MG, Critchley HOD, Broder MS, Fraser IS. FIGO classification system (PALM-COEIN) for causes of abnormal uterine bleeding in nongravid women of reproductive age. *Int J Gynecol Obstet.* 2011;113(1):3–13.

[10] Wood C. Adenomyosis: Difficult to Diagnose, and Difficult to Treat. *Diagn Ther Endos*c. 2001;7(2):89–95.

[11] Gordts S, Grimbizis G, Campo R. Symptoms and classification of uterine adenomyosis, including the place of hysteroscopy in diagnosis. *Fertil Steril.* 2018;109(3):380–388.e1.

[12] Zia A, Rajpurkar M. Challenges of diagnosing and managing the adolescent with heavy menstrual bleeding. *Thromb Res.* 2016;143(2016):91–100.

[13] Stewart EA. Epidemiology, clinical manifestations, diagnosis, and natural history of uterine leiomyomas. In: Basow D, editor. *UpToDate*. Waltham (Mass): UpToDate; 2008;2008.

[14] Vilos GA, Allaire C, Laberge PY, Leyland N, Vilos AG, Murji A, et al. The Management of Uterine Leiomyomas. *J Obstet Gynaecol* Canada. 2015;37(2):57–178.

[15] *Linee Guida Sulla Prevenzione E Trattamento Fibromiomatosi SIGO*:1–8 [*SIGO Fibromyomatosis Prevention and Treatment Guidelines*].

[16] SOGC Clinical Practice Guideline No. 318, February 2015 Replaces, No. 128, May 2003) *The Management of Uterine Leiomyomas* George A.Vilos, MD, London ON Catherine Allaire, MD, Vancouver BC Philippe-Yves aberge, MD, Quebec QC Nicholas Leyland, MD, MHCM, Hamilton ON. 2015;(318):2015.

[17] Islam MS, Ciavattini A, Petraglia F, Castellucci M, Ciarmela P. Extracellular matrix in uterine leiomyoma pathogenesis: A potential target for future therapeutics. *Hum Reprod Update.* 2018;24(1):59–85.

[18] Sohn GS, Cho S, Kim YM, Cho C-H, Kim M-R, Lee SR. Current medical treatment of uterine fibroids. *Obs Gynecol Sci.* 2018;61612192(2):192–201.

[19] Day Baird D, Dunson DB, Hill MC, Cousins D, Schectman JM. High cumulative incidence of uterine leiomyoma in black and white women: ultrasound evidence. *Am J Obstet Gynecol* 2003;188:100 – 7. 2003;2003.

[20] Kundu S, Iwanuk C, Staboulidou I, Garcia-Rocha GJ, Soergel P, Hertel H, et al. Morbidity, fertility and pregnancy outcomes after myoma enucleation by laparoscopy versus laparotomy. *Arch Gynecol* Obstet. 2018;297(4):969–76.

[21] Marjoribanks J, Lethaby A, Farquhar C. Surgery versus medical therapy for heavy menstrual bleeding (Review) *Summary of Findings for the Main Comparison.* 2016;(1).

[22] Dowlut-McElroy T, Williams KB, Carpenter SL, Strickland JL. Menstrual Patterns and Treatment of Heavy Menstrual Bleeding in Adolescents with Bleeding Disorders. *J Pediatr Adolesc Gynecol.* 2015;28(6):499–501.

[23] Islam MS, Protic O, Giannubilo SR, Toti P, Tranquilli AL, Petraglia F, et al. Uterine leiomyoma: Available medical treatments and new possible therapeutic options. *J Clin Endocrinol Metab*. 2013;98(3):921–34.

[24] Maybin JA, Critchley HOD. Medical management of heavy menstrual bleeding. *Womens Health* (Lond Engl). 2016;12(1):27–34.

[25] Chen YJ, Li YT, Huang BS, Yen MS, Sheu BC, Chow SN, et al. Medical treatment for heavy menstrual bleeding. *Taiwan J Obstet Gynecol.* 2015;54(5):483–8.

[26] McLucas B. Diagnosis, imaging and anatomical classification of uterine fibroids. *Best Pract Res Clin Obstet Gynaecol*. 2008;22(4):627–42.

[27] Van Den Bosch T, Dueholm M, Leone FPG, Valentin L, Rasmussen CK, Votino A, et al. Terms, definitions and measurements to describe sonographic features of myometrium and uterine masses: A consensus opinion from the Morphological Uterus Sonographic Assessment (MUSA) group. *Ultrasound Obstet Gynecol.* 2015;46(3):284–98.

[28] Di Spiezio Sardo A, Calagna G, Santangelo F, Zizolfi B, Tanos V, Perino A, et al. The Role of Hysteroscopy in the Diagnosis and Treatment of Adenomyosis. *Biomed Res Int.* 2017;2017.

[29] Pop-Trajković-Dinić S, Ljubić A, Kopitović V, Antić V, Stamenović S, Pjević AT. The role of hysteroscopy in diagnosis and treatment of postmenopausal bleeding. *Vojnosanit Pregl.* 2013;70(8):747–50.

[30] by Dove Press published. IJWH-98579-*management-of-abnormal-uterine-bleeding---focus-on-ambulator*. 2018;127–36.

[31] Lahteenmaki P, Rauramo I, Backman T. The levonorgestrel intrauterine system in contraception. *Steroids.* 2000;65(10–11):693–7.

[32] Xie ZW, Zhang YN, Wan S, Xu WZ, Chen J. Levonorgestrel-releasing intrauterine device is an efficacious contraceptive for women with leiomyoma. *J Int Med Res.* 2012;40(5):1966–72.

[33] Zapata LB, Whiteman MK, Tepper NK, Jamieson DJ, Marchbanks PA, Curtis KM. Intrauterine device use among women with uterine fibroids: a systematic review. *Contraception*. 2010;82(1):41–55.

[34] Soysal S, Soysal ME. The efficacy of levonorgestrel-releasing intrauterine device in selected cases of myoma-related menorrhagia: A prospective controlled trial. *Gynecol Obstet Invest*. 2005;59(1):29–35.

[35] Éticos A, Uso DEL, Diu DEL, Miranda MT, Simó PAUA. Aspectos éticos del uso del DIU Mirena ® en el tratamiento de la hemorragia menstrual severa [Ethical Aspects of the Use of Mirena(r) Iud in the Treatment of Heavy Menstrual Bleeding]. *Cuadernos de Bioética.* 2018;29(96):159–76.

[36] Kriplani A, Awasthi D, Kulshrestha V, Agarwal N. Efficacy of the levonorgestrel-releasing intrauterine system in uterine leiomyoma. *Int J Gynecol Obstet.* 2012;116(1):35–8.

[37] Oliveira N, Rosado V, Machado AI, Marques C. Levonorgestrel intrauterine device effectiveness in heavy menstrual bleeding treatment in obese women. *Acta Obstet Ginecol Port* 2014;8(4):347–53.

[38] Saito-Tom LY, Soon RA, Harris SC, Salcedo J, Kaneshiro BE. Levonorgestrel Intrauterine Device Use in Overweight and Obese Women. *Hawai'i J Med Public Heal*. 2015;74(11):369–74.

[39] Saito-Tom L, Ahn HJ, Kaneshiro B. Levonorgestrel Intrauterine Device Complications among Obese Women in a Multiracial Population [21F]. *Obstet Gynecol.* 2017;129:66S–67S.

[40] Pakrashi T, Taylor JE, Nelson A, Archer DF, Jacot T. The Effect of Levonorgestrel on Fibrinolytic Factors in Human Endometrial Endothelial Cells. *Reprod Sci.* 2016;23(11):1536–41.

[41] Herman MC, van den Brink MJ, Geomini PM, van Meurs HS, Huirne JA, Eising HP, et al. Levonorgestrel releasing intrauterine system (Mirena) versus endometrial ablation (Novasure) in women with heavy menstrual bleeding: A multicentre randomised controlled trial. *BMC Womens Health.* 2013;13(1):1.

[42] Buttini MJ, Jordan SJ, Webb PM. The effect of the levonorgestrel releasing intrauterine system on endometrial hyperplasia: An Australian study and systematic review. *Aust New Zeal J Obstet Gynaecol.* 2009;49(3):316–22.

[43] Kaunitz AM, Inki P. The levonorgestrel-releasing intrauterine system in heavy menstrual bleeding: A benefit-risk review. *Drugs.* 2012;72(2):193–215.

[44] Katz TA, Yang Q, Treviño LS, Walker CL, Al-Hendy A. Endocrine-disrupting chemicals and uterine fibroids. *Fertil Steril.* 2016;106(4):967–77.

[45] Wong JYY, Gold EB, Johnson WO, Lee JS. Circulating sex hormones and risk of uterine fibroids: Study of women's health across the nation (swan). *J Clin Endocrinol Metab.* 2016;101(1):123–30.

[46] Luciano DE, Exacoustos C, Albrecht L, LaMonica R, Proffer A, Zupi E, et al. Three-dimensional ultrasound in diagnosis of adenomyosis: Histologic correlation with ultrasound targeted biopsies of the uterus. *J Minim Invasive Gynecol.* 2013;20(6):803–10.

[47] Vannuccini S, Luisi S, Tosti C, Sorbi F, Petraglia F. Role of medical therapy in the management of uterine adenomyosis. *Fertil Steril.* 2018;109(3):398–405.

[48] Livia M. Focal adenomyosis (intramural endometriotic cyst) in a very young patient -differential diagnosis with uterine fibromatosis. *J Med Life.* 2016;9(2):180–2.

[49] Levgur M. Therapeutic options for adenomyosis: A review. *Arch Gynecol Obstet.* 2007;276(1):1–15.

[50] Krentel H, Cezar C, Becker S, Sardo ADS, Tanos V, Wallwiener M, et al. From Clinical Symptoms to MR Imaging: Diagnostic Steps in Adenomyosis. *Biomed Res Int*. 2017;2017.

[51] Minghan C, Shili S, Baihua D. Morphological and Ultrastructural Changes in Human Endometrium Following Low-Dose Levonorgestrel Contraceptive. *J Obstet Gynecol India.* 2015;65:323–7.

[52] Tosun AK, Tosun I, Suer N. Comparison of levonorgestrel-releasing intrauterine device with oral progestins in heavy menstrual bleeding (HMB) cases with uterine leiomyoma (LNG-IUD and oral progestin usage in myoma uteri). *Pakistan J Med Sci.* 2014;30(4).

In: Uterine Fibroids
Editors: S. Ferrero and F. Barra

ISBN: 978-1-53615-046-9

Chapter 10

NON-INVASIVE PROCEDURES FOR UTERINE MYOMAS

Giulio Bovio**, MD, Nicola Camisassi, MD, Francesco Petrocelli, MD and Alice Utili, MD
Vascular and Interventional Radiology Department,
IRCCS Ospedale Policlinico San Martino, Genoa, Italy

ABSTRACT

Uterine fibroid embolization (UFE) has become established as an accepted minimally invasive treatment for women with symptomatic uterine fibroids, having shown to reduce pain, bulk symptoms (pressure and abdominal wall distortion), and menorrhagia in most cases. The aim of this appendix is to introduce the role of UFE in the management of patients with fibroids.

Keywords: uterine fibroids, uterine fibroid embolization, minimally invasive treatment

1. INTRODUCTION

Uterine fibroid embolization (UFE) has become established as an accepted minimally invasive treatment for patients with symptomatic uterine fibroids. UFE has been shown to reduce pain, bulk symptoms (pressure and abdominal wall distortion), and menorrhagia in most cases [1].

* Corresponding Author's E-mail: giulio.bovio@hsanmartino.it.

The safety and efficacy of the procedure have been extensively studied, and although hysterectomy remains the most common intervention for fibroids, uterine embolization has emerged as one of the most important uterine-sparing options [2].

Relatively few absolute contraindications exist: pregnancy, known or suspected gynecologic malignancy, and current uterine or adnexal infection. Both the interventional radiologist and the gynecologist must fully evaluate each single patient before recommending UFE as a treatment for symptomatic fibroids.

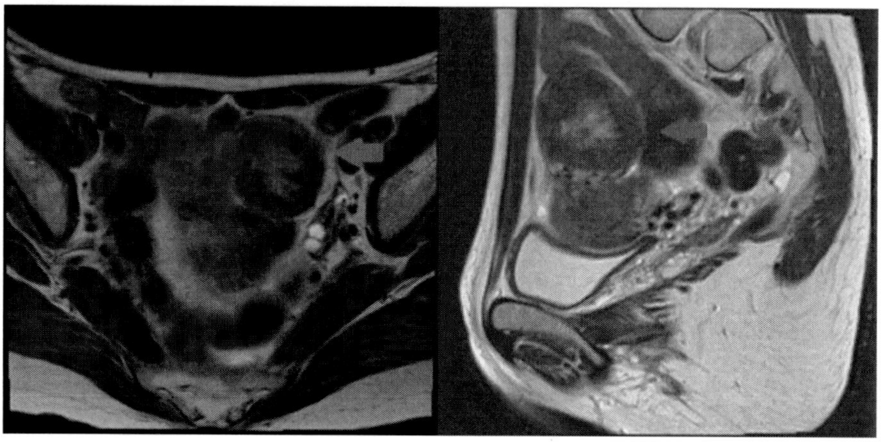

Figure 1. Axial (left) and sagittal T2-weighted turbo spin-echo (right) images of the pelvis show a left subserosal fibroid (arrows).

Once the pathology has been assessed from the clinical point of view and through intracavitary ultrasound, magnetic resonance (MR) imaging should be used to evaluate patients before and after the procedure. Its superior spatial resolution and multiplanar capability enable the interventional radiologist to accurately assess fibroid location within the uterus and fibroid number and size (Figure 1); furthermore, MR imaging can demonstrate the vascularity of fibroids on contrast material–enhanced images and allows determination of whether embolization is a reasonable treatment option [2].

2. Indications

Both single and multiple fibroids can be treated with UFE and all fibroid locations (submucosal, intramural, and subserosal) are eligible for embolization. Certain anatomic fibroid subtypes deserve special consideration: intracavitary fibroids are more likely to be expelled in the weeks and months after embolization and this may lead to some post-procedural complications; pedunculated subserosal fibroids, particularly those with a narrow attachment to the uterus have been suggested as a contraindication to UFE because of the potential risk of detachment [3]. Another class of fibroids, cervical fibroids, has also been investigated. In comparison with other fibroid subtypes, cervical fibroids appear to be resistant to complete hemorrhagic infarction after UFE, although the data are limited. Incomplete infarction may be due to an additional or alternative blood supply to the cervix [4].

The primary symptom for which women seek treatment for fibroids is menorrhagia [5]. Symptomatic fibroids typically cause heavy menstrual cycles, with an increase in the length of the cycle and the number of days of heavy bleeding. Bleeding between menstrual periods (metrorrhagia) is less typical and raises the possibility of other diagnoses, such as a cervical lesion, endometrial polyp, or carcinoma. Other symptoms include pelvic pain, pressure, and urinary symptoms, such as urinary frequency or retention. Women with fibroid-induced infertility who are not candidates for surgery may also be considered for UFE, but the decision as to whether uterine embolization is the best choice in any given patient is complex [2]. There are a few absolute and relative contraindications to UFE. The first absolute contraindication is current pregnancy which has to be excluded in every patient undergoing UFE. Another absolute contraindication is a known or suspected gynecologic malignancy. Therefore, complex cystic masses suspicious for ovarian malignancy need to be diagnosed before UFE. Although rare, leiomyosarcoma has to be excluded too and this may be difficult because of the overlap with the MR imaging appearance of fibroids and definitive diagnosis may require biopsy or surgical resection [6-7]. Finally, current uterine or adnexal infection is also a contraindication to UFE, at least until treated. Once the infection has been treated, there should not be any barrier to UFE. There are also relative contraindications to consider. These include contrast material allergy, coagulopathy, and renal failure.

3. Procedure

UFE is an angiographic procedure that is typically performed by using a unilateral femoral artery approach. Some operators use a bilateral femoral artery approach [8]. Regardless of access, in all cases, bilateral uterine artery catheterization and embolization are needed, since most uterine fibroids receive blood supply from both uterine arteries and, in the other cases, the unilateral embolization can give rise to the opening of intra-uterine anastomosis leading to the fibroid revascularization. At first an aortography at the renal arteries plane has to be performed (Figure 2) to exclude the presence of any uterine branch coming from the ovarian arteries, then, under fluoroscopy, the left internal iliac (hypogastric) artery is accessed with a catheter. Thereafter, many operators catheterize the uterine artery with a microcatheter. After uterine arteriography, embolic material is injected into the uterine artery to occlude the vessels of the fibroid (Figures 3 A-B).

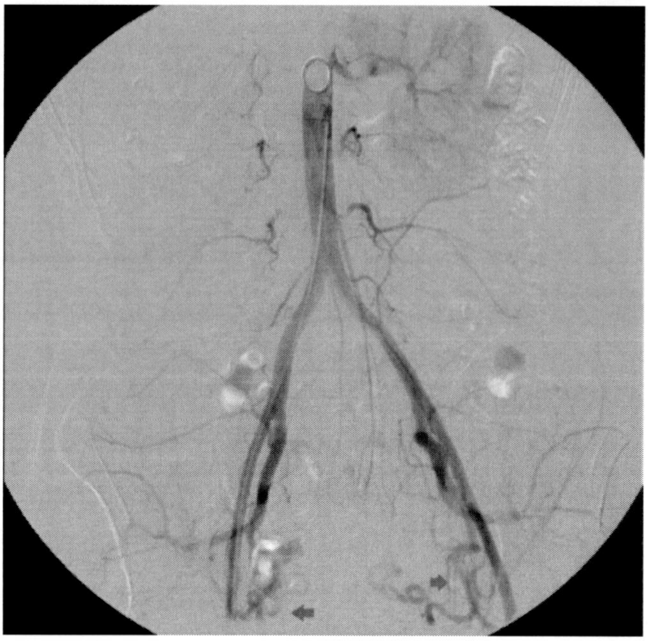

Figure 2. Abdominal aortography. Digital subtraction angiographic image obtained in the arterial phase shows bilateral hypertrophy of the uterine arteries (arrows) and the absence of uterine branches from the left ovarian artery feeding the fibroid.

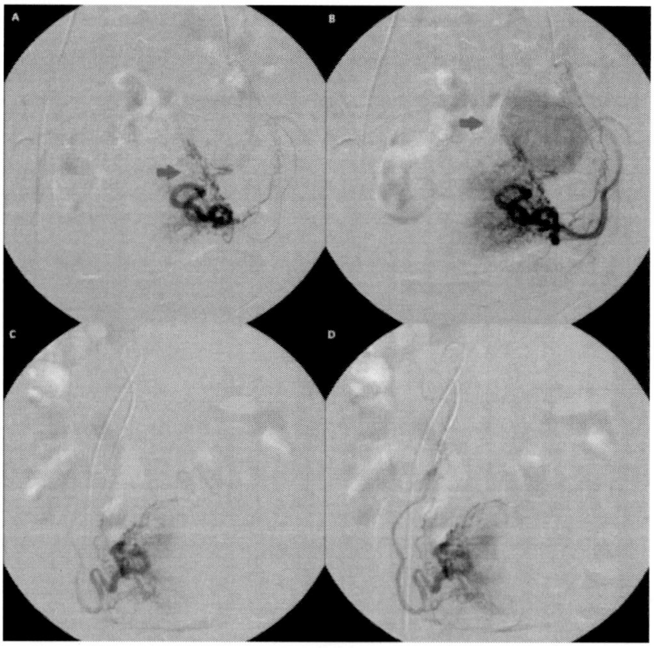

Figure 3. Two consecutive uterine angiograms confirm the presence of enlarged vessels feeding a large fibroid projecting from the left side of the uterus (arrows, A-B); the right uterine angiogram and the injection of embolic material is performed as well to avoid the opening of intra-uterine anastomoses which may lead to the fibroid revascularization (C-D).

This procedure is repeated in the contralateral uterine artery as well (Figures 3 C-D). Because there are enlarged vessels feeding the fibroid, there is preferential flow to these vessels early in the embolization process. The goal is to occlude the vessels of the fibroid but not to completely occlude the uterine artery. Commonly, there is still sluggish flow in the uterine arteries at the conclusion of the embolization procedure [9]. From a technical perspective, the choice of embolic material and the end point of embolization have been a subject of great interest to interventionalists in this field. Spies et al. [9] compared the outcomes of UFE for uterine fibroids with use of tris-acryl gelatin microspheres (TAGM) versus polyvinyl alcohol (PVA) particles concluding that the use of PVA particles results in an unacceptably high rate of failed tumor infarction in UFE. A well-planned protocol for postprocedural care is important to ensure that patients have a positive experience recovering from the embolization. Most patients will have moderate pain for several hours after UFE. The pain is due to ischemia [10], but if not properly controlled, it can progress to severe pain and can be difficult to manage.

4. Adverse Effects

Given the broad range of practice settings in which UFE is performed, it has proved to be remarkably safe. The major complications of UFE are venous thromboembolism, fibroid expulsion, ovarian failure and amenorrhea. Venous thromboembolism is the most serious adverse event with a rate of one pulmonary embolus in 400 patients in one study [11]. Fibroid expulsion is a troublesome complication that may occur after uterine embolization, which can result in substantial pain, vaginal discharge, bleeding, and infection. Overall, it occurs in about 5% of patients, although the frequency depends on the location of the fibroid [12]. Hysterectomy may be necessary if the fibroid cannot be removed transvaginally or if infection cannot be cleared. The last important although infrequent adverse outcome of UFE is ovarian failure, with amenorrhea the result. It is believed to be caused by occlusion of ovarian vessels via tubal branches fed by the uterine arteries [13].

5. Outcomes

Patients can reasonably expect resolution of symptoms such as menorrhagia, pelvic pressure, and pelvic pain, within one year after the procedure; often most of the improvement is reasonable to be expected in the first six months. Non-responding cases might undergo contrast material enhanced MRI examination to demonstrate the effective decrease in the size of fibroids (Figure 4) and the absence or presence of any residual vascularization. UFE outcomes have been well documented. Early studies showed technically successful procedures with menorrhagia control in 90%–92% of patients after 12 months and improvement in bulk symptoms in 88%–96% of patients at 12 months [14-15]. More recently, several randomized studies that compared UFE outcomes and surgical outcomes after long-term follow-up have been published. According with the literature, the efficacy of embolization and of hysterectomy by laparotomy for compression symptoms and pelvic pain do not differ at 12 or 24 months but the duration of hospitalization, convalescence and sick-leave is shorter after embolization than after hysterectomy by laparotomy, and the cost of embolization is less at 12 months and at 24 months, even considering the cost of the follow-up imaging and revision surgery [16]. Studies comparing embolization with vaginal or laparoscopic hysterectomy have not been published yet. Regarding the comparison between embolization and myomectomy, they showed to have the same efficacy for either bleeding or compression symptoms at 6-26 months after treatment. Also in this case the durations of hospitalization and convalescence as well as of sick-leave are shorter after embolization than after either type of myomectomy [16]. At the report two years after treatment of a randomized study of 121 patients compared myomectomy with UFE for treatment of fibroids, myomectomy had better reproductive outcomes, as 78% of myomectomy patients became pregnant compared with 50% of UFE patients [17]. UFE was also associated with a greater likelihood of not delivering and of spontaneous abortion. Even if longer-term data from this study are not yet available, patients must be informed of the risks in case they decide they want to become pregnant after embolization. Although the evidence is still limited, in sum, UFE should not be first-line treatment for women with infertility due to fibroids or who have a strong desire to become pregnant. However, it is still an option for patients who are poor surgical risks due to comorbidities, prior surgery, or the extent of the fibroids. The evidence also suggests that successful pregnancy is possible after UFE; for those who choose not to have surgery, that option is not foreclosed. Women should be appropriately counseled about their choices at the time of the consultation, when the extent of fibroids, patient preferences, and reproductive status can be considered as a whole [2].

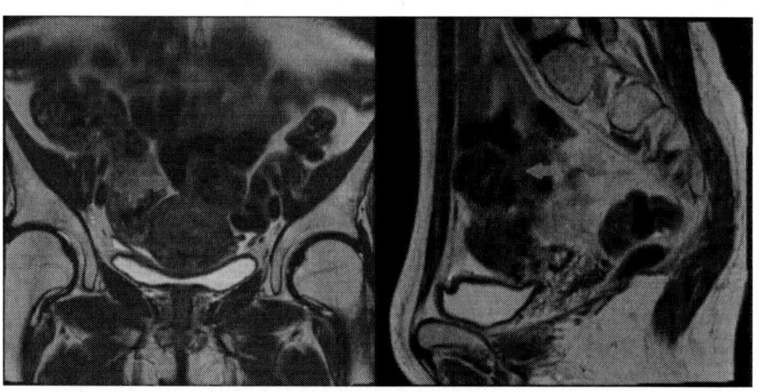

Figure 4. Axial (left) and sagittal T2-weighted turbo spin-echo (right) images obtained after UFE show decrease in the size of the fibroid (arrows).

REFERENCES

[1] Spies JB, Myers ER, Worthington-Kirsch R, et al. The FIBROID Registry: symptom and quality-of life status 1 year after therapy. *Obstet Gynecol.* 2005; 106(6):1309–1318.

[2] Bulman JC, Ascher SM, Spies JB. Current concepts in uterine fibroid embolization. *Radio Graphics*. 2012; 32:1735–1750.

[3] Andrews RT, Spies JB, Sacks D, et al. Patient care and uterine artery embolization for leiomyomata. *J VascInterv Radiol.* 2004; 15(2 pt 1):115–120.

[4] Kim MD, Lee M, Jung DC, et al. Lim ited efficacy of uterine artery embolization for cervical leiomyomas. *J VascInterv Radiol*. 2012; 23(2):236–240.

[5] Parker WH. Etiology, symptomatology, and diagnosis of uterine myomas. *Fertil Steril.* 2007;87(4):725–736.

[6] Leibsohn S, d'Ablaing G, Mishell DR Jr, Schlaerth JB. Leiomyosarcoma in a series of hysterectomies performed for presumed uterine leiomyomas. *Am J Obstet Gynecol.* 1990;162(4):968–974; discussion 974–976.

[7] Tanaka YO, Nishida M, Tsunoda H, Okamoto Y, Yoshikawa H. Smooth muscle tumors of uncertain malignant potential and leiomyosarcomas of the uterus: MR findings. *J Magn Reson Imaging*. 2004; 20(6):998–1007.

[8] Costantino M, Lee J, McCullough M, Nsouli-Maktabi H, Spies JB. Bilateral versus unilateral femoral access for uterine artery embolization: results of a randomized comparative trial. *J Vasc Interv Radiol.* 2010; 21(6):829–835.

[9] Spies JB, Allison S, Flick P, et al. Polyvinyl alcohol particles and tris-acryl gelatin microspheres for uterine artery embolization for leiomyomas: results of a randomized comparative study. *J Vasc Interv Radiol.* 2004;15(8):793–800.

[10] Ruuskanen A, Sipola P, Hippeläinen M, Wüstefeld M, Manninen H. Pain after uterine fibroid embolization is associated with the severity of myometrial ischaemia on magnetic resonance imaging. *Eur Radiol.* 2009;19(12):2977–2985.

[11] Czeyda-Pommersheim F, Magee ST, Cooper C, Hahn WY, Spies JB. Venous thromboembolism after uterine fibroid embolization. *Cardiovasc Intervent Radiol.* 2006;29(6):1136–1140.

[12] Shlansky-Goldberg RD, Coryell L, Stavropoulos SW, et al. Outcomes following fibroid expulsion after uterine artery embolization. *J VascInterv Radiol.* 2011;22(11):1586–1593.

[13] Ryu RK, Chrisman HB, Omary RA, et al. The vascular impact of uterine artery embolization: prospective sonographic assessment of ovarian arterial circulation. *J Vasc Interv Radiol*. 2001;12(9): 1071–1074.

[14] Hutchins FL Jr, Worthington-Kirsch R, Berkowitz RP. Selective uterine artery embolization as primary treatment for symptomatic leiomyomata uteri. *J Am Assoc Gynecol Laparosc*. 1999;6(3):279–284.

[15] Walker W, Green A, Sutton C. Bilateral uterine artery embolisation for myomata: results, complications and failures. *Min Invas Ther & Allied Technol.* 1999;8(6):449–454.

[16] Marret H, Fritel X, Ouldamer L, Pelage JP, Fernandez H et al. Therapeutic management of uterine fibroid tumors: updated French guidelines. *European Journal of Obstetrics & Gynecology and Reproductive Biology.* 2012;165: 156–164.

[17] Mara M, Maskova J, Fucikova Z, Kuzel D, Belsan T, Sosna O. Midterm clinical and first reproductive results of a randomized controlled trial comparing uterine fibroid embolization and myomectomy. *Cardiovasc Intervent Radiol.* 2008;31(1):73–85.

In: Uterine Fibroids
Editors: S. Ferrero and F. Barra
ISBN: 978-1-53615-046-9

Chapter 11

UTERINE MYOMAS AND FERTILITY

Chiara Bondi[1,2], MD, Fabio Barra[1,2], MD and Simone Ferrero[1,2,*], MD, PhD

[1]Obstetrics and Gynecology, Department of Neurosciences, Rehabilitation, Ophthalmology, Genetics, Maternal and Child Health (DiNOGMI), University of Genoa, Italy

[2]Academic Unit of Obstetrics and Gynecology, IRCCS Ospedale San Martino, Genoa, Italy

ABSTRACT

Three important statistics help us better understand the current impact of myomas on fertility: overall, infertility afflicts up to 10 - 15% of couples of reproductive ages; about 10 - 15% of women exhibit uterine myomas; myomas are the single sufficient cause of infertility in 1 - 2.5% of the non-conceiving population.

It has been demonstrated that uterine myomas not only cause distortions of the uterine cavity but also alterations of the endometrial milieu due to high production of pro inflammatory mediators, with subsequent unfavorable molecular and histological effects on embryo implantation.

It is possible to distinguish myomas into three types (submucosal, intramural and subserosal), which can require different surgical therapies. Overall, hysteroscopic myomectomy for submucosal myomas seems increase pregnancy rate. The operative management of intramural myomas remains more controversial, although it appears indicated in case of myomas sized more than 4cm or when multiple attempts of assisted reproductive technology have failed. The impact of subserosal myomas on fertility does not seem relevant.

* Corresponding Author's E-mail: simoneferrero@me.com.

Further studies are necessary for investigating therapeutic indications for myomas in infertile patients. Overall, treatments should be individualized in relation to multiple factors such as myomas size and location, patient's case history, available techniques.

Keywords: uterine myomas, fertility, myomectomy, submucosal myomas, intramural myomas

EPIDEMIOLOGY

Infertility is a widespread problem of modern society, affecting about 10 - 15% of reproductive-aged couples. It is known to be due to different causes that can concern both male and female. The male etiology occurs in about a quarter of cases; the remaining 70 - 75% of female cases are due to dysfunctional ovulation (25%), uterine or tubal causes (20%), other (10%) and unexplained (15%) etiologies [1, 2].

Myomas affect about 35-77% of women of reproductive ages, although their prevalence may be likely higher because of asymptomatic tumors [3]. Among the infertile population, myomas are detected in 5-10% of the cases and they represent the only explicable reason of infertility in 1-2.5% of patients [4].

IMPACT OF MYOMAS ON FERTILITY

It has been demonstrated that uterine factor represents 5% of causes of infertility. Besides the presence of voluminous uterine myomas and polyps, there are other possible uterine causes, such as congenital malformations (uterine agenesis), anomalies of position (fixed uterine retroversion associated with gynecological diseases like endometriosis, chronic salpingitis, etc.), inflammatory processes, extensive uterine synechiae (for example, in Asherman's syndrome) and injuries due to trauma.

Specifically, the presence of uterine myomas determines an abnormal uterine contractility, which can cause torsion or crushing of the cervical canal hindering a correct implant and/or embryo development. Moreover, according to Richards and coworkers, it has been shown how intramural or submucosal myomas are able to alter calcium metabolism, promoting an increase in its intracellular concentrations that cause myometrial irritability [5].

Furthermore, endometrial erosion seems to alter the characteristics of intrauterine fluid by releasing inflammatory mediators and other vasoactive amines; this process may make embryo implantation more difficult [6]. Ben-Nagi et al. showed a reduction in levels of "pro-implant" cytokines, such as interleukin 10 (IL-10) and glycodelin, in the midluteal uterine washing of women with submucosal myomas [7]. The same trend was detected in the expression of some endometrial genes (HOXA10, HOXA11 and BTEB1) favoring endometrial receptivity for blastocysts; they seem to be decreased in infertile women with submucosal myomas during the follicular phase; in particular, it has been shown that these genetic expressions may not only affect the endometrial area above the myoma, but the whole uterine cavity [8]. Myomas may also cause alterations in the Endo-Myometrial Junctional (EMJ) Zones, in particular, reducing the activity of macrophages and uterine natural killers (NK). This seems to hamper an adequate decidualization [9]. In patients with myomas objective histological changes (such as elongation and distortion of the glands, cystic glandular hyperplasia, polyposis and endometrial venule ectasia) have been demonstrated; these changes may decrease the overall endometrial receptivity for blastocysts [10]. Furthermore, the partial interruption of blood circulation at the endometrial level, in particular, in presence of submucosal myomas, may highly decrease the chances of embryo survival [11]. The presence of myomas can also obstruct the fallopian tubes and distortion of uterine cavity. Moreover, myomas can also affect both transport of sperms [12].

Already in 1999, Bulletti and colleagues performed a study on the etiological role of myomas in causing infertility by compering infertile women with or without myomas: it was shown a better rate of spontaneous conception in healthy women (11% in presence of myomas versus 25% without myomas). Additionally, an increased pregnancy rate after their removal was reported (from 25 to 42%) [13].

Other studies showed how myomas (especially submucosal ones) can negatively influence the outcomes of assisted reproductive technology (ART) [14].

DIAGNOSIS

The main used diagnostic methods for assessing of uterine myomas are transvaginal ultrasonography (TVS), hysteroscopy, saline infusion-TVS (S-TVS, known also as hysterosonography), hysterosalpingography, magnetic resonance imaging (MRI) and, only in selected cases, laparoscopy.

TVS is widely used for studying uterine anatomy, especially during the luteal phase to analyze the relation between endometrial thickness and myometrium. Despite of not being widespread, the use of 3D-TVS has demonstrated a diagnostic accuracy of 84.1% for evaluating intrauterine pathology of infertile women [15].

Hysteroscopy is the primary method for defining intrauterine lesions either in office or operative setting (depending on extent and characteristics of each lesion) (Figure 1).

The S-TVS expands the uterine cavity, accurately detecting the limits between endometrium and myometrium. S-TVS has a sensitivity of 75% and a specificity of 90% for diagnosing endometrial defects; moreover, a positive predictive value of 50% and a negative predictive value of 95% have been described in favor of this technique compared to traditional hysterosalpingography [16].

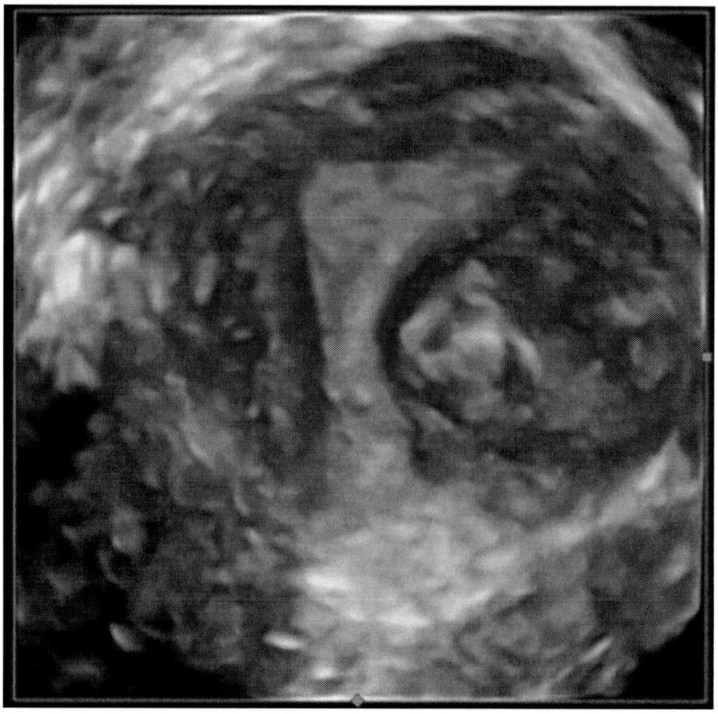

Figure 1. Hysteroscopic view of a submucosal myoma (3.0 x 2.6cm) impacting the endometrial surface.

S-TVS is also useful for differencing pedunculated leiomyomas from polyps. In particular, it is highly appropriated for the evaluation of myomas (submucosal and intramural) imprinting the endometrial cavity.

Overall, the evaluation of myomas infiltration degree and myometrial thickness should be performed by hysteroscopic examination associated with TVS or S-TVS [17].

Hysterosalpingography is an optimal modality for studying congenital uterine anomalies, having a sensitivity of about 98%, a specificity of 35%, a positive predictive value of 70% and a negative predictive value of 8% [18].

MRI is used for completing diagnostic assessment of myomas, despite of being sometimes used also to treat them.

Customized Treatment for Improving Fertility: Which Choice is the Most Appropriate?

Numerous drugs have been investigated for the preoperative treatment of uterine myomas [19-23]. However, long-term medical treatment should not be recommended as first-line treatment for infertile women with myomas because of suppression of ovulation and other eventual hormonal alterations (including the reduction of estrogens) induced by drugs employed in this setting [24-25].

Overall, the impact of myomectomy on infertility is not clear. In fact, in the few studies performed on this topic, there are a relevant clinical variability of myomas (for localization, extension and number) and techniques employed (surgical and not only). Similarly, the comparison between laparoscopic and open approaches is difficult, because these surgical options are operator-dependent and characterized by multiple variables (for example, the not routinely use of antiadhesion agents). However, both techniques seem to be equally effective in fertility restoration, although laparoscopy is known to be associated with better postoperative course and less morbidity.

It is necessary to remember that the submucosal myomas are preferentially managed by hysteroscopy within 5cm of diameter. Above this size, it is recommended to perform the hysteroscopic approach in more surgical-steps (according to The Society of Obstetricians and Gynecologists of Canada [SOGC] guidelines of March 2015). Currently, there are conflicting opinions about the optimal management of intramural myomas, as few studies have been performed in this setting [26-28], and some of these contain important bias. First of all, some patients with submucosal myomas are mistakenly included into the analyzed population; moreover, not all the intramural myomas are correctly recognized (the largest ones are often subjected to major surgeon techniques, thus avoiding the hysteroscopic approach). Furthermore, there are no specific studies aiming to analyze the distance between fibroid edge and endometrium. Overall, at the moment the surgical options for these patients should be expertly individualized.

Myomectomy may have an impact on fertility depending from the specific location of the lesion. Casini et al. demonstrated an improvement in the clinical pregnancy rate after excision of submucosal myomas compared to women undergoing expectant management (43.3% versus 27.2%). The same authors reported positive outcomes about the excision of intramural myomas compared to women undergoing expectant management (pregnancy rate of 56.5% versus 41%) [29]. In 2015, Galliano et al. emphasized the correct execution of myomectomy for intramural myomas (according to FIGO stages from 3 to 6), in particular when they have size greater than 4cm. The authors suggested the removal of smaller myomas only in case of multiple IVF failures [12].

The impact on fertility of subserosal myomas seems to be insignificant. Thus, their removal is indicated only in the case of causing important clinical symptoms, provoking complications during pregnancy or coexisting with other myoma types.

Since the size of the fibroid seems to have a proportionally negative impact on the efficacy of ART therapies, the removal of intramural or submucosal myomas of dimensions greater than 5cm is routinely recommended [30]. Despite this, Metwally et al. claim that the value of current studies on this topic is too limited to draw accurate conclusion [31]. Pritts et al. underscored the importance of the proximity of the myoma to the endometrium for worsening the fertility; thus, these authors suggested the need of an accurate uterine cavity evaluation in presence of submucosal myomas [32]. According to the ASMR (American Society for Reproductive Medicine), particular attention should be payed to those patients who, despite of having submucosal myomas, do not have a relevant distortion of the uterine cavity (in these cases, myomectomy could represent an overtreatment with the subsequent risk of developing adhesion) [33].

Clearly, all these assumptions are valid for women seeking a pregnancy without other the concomitant presence of additional infertility factors.

Conclusion

Until now, the relation between myomas and infertility remains very debated; this is essentially due to sufficient controlled randomized studies on this topic.

At the moment, it is critical to correctly define the size, numbers and location of myomas in order to understand how they may influence fertility outcomes in each patient.

It seems that some infertile women can benefit from removal of intracavitary myomas, especially in the cases of submucosal myomas, with a size greater than 5cm or more than two or three. The effect of intramural myomas is more uncertain (even if those larger than 4cm have largely demonstrated to imprint the uterine cavity, thus reducing pregnancy outcomes). Instead, subserosal myomas do not seem to affect fertility of patients (especially, in case of not being too bulky) [34].

References

[1] American Society for Reproductive Medicine. Aging and infertility in women. *Fertil. Steril.,* 2006a; 86 (Suppl. 4): S248.

[2] Ferrero, S., Abbamonte, L. H., Giordano, M., Parisi, M., Ragni, N. Uterine myomas, dyspareunia, and sexual function. *Fertility and Sterility*, 2006.

[3] Cramer, S., Patel, A. The frequency of uterine leiomyomas. *Am. J. Clin. Pathol.*, 1990; 94: 435 - 8.

[4] Cook, H., Ezzati, M., Segars, J., et al. The impact of uterine leiomyomas on reproductive outcomes. *Minerva Ginecol.,* 2010; 62: 225 - 36.

[5] Richards, P. A., Richards, P. D. G., Tiltman, A. J. The ultrastructure of fibromyomatous myometrium and its relationship to infertility. *Hum. Reprod. Update*, 1998; 4(5):520 - 5.

[6] Mukhopadhaya, N., Pokuah Asante, G. P., Manyonda, I. T. Uterine fibroids: impact on fertility and pregnancy loss. *Obstet. Gynaecol. Reprod. Med.,* 2007; 17:311e7.

[7] Ben-Nagi, J., Miell, J., Mavrelos, D., Naftalin, J., Lee, C., Jurkovic, D. Endometrial implantation factors in women with submucous uterine fibroids. *Reprod. Biomed. Online*, 2010; 21(5):610 - 5.

[8] Rackow, B., Taylor, H. Submucosal uterine leiomyomas have a global effect on molecular determinants of endometrial receptivity. *Fertil. Steril.,* 2010; 93:2027 - 34.

[9] Kitaya, K., Yasuo, T. Leukocyte density and composition in human cycling endometrium with uterine fibroids. *Hum. Immunol.,* 2010; 71:161 - 63.

[10] Somigliana, E., Vercellini, P., Daguati, R., et al. Fibroids and female reproduction: a critical analysis of the evidence. *Hum. Reprod. Update,* 2007; 13:465 - 76.

[11] Farhi, J., Ashkenazi, J., Feldberg, D., Dicker, D., Orvieto, R. and Ben Rafael, Z. Effect of uterine leiomyomata on the results of in vitro fertilization treatment. *Hum. Reprod.,* 1995; 10: 2576 - 78.

[12] Galliano, D., Bellver, J., Díaz-García, C., et al. ART and uterine pathology: how relevant is the maternal side for implantation? *Hum. Reprod. Update,* 2015; 21:13e38.

[13] Bulletti, C., De Ziegler, D., Polli, V., et al. The role of leiomyomas in infertility. *J. Am. Assoc. Gynecol. Laparosc.*, 1999; 6:441 - 5.

[14] Savasi, V., Leone, F. P., Fusè, F., Parisi, F., Cetin, I. Assisted reproductive technologies and uterine factors influencing their success. *Minerva Ginecol.,* 2013; 65(5):505 - 524.

[15] Apirakviriya, C., Rungruxsirivorn, T., Phupong, V., Wisawasukmongchol, W. Diagnostic accuracy of 3D-transvaginal ultrasound in detecting uterine cavity abnormalities in infertile patients as compared with hysteroscopy. *European Journal of Obstetrics and Gynecology and Reproductive Biology,* 2016;200:24-28.

[16] Soares, S., Barbosa dos Reis, M., Camargos, A.: Diagnostic accuracy of sonohysterography, transvaginal sonography, and hysterosalpingography in patients with uterine cavity diseases. *Fertil. Steril.*, 2000; 73: 406.

[17] SOGC Clinical Practice Guideline. The Management of Uterine Fibroids in Women With Otherwise Unexplained Infertility. *J. Obstet. Gynaecol. Can.,* 2015; 37(3): 277 - 85.

[18] Hoffman, L. B., Schorge, J. O., Shaffer, J. I. et al. Evaluation of the Infertile Couple. In: *Williams Gynecology, Mc Graw Hill Medical*- Second edition 2012; Chapter 19: 506 - 28.

[19] Ferrero, S., Alessandri, F., Vellone, V. G., Venturini, P. L., Leone Roberti Maggiore, U. Three-month treatment with ulipristal acetate prior to laparoscopic myomectomy of large uterine myomas: a retrospective study. *Eur. J. Obstet. Gynecol. Reprod. Biol.,* 2016; 205:43 - 7.

[20] Ferrero, S., Racca, A., Tafi, E., Alessandri, F., Venturini, P. L., Leone Roberti Maggiore, U. Ulipristal Acetate Before High Complexity Hysteroscopic

Myomectomy: A Retrospective Comparative Study. *J. Minim. Invasive Gynecol.*, 2016; 23(3):390 - 5.

[21] Ferrero, S., Scala, C., Barra, F. Regarding "Does Ulipristal Acetate Affect Surgical Experience at Laparoscopic Myomectomy?". *J. Minim. Invasive Gynecol.*, 2018; 25(3):541.

[22] Ferrero, S., Vellone, V. G., Barra, F. Pharmacokinetic drug evaluation of ulipristal acetate for the treatment of uterine fibroids. *Expert Opin. Drug Metab. Toxicol.*, 2018; 14(1):107 - 16.

[23] Ferrero, S., Vellone, V. G., Barra. F., Scala, C. Ulipristal Acetate before Hysteroscopic and Laparoscopic Surgery for Uterine Myomas: Help or Hindrance? *Gynecol. Obstet. Invest.*, 2018:1 - 13.

[24] Tafi, E., Scala, C., Leone Roberti Maggiore, U., Bizzarri, N., Candiani, M., Venturini, P. L., et al. Drug safety evaluation of ulipristal acetate in the treatment of uterine fibroids. *Expert Opin. Drug Saf.*, 2015; 14(6):965 - 77.

[25] Sohn, G. S., Cho, S., Kim, Y. M., Cho, C. H., Kim, M. R., Lee, S. R., et al. Current medical treatment of uterine fibroids. *Obstet. Gynecol. Sci.*, 2018; 61(2):192 - 201.

[26] Alessandri, F., Lijoi, D., Mistrangelo, E., Ferrero, S., Ragni, N. Randomized study of laparoscopic versus minilaparotomic myomectomy for uterine myomas. *J. Minim. Invasive Gynecol.*, 2006; 13(2):92 - 7.

[27] Alessandri, F., Remorgida, V., Venturini, P. L., Ferrero, S. Unidirectional barbed suture versus continuous suture with intracorporeal knots in laparoscopic myomectomy: a randomized study. *J. Minim. Invasive Gynecol.*, 2010; 17(6):725 - 9.

[28] Flyckt, R., Coyne, K., Falcone, T. Minimally Invasive Myomectomy. *Clin. Obstet. Gynecol.*, 2017; 60(2):252 - 72.

[29] Casini, M., Rossi, F., Agostini, R., et al. Effects of the position of fibroids on fertility. *Gynecol. Endocrinol.*, 2006; 22:106 - 9.

[30] Bulletti, C., DE Ziegler, D., Levi Setti, P., et al. Myomas, pregnancy outcome, and in vitrofertilization. *Ann. NY Acad. Sci.*, 2004; 1034: 84 - 92.

[31] Metwally, M., Farquhar, C. M., Li, T. C. Is another meta-analysis on the effects of intramural fibroids on reproductive outcomes needed? *Reprod. Biomed. Online*, 2011;23(1): 2 - 14.

[32] Pritts, E. A., Parker, W. H., Olive, D. L. Fibroids and infertility: an updated systematic reviewof the evidence. *Fertility and Sterility*, 2009; 91(4): 1215 - 23.

[33] Practice Committee of the American Society for Reproductive Medicine. Removal of myomas in asymptomaticpatients to improve fertility and/or reduce miscarriage rate: a guideline. *Fertility and Sterility*, 2017; 108(3):416 - 25.

[34] Zepiridis, L. I., Grimbizis, G. F., Tarlatzis, B. C. Infertility and uterine fibroids. *Best Practice and Research Clinical Obstetrics and Gynaecology*, 2016.

In: Uterine Fibroids
Editors: S. Ferrero and F. Barra

ISBN: 978-1-53615-046-9

Chapter 12

UTERINE MYOMAS AND SEXUAL FUNCTION

Stefano Ciccarelli[1,2], MD, Fabio Barra[1,2], MD and Simone Ferrero[1,2,*], MD, PhD

[1]Obstetrics and Gynecology, Department of Neurosciences, Rehabilitation, Ophthalmology, Genetics, Maternal and Child Health (DiNOGMI), University of Genoa, Genoa, Italy

[2]Academic Unit of Obstetrics and Gynecology, IRCCS Ospedale San Martino, Genoa, Italy

ABSTRACT

An association between uterine myomas and sexual dysfunction, and in particular deep dyspareunia, has been suggested by recent epidemiological studies. This association has been suggested to be stronger in case of fundal uterine myomas.

However, available data in the literature are scanty and controversial. Likewise, the role of treatment of myomas on ameliorating sexual function is poorly understood: regarding to this, myomectomy and artery embolization seem to improve the dyspareunia of women affected by uterine myomas. Otherwise, case reports have shown that sexual dysfunction can also occur after the surgical treatment of these benign tumors.

Keywords: uterine myomas, treatment, sexual dysfunction, dyspareunia

[*] Corresponding Author's E-mail: simoneferrero@me.com.

1. Introduction

Uterine myomas, which are the most common benign tumors of women, are often associated with relevant symptoms like abnormal uterine bleeding, pelvic pain or pressure, reduced urinary capacity of bladder, constipation and reproductive dysfunction [1]. More recently, particular attention has been given to the association between myomas and quality of life of patients, [2] with particular regard to their impact on sexual function.

Table 1 shows the main results from selected published studies that considered the frequency of dyspareunia or other sexual dysfunction in women affected by myomas in comparison with women without this condition; the results on this topic are controversial [2-7]. For example, no relation between deep dyspareunia and presence of myomas emerged in a study conducted at our institution (Genoa, Italy) by Ferrero et al. [5]. Otherwise, a strong association has been reported in another population study done by Lippman et al. [7].

These discrepancies may be partly due to the different designs and methodological pitfalls of these observational studies.

First of all, it is important to under light the difficulty of assessing prevalence of sexual dysfunction at baseline among women with myomas; in fact, these studies tend to use heterogenous patients' population and diagnostic criteria.

For example, in the study by Ferrero et al., only women undergoing surgery for benign gynecological conditions were enrolled [5]. Conversely, in another multi-countries study, the diagnosis of myomas was self-reported by the patients [2].

Moreover, different control groups have been employed in these articles: in the study by Ferrero et al., patients with myomas were compared to women scheduled for surgery for ovarian cysts [5]; Lipman et al. did a comparison between women with familiar or sporadic myomas [6]; in another study, patients with lifelong diagnosis of myomas were compared to women without diagnosis of this benign condition [2].

The diagnostic criteria of dyspareunia and sexual dysfunction also differ among these data: some studies used a simple yes/no question [3], others the VAS (Visual Analogue Scale) pain scale [5, 7] and others standardized questionnaires such as the GSSI (Global Sexual Satisfaction Index) and the FSFI (Female Sexual Function Index) [4]. For example, the mean FSFI scores in women with myomas is affected by menstrual cycle; thus, by using this tool in a small study, nearly half of the women included reported a different grade of sexual dysfunction in relation to the menstrual period [8].

Although it is known that uterine myomas are associated to sexual dysfunction, it does not seem to have a direct effect on either the arousal or orgasmic phases. However, deep dyspareunia is thought to precede and worsen other common sexual dysfunctions in these patients (in particular, loss of desire, the most common sexual dysfunction observed among post-menopausal women).

Table 1. Findings from selected studies on the association between uterine myomas and sexual function

	Study Design	Population and Number of Patients	Dyspareunia Assessment	Results
Moshesh et al. [3] (2014)	Cross sectional study	827 women aged 35–49 randomly selected from the membership rolls of a prepaid health plan.	Questionnaire on symptoms with questions about DD	UM were associated with DD (OR = 1.7)
Zimmermann et al. [2] (2012)	Population-based cross-sectional study	21,479 women across 8 countries	Simple yes/no question	women with UM reported significantly more pain during sexual intercourse (23.5% vs. 9.1%)
Ertunc et al. [4] (2009)	Case control study	80 women with UM and 75 control women.	FSFI	Women with UM had lower FSFI pain and satisfaction scores than women without UM.
Ferrero et al. [5] (2006)	Cross sectional study.	305 premenopausal women scheduled for surgery for benign gynecological conditions (214 women with UM with or without ovarian cysts and 91 with other conditions)	DD by VAS SF by GSSA	No association between UM and dyspareunia and sexual function
Osoko et al. [6] (2005)	Case-control study	Women with (n = 45) and without family history of UM (n = 255)	Questionnaire on symptoms with questions on dysmenorrhea	Incidence of DD in women with familiar UM was 43.2% vs 27.9% in women with sporadic UM (P = 0.012)
Lippman et al. [7] (2003)	Population-based cross-sectional study	Population sample from the Seveso Women's Health Study conducted in 1976	DD severity (VAS scale). Self-report of the avoiding intercourse because of pain.	Women with UM were more likely to report mild and severe DD (OR mild = 1.4, OR severe 1.8)
Lippman et al. [7] (2003)	Population-based cross-sectional study	Population sample from the Seveso Women's Health Study conducted in 1976	DD severity (VAS scale). Self-report of the avoiding intercourse because of pain.	Women with UM were more likely to report mild and severe DD (OR mild = 1.4, OR severe 1.8)

DD = deep dyspareunia, SF = sexual function, UM = uterine myomas, FSFI = Female sexual function index, OR = odds ratio, VAS = visual analogue scale, GSSA = Global Sexual Satisfaction Index.

Different myomas and patients' characteristics may differently influence sexual function. For example, in a study including 111 premenopausal women affected by myomas consulting for routine examination, uterine retroversion was associated with a higher prevalence of dyspareunia (66.7% versus 42.1%, p = 0.03) and a higher VAS score for dyspareunia (2.7+/-2.6 versus 1.6+/-2.4, p = 0.04) [9]. Moreover, fundal myomas have been reported to be strongly associated with dyspareunia in two other studies [4, 5]. Specifically, in the study by Ertung et al., fundal and posterior myomas were associated with pain, whereas only posterior myomas were related to a decrease in overall FSFI scores [4].

Another interesting finding also emerged in a comparative study conducted by Osoko et al., in which women with myomas with (n = 45) and without (n = 255) family history of myomas were considered. Familial prevalence of myomas was associated with a higher incidence of deep dyspareunia (43.2% versus 27.9%; P = 0.012). Moreover, there was an increased expression of angiogenetic substances such as VEGF-A (vascular endothelial growth factor-A) in myoma tissue of patients with familial myomas compared to those without familial myomas (64% versus 28%). Moreover, women with a uterine volume over 200 cm had significantly lower mean FSFI and pain [6], as also emerged in the study by Ertung et al. [4]. However, uterine volume was not associated with severity of dyspareunia in another study [3].

Patients may undergo several treatments in order to alleviate myomas-related symptoms and to improve general quality of life. In general, positive postoperative sexual function and good quality of life are considered important outcomes for procedure aiming to treat myomas. In the study by Ertung et al. [4], the mean FSFI of the patients improved significantly after undergoing myomectomy. Similarly, postoperative FSFI domain scores (desire, lubrication, arousal, orgasm, satisfaction, pain) were also significantly higher than preoperative scores in a study which included 95,129 patients undergoing laparoscopic myomectomy [10]. Likewise, an improved sexual function has been reported after artery embolization [11] or high-intensity focused ultrasound treatment for myomas [12].

Otherwise, case reports have shown that sexual dysfunction can occur after the invasive treatment of uterine myomas [13]. Anyway, this important adverse effect is relatively understudied and new studies on this topic are needed.

In conclusion, the association between uterine myomas and sexual function is a issue of recent interest in the gynecological literature. Overall, published studies offer limited and data mainly due to methodological problems (for example, difference in the study design and diagnostic criteria). In the near future, findings from different populations and based on more standardized criteria may provide a more detailed picture of the association between myomas and sexual function as well as the impact of their treatment on ameliorating patients' quality of life.

REFERENCES

[1] Stovall, D. W. Clinical symptomatology of uterine leiomyomas. *Clin. Obstet. Gynecol.*, 2001;44:364 –71.

[2] Zimmermann, A., Bernuit, D., Gerlinger, C., Schaefers, M., Geppert, K. Prevalence, symptoms and management ofuterine fibroids: an international internet-based survey of 21,746 women. *BMC Women's Health,* 2012;12:6.

[3] Moshesh, M., Olshan, A. F., Saldana, T., Baird, D. Examining the relationship between uterine fibroids and dyspareunia among premenopausal women in the United States. *J. Sex. Med.,* 2014; 11(3):800-8.

[4] Ertunc, D., Uzun, R., Tok, E. C., Doruk, A., Dilek, S. The effect of myoma uteri andmyomectomy on sexual function. *J. Sex. Med.,* 2009; 6(4):1032-1038.

[5] Ferrero, S., Abbamonte, L. H., Giordano, M., Parisi, M., Ragni, N., Remorgida, V. Uterine myomas, dyspareunia, and sexual function. *Fertil. Steril.,* 2006; 86:1504–10.

[6] Okolo, S. O., Gentry, C. C., Perrett, C. W., Maclean, A. B. Familial prevalence of uterine fibroids is associated with distinct clinical and molecular features. *Hum. Reprod.*, 2005;20:2321–4.

[7] Lippman, S. A., Warner, M., Samuels, S., Olive, D., Vercellini, P., Eskenazi, B. Uterine fibroids and gynecologic pain symptoms in a population-based study. *Fertil. Steril.,* 2003; 80:1488–94.

[8] Laughlin-Tommaso, S. K., Borah, B. J., Stewart, E. A. The effect of menses on standardized assessment of sexual dysfunction among women with uterine fibroids: a cohort study. *Fertil. Steril.*, 2015; 104(2): 435–439.

[9] Fauconnier, A., Dubuisson, J. B., Foulot, H., Deyrolles, C., Sarrot, F., Laveyssière, M. N., Jansé-Marec, J., Bréart, G. Mobile uterine retroversion is associated with dyspareunia and dysmenorrhea in an unselected population of women. *Eur. J. Obstet. Gynecol. Reprod. Biol.*, 2006;127(2):252-6.

[10] Radosa, J. C., Radosa, C. G., Mavrova, R., Wagenpfei Hamza, S. A., Joukhadar, R., Baum, S. Karsten, Juhasz-Boess, I., Solomayer, E. F., Radosa, M. P. Postoperative Quality of Life and Sexual Function in Premenopausal Women Undergoing Laparoscopic Myomectomy for Symptomatic Fibroids: A Prospective Observational Cohort Study. *PLoS ONE,* 2016.

[11] Voogt, M. J., De Vries, J., Fonteijn, W., Lohle, M., Boekkooi, P. F. *Sexual functioning and psychological well-being after uterine artery embolization in women with symptomatic uterine fibroids.* 2009;92(2):756-61.

[12] Wang, X. 1., Qin, J., Wang, L., Chen, J., Chen, W., Tang, L. Effect of high-intensity focused ultrasound on sexual function in the treatment of uterine fibroids: comparison to conventional myomectomy. *Arch. Gynecol. Obstet.,* 2013; 288(4):851-8.

[13] Louie, A. R., Armstrong, J. A., Findeiss, L. K., Goodwin, S. C. Comparison of Sexual Dysfunction Using the Female Sexual Function Index following Surgical Treatments for Uterine Fibroids Case Reports in *Obstetrics and Gynecology Volume*, 2012; 2012:368136.

In: Uterine Fibroids
Editors: S. Ferrero and F. Barra

ISBN: 978-1-53615-046-9

Chapter 13

Office Hysteroscopic Myomectomy Using the Versapoint Bipolar Electrode

***Simone Ferrero*[1,2,*]*, MD, PhD, Carolina Sala*[1,2]*, MD and Fabio Barra, MD*[1,2]**

[1]Academic Unit of Obstetrics and Gynecology,
IRCCS Ospedale Policlinico San Martino, Genoa, Italy
[2]Department of Neurosciences, Rehabilitation, Ophthalmology, Genetics,
Maternal and Child Health (DiNOGMI),
University of Genoa, Genoa, Italy

Abstract

Submucosal myomas are usually treated by hysteroscopic resection under general anesthesia. However, in the last twenty years, the Versapoint Bipolar Electrosurgical System has been used to treat small submucosal myomas (largest diameter < 2cm). The Versapoint bipolar electrode has several advantages over conventional hysteroscopic surgery. It does not require cervical dilation, thus decreasing the risk of cervical incompetence, cervical lacerations, and uterine perforation. It can be used with physiological saline as distention medium, thus decreasing the risk of fluid overload.

Furthermore, it allows avoiding the risks of anesthesia and the inconvenience of the operating room. The Twizzle electrode is used to divide the myoma in two half-spheres. Subsequently, each fragment is further sliced until it can be pulled out through the uterine cavity using grasping forceps with teeth.

---

[*] Corresponding Author's E-mail: simoneferrero@me.com.

Keywords: hysteroscopy, myoma, myomectomy, submucosal myomas, Versapoint

INTRODUCTION

Submucous myomas are located under the mucosal layer and they protrude into the uterine cavity. These myomas may cause several symptoms including heavy menstrual bleeding, recurrent miscarriages, infertility and dysmenorrhea. A classification of submucous myomas depends on the degree of invasion of the tumor in the uterine wall. Type 0 myomas (Figure 1) are entirely located in the uterine cavity and they do not invade the myometrium; type I myomas invades for less than 50% the uterine wall and type II myomas invades for more than 50% the uterine wall.

While intramural and subserosal myomas are usually treated by minilaparotomy or laparoscopy [1, 2]; submucosal myomas are commonly treated by hysteroscopic resection under general anesthesia [3, 4]. When multiple submucosal myomas are present, a preoperative hormonal treatment may facilitate surgery and increases the chances of a complete hysteroscopic resection in one procedure [5, 6].

However, when these myomas are small they can be excised by using small diameter hysteroscopic sheaths (5mm) that include a working channel and continuous flow features.

This technology allows avoiding the use of general anesthesia and operative room [7].

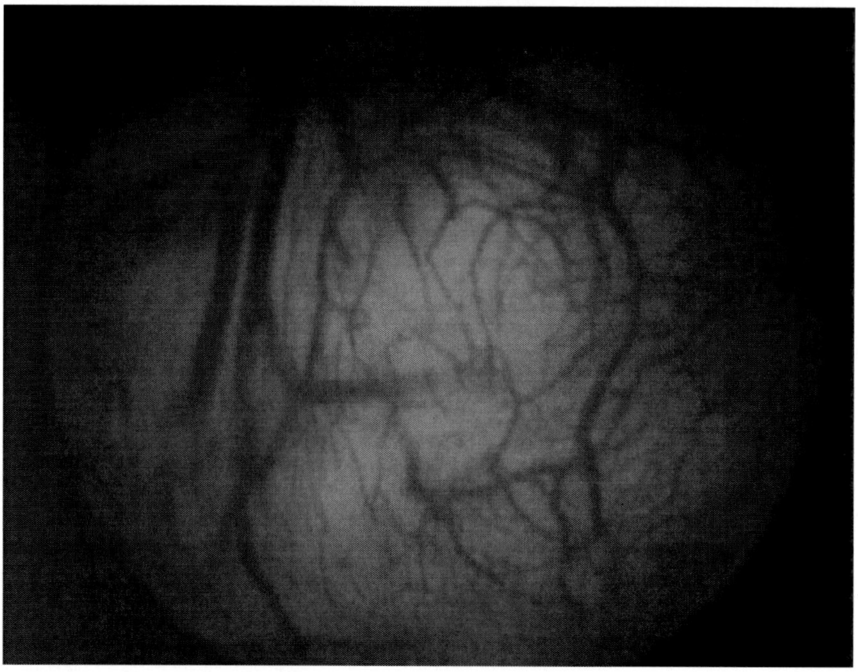

Figure 1. Submucosal type 0 myoma.

SURGICAL TECHNIQUE

One of devices most commonly used during office hysteroscopy for the treatment of uterine myomas is the Versapoint Bipolar Electrosurgical System (Gynecare, Ethicon Inc., NJ, USA), an electrosurgical generator dedicated to hysteroscopic procedures. It can work with two different small caliber electrodes (1.7mm): the Twizzle that allows a precise vaporization and resembles cutting; the Spring that is used for diffuse tissue vaporization. An obvious advantage of this device is that it can be used with physiological saline as distention medium, thus decreasing the risk of fluid overload when compared with the use of hypotonic nonionic media (such as glycine, sorbitol or mannitol). The Versapoint Bipolar Electrosurgical System can be used with small hysteroscopes (5mm diameter) and, thus, it does not require to dilate the uterine cervix.

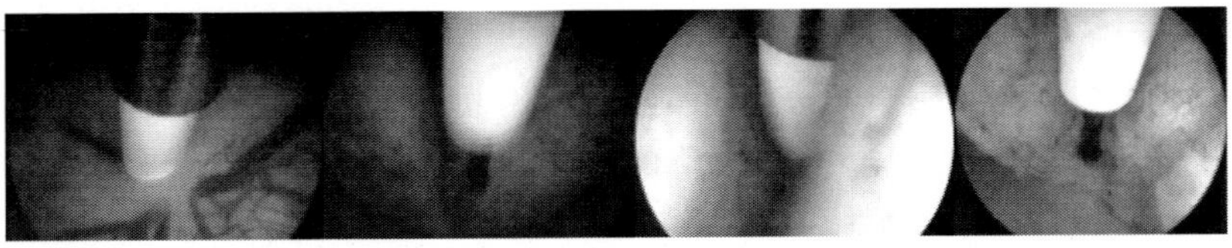

Figure 2. The myoma is divided in two half-spheres by using the Versapoint Twizzle electrode.

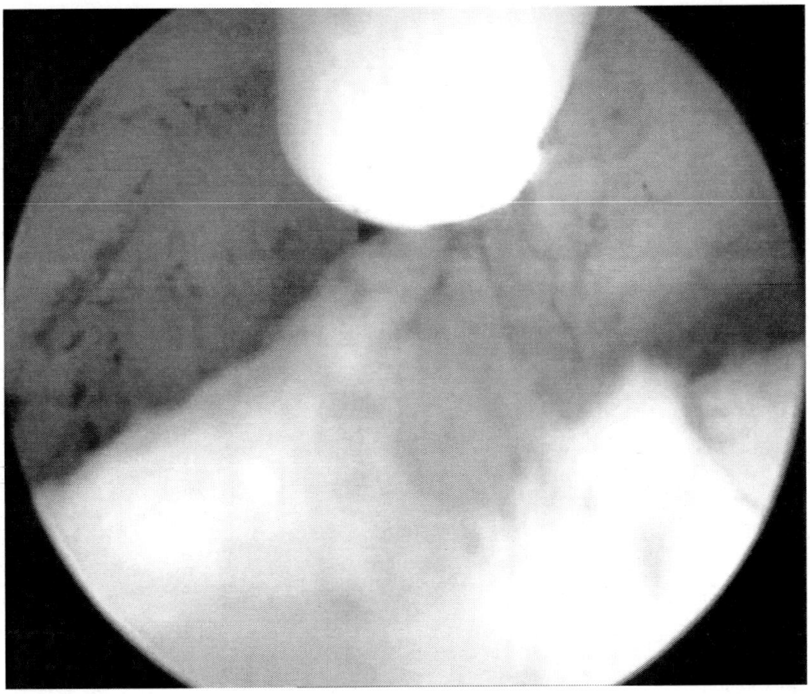

Figure 3. The half-myoma is further sliced in two fragments by using the Versapoint Twizzle electrode.

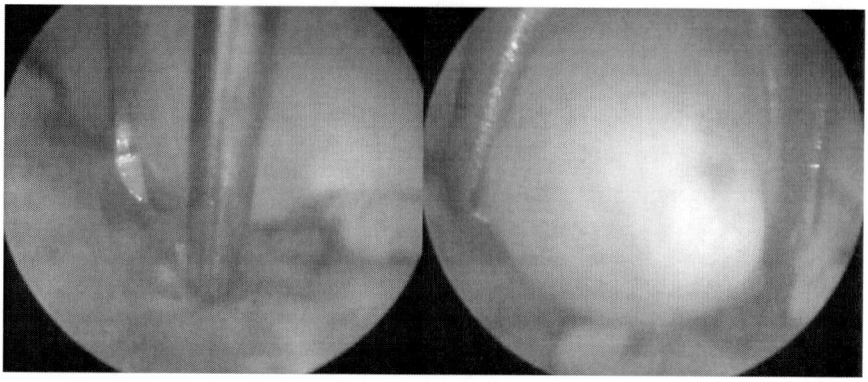

Figure 4. Grasping forceps are used to pull out the myoma fragments.

At the beginning of the procedure the myoma is separated from the capsule using grasping forceps or scissors in order to avoid any myometrial stimulation. Since one the most difficult steps in the treatment of submucosal myomas is the extraction from the uterine cavity, the myoma is initially divided in two half-spheres by using the Versapoint Twizzle electrode and then each of these fragments is further sliced until it can be pulled out through the uterine cavity using a grasping forceps with teeth (Figure 2-3-4) [8].

The patient should be informed that mild uterine cramping and vaginal bleeding may occur during the first week after the procedure.

Clinical Studies

The use of the Versapoint bipolar electrode for office hysteroscopic myomectomy was originally described in small series about 20 years ago [9-11]. In 2002, Shi et al. described their experience of hysteroscopic myomectomies performed using the Versapoint system in a prospective study including 94 women. The patients were treated under continuous epidural anesthesia. All the myomas were completely resected in one procedure, apart from some residual myomas in the five patients with more than two submucosal myomas. Four patients had blood loss >100ml during surgery but no other complication occurred [12]. Another study by Clark et al. investigated the clinical efficacy and safety of the hysteroscopic treatment of submucosal myomas performed using the Versapoint system in 37 symptomatic women. The myomas extending into the myometrium were only partially excised while small submucosal myomas (sessile, diameter < 1 cm) were ablated if excision was considered unfeasible. The treatment was successful in all the patients; in fact, no patient required to repeat the procedure. There were no serious complications. The amount of abnormal uterine bleeding was significantly decreased at 6 months compared to immediately prior to treatment; 92% of the patients were satisfied with the treatment [13]. In an observational study, Bettocchi et al. reported their experience in the office hysteroscopic treatment of benign intrauterine pathologies in 501 women. The procedures were performed with or without anesthesia. The study included 49 submucosal myomas <2cm and 21-partial intramural myomas with a submucosal section <1.5cm. The largest diameter of the 49 submucosal myomas ranged between 0.5 and 2.0 cm; the average operative time was 22 minutes due to the need to slice the myoma prior to removal from the uterine cavity. The 21-partial intramural myomas were preoperatively treated with gonadotropin releasing hormone analogues. Their diameter ranged between 0.6 and 1.5cm and the operative time was 31 minutes. The hysteroscopic treatment was successful in all the patients and there was no major complication [8].

CONCLUSION

The Versapoint bipolar electrode is an effective alternative to conventional hysteroscopic surgery in the treatment of small submucosal myomas (largest diameter < 2 cm). Theoretically, the Versapoint bipolar electrode could also be used to treat larger myomas (diameter > 2 cm); however, these procedures are time-consuming and yield lower quality results [8]. This device can be used with physiological saline as distention medium, thus decreasing the risk of fluid overload [14]. It is well tolerated and safe, in fact most of the studies do not report major complications (such as vagal reflex and uterine perforation) [8, 12, 13]. An advantage of the Versapoint bipolar electrode is that it does not require cervical dilation, thus decreasing the risk of cervical incompetence, cervical lacerations, and uterine perforation [15]. A final advantage of the Versapoint is that it allows to avoid the risks of anesthesia and the inconvenience of the operating room [7]. A drawback of Versapoint is the increased cost compared to other devices.

REFERENCES

[1] Alessandri, F., Lijoi, D., Mistrangelo, E., Ferrero, S., Ragni, N. Randomized study of laparoscopic versus minilaparotomic myomectomy for uterine myomas. *J. Minim. Invasive Gynecol.,* 2006;13(2):92-7.

[2] Alessandri, F., Remorgida, V., Venturini, P. L., Ferrero, S. Unidirectional barbed suture versus continuous suture with intracorporeal knots in laparoscopic myomectomy: a randomized study. *J. Minim. Invasive Gynecol.,* 2010;17(6):725-9.

[3] Thubert, T., Foulot, H., Vinchant, M., Santulli, P., Marzouk, P., Borghese, B., et al. Surgical treatment: Myomectomy and hysterectomy; Endoscopy: A major advancement. *Best Pract. Res. Clin. Obstet. Gynaecol.*, 2016;34:104-21.

[4] Mazzon, I., Bettocchi, S., Fascilla, F., D. Dep, Palma, F., Zizolfi, B., et al. Resectoscopic myomectomy. *Minerva ginecologica*, 2016; 68(3):334-44.

[5] Ferrero, S., Racca, A., Tafi, E., Alessandri, F., Venturini, P. L., Leone Roberti Maggiore, U. Ulipristal Acetate Before High Complexity Hysteroscopic Myomectomy: A Retrospective Comparative Study. *J. Minim. Invasive Gynecol.*, 2016;23(3):390-5.

[6] Bizzarri, N., Ghirardi, V., Remorgida, V., Venturini, P. L., Ferrero, S. Three-month treatment with triptorelin, letrozole and ulipristal acetate before hysteroscopic resection of uterine myomas: prospective comparative pilot study. *Eur. J. Obstet. Gynecol. Reprod. Biol.,* 2015;192:22-6.

[7] Salazar, C. A., Isaacson, K. B. Office Operative Hysteroscopy: An Update. *J. Minim. Invasive Gynecol.*, 2018;25(2):199-208.

[8] Bettocchi, S., Ceci, O., Di Venere, R., Pansini, M. V., Pellegrino, A., Marello, F., et al. Advanced operative office hysteroscopy without anaesthesia: analysis of 501 cases treated with a 5 Fr. bipolar electrode. *Human Reproduction*, 2002; 17(9):2435-8.

[9] Kung, R. C., Vilos, G. A., Thomas, B., Penkin, P., Zaltz, A. P., Stabinsky, S. A. A new bipolar system for performing operative hysteroscopy in normal saline. *J. Am. Assoc. Gynecol. Laparosc.,* 1999;6(3):331-6.

[10] Toth, D., Kuzel, D., Fucikova, Z., Hruskova, H., Cibula, D., Zivny, J. [Initial experience with the Versapoint bipolar electrode in hysteroscopic tissue vaporization]. *Ceska Gynekol.*, 2000;65(4):269-72.

[11] Loffer, F. D. Preliminary experience with the VersaPoint bipolar resectoscope using a vaporizing electrode in a saline distending medium. *J. Am. Assoc. Gynecol. Laparosc.*, 2000;7(4):498-502.

[12] Shi, Y. P., Xie, H. L., Feng, Z. C., Wang, Y. B. Hysteroscopic myomectomy using the Versapoint system in a normal saline field: report of 94 cases. *Gynaecological Endoscopy*, 2002;11:257-60.

[13] Clark TJ, Mahajan D, Sunder P, Gupta JK. Hysteroscopic treatment of symptomatic submucous fibroids using a bipolar intrauterine system: a feasibility study. *Eur J Obstet Gynecol Reprod Biol.* 2002;100(2):237-42.

[14] Berg A, Sandvik L, Langebrekke A, Istre O. A randomized trial comparing monopolar electrodes using glycine 1.5% with two different types of bipolar electrodes (TCRis, Versapoint) using saline, in hysteroscopic surgery. *Fertil Steril.* 2009;91(4):1273-8.

[15] Roy, K. K., Metta, S., Kansal, Y., Kumar, S., Singhal, S., Vanamail, P. A Prospective Randomized Study Comparing Unipolar Versus Bipolar Hysteroscopic Myomectomy in Infertile Women. *J. Hum. Reprod. Sci.,* 2017.

In: Uterine Fibroids
Editors: S. Ferrero and F. Barra
ISBN: 978-1-53615-046-9

Chapter 14

RISK OF SARCOMA DISSEMINATION DURING LAPAROSCOPIC MYOMECTOMY

Matteo Tantari[1,2], MD, Fabio Barra[1,2], MD, Stefano Di Domenico[3], MD, Valerio Gaetano Vellone[3], MD, Franco De Cian[3], MD and Simone Ferrero[1,2,*], MD, PhD

[1]Academic Unit of Obstetrics and Gynecology,
IRCCS Ospedale Policlinico San Martino, Genoa, Italy
[2]Department of Neurosciences, Rehabilitation, Ophthalmology, Genetics,
Maternal and Child Health (DiNOGMI),
University of Genoa, Italy
[3]Department of Surgical and Diagnostic Sciences,
IRCCS Ospedale Policlinico San Martino, Genoa, Italy

ABSTRACT

Patients with symptomatic fibroids are commonly treated with surgical approaches, such as hysterectomy or myomectomy. In these women, the risk of unexpected malignant diseases must be considered, in particular, after the previous safety communication by the Food and Drug Administration in 2014. In fact, it has been reported that during the procedure of tissue retrieval performed by morcellation is higher the risk of tumor cell dispersion, which may disseminate in the peritoneal space. The aim of this appendix is to examine the literature searching for the data on risk of morcellating of uterine leiomyosarcoma in patients undergoing myomectomy for benign uterine myomas and on

* Corresponding Author's E-mail: simoneferrero@me.com.

recent techniques able to prevent the possible dissemination of tumor cells during the procedure.

Keywords: uterine fibroid, myomectomy, morcellation, leiomyosarcoma

INTRODUCTION

For extracting myomas during minimally invasive myomectomies, the most used technique in recent years is the power morcellation. By performing morcellation, the goal is to crush the fibroid, reducing it to smaller parts, and, thus, allowing its total extraction. When the myoma extraction is performed without any morcellation, usually a larger incision is required often converting the access to minilaparotomy.

Currently, morcellation should be performed by using endo-bag, as itcan prevent eventual tumor cell dissemination, occurring in case of inadvertent leiomyosarcoma (LMS) morcellation. Power morcellation has been described for the first time in 1993; the Food and Drug Administration (FDA) approval has been obtained in 1995 [1,2]. This procedure is usually performed via a 12-20 mm trocar, or through vaginal route, depending on surgeon's preference [3,4].

Since its initial introduction, many technological improvements have been done for power morcellation (for example, smaller blade diameter or different cutting speeds). Anyway, it has been demonstrated that they did not provide significant advantages [3,5].

Another alternative approach to power morcellation is the hand morcellation (or mechanical tissue extraction) [6], but an important disadvantage of this technique is that it required a larger incision compared with that of power morcellation.

Recently, different methods have been proposed in order to reduce the risks related with the inadvertent dissemination of tissue fragments during myomas extraction by laparoscopic power morcellation; these methods include the use of trans-abdominal mini-laparotomy manual contained morcellation, trans-vaginal manual contained morcellation and Contained Tissue Extraction (CTE) System (Olympus America, Inc., Center Valley, Pennsylvania) [7,8].

Overall, the reported incidence of unexpected malignancies is 0.6% of the total myomas or uterine specimens [9]; this is a not negligible risk when is performed myomectomy, a common surgical procedure that is routinely performed by gynecologists. For this reason, in 2014, after a safety communication against power morcellation proposed by the FDA, the use of this technique has been prohibited or abandoned in several American centers for the relevant risk of unnoticed morcellation of occult LMS [10]. After this recommendation, in a retrospective review conducted in a single center on 189 cases was noted a 19% reduction in minimally invasive procedures for performing myomectomy [11].

The incidence of LMS is approximately 1.5% of all uterine malignant neoplasms; anyway, the aggressiveness of this disease leads to a 5-year survival of only 66% (Figure 1) [12]. Unfortunately, cytology obtained from peritoneal washing does not detect with high accuracy the eventual disseminated cells after power myomas morcellation [13]. The definitive diagnosis of LMS is histological, as most tumors often suggestive microscopic features such as diffuse atypia, high mitotic count and tumor cell necrosis (Figure 1).

A study investigated the incidence of LMS in 2790 patients undergoing hysterectomies or myomectomies for presumed benign disease. The surgical myomectomies were performed by any route: there were observed 1878 cases of myomas; anyway, there were no initially detected cases of LMS and 11 cases of unexpected malignancy during the procedures [9]. Another study revealed an incidence of 1/3906 cases of LMS after laparoscopic myomectomy and power morcellation [14].

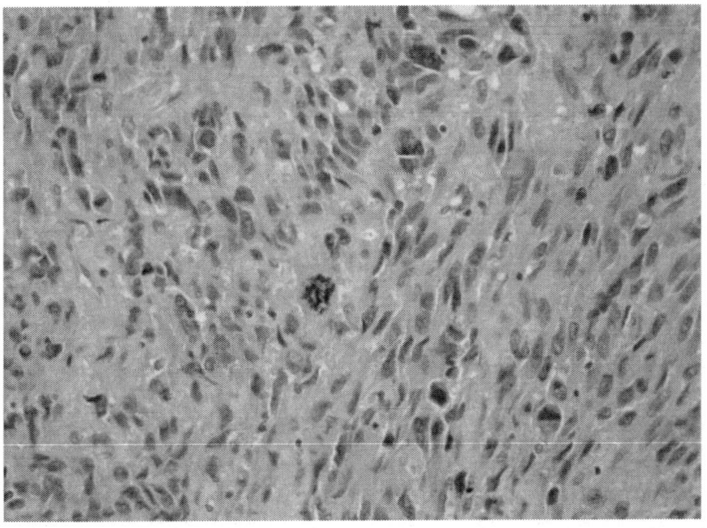

Figure 1. Uterine spindle cell leiomyosarcoma. Characteristic diagnostic hallmarks are present: severe cytological atypia, brisk mitotic activity (>10 mitoses/10hpf) with atypical mitoses. (hematoxylin/eosin; 400X).

Although the use of morcellation is lower in many American centers than in the past, some institutions support its use in selected patients after careful diagnostic procedures [4]. The diagnostic procedure has to be based on the ultrasonographic data, including the doppler velocimetry, in order to analyze vascularization of the uterine formation, presence of eventual necrosis and eventual increase of the endometrial thickness [4]. Even if magnetic resonance imaging (MRI) had a high diagnostic accuracy for detecting new uterine formations, at the moment, it is still difficult to distinguish a benign from a malignant neoplasm, and, thus, it not systematically employed in the preoperative work-up of myomas (considering also its cost) [15].

The current recommendations of the European Society of Gynecological Oncology (ESGO) suggest the use of morcellation only in patients with strongly desire to conceive and without risk factors for LMS [16]. To avoid the problem of intraperitoneal cellular diffusion during morcellation, contained methods can be used. Moreover, an extensive peritoneal lavage associated with careful removal of all the fragment should be performed [17]. Currently, most of them use a laparoscopic port with diameter of approximately 20-30 mm in length; by this incision it is possible to insert a containment bag into the peritoneal cavity and thus morcellate the myoma directly inside of the bag under direct visualization (Figure 2) [18].

Other studies on power morcellation in endo-bag supported its use to minimize the risk of inadvertent tissue dissemination [6, 19, 20]. However, the real advantages on survival benefits of bag morcellation still have to be established [4], even if performed by innovative devices, such as PneumoLiner or Tissue Containment System that are approved by the FDA for mechanical morcellation.

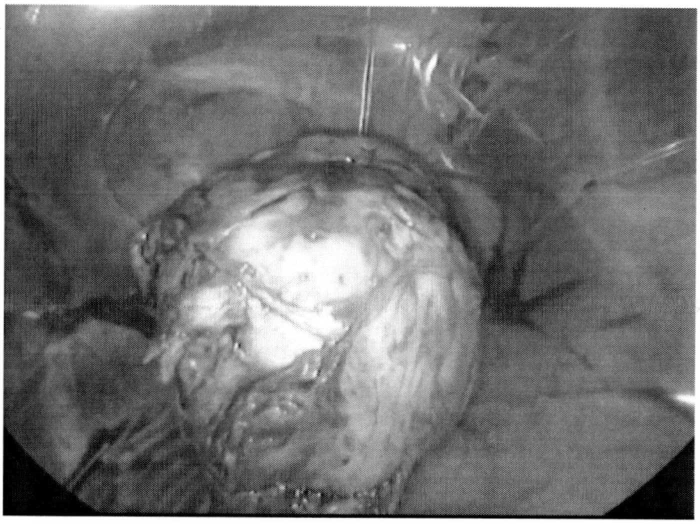

Figure 2. Uterine myomas inside containment bag for preparing a safety morcellation.

Another possible complication of tissue dissemination is subsequent parasitic leiomyomas and pelvic adenomyotic lesions [17, 21]. A partial resolution to this problem can be represented by extensive peritoneal lavage standing the patient in Trendelemburg position in order to better examine the abdominal cavity [22].

Conclusion

Patients with LMS have a poor prognosisdue tothe higher biological aggressiveness of these tumors in comparison to other gynecological malingnat tumors [23-25]; new treatment options are demanding for this group of women, who, at the moment, tend to have limited therapeutic options [26].

Laparoscopic tissue morcellation can be performed in patients with presumed "low risk" of malignant disease during diagnostic preoperative procedures. Anyway, the use of morcellation containment bags should be strongly recommended to prevent eventual tissue dissemination. An accurate counseling with the patient must be conducted prior surgery about the possible risk associated with the use of morcellation, including the incidence of occult malignant diseases that may be disseminated during the procedure. Nevertheless, further studies must be conducted on this topic to improve data on LMS risk and management of patients with diagnosis of presumed uterine leiomyomas.

REFERENCES

[1] Steiner R.A. Wight E. Tadir Y. Haller U. Electrical cutting device for laparoscopic removal of tissue from the abdominal cavity. *Obstet Gynecol.* 1993;471–4.

[2] Adelman MR. The morcellation debate: The history and the science. *Clin Obstet Gynecol.* 2015;58(4):710–7.

[3] Taylan E, Sahin C, Zeybek B, Akdemir A. Contained Morcellation: Review of Current Methods and Future Directions. *Front Surg.* 2017;4.

[4] AAGL Practice Report: Morcellation During Uterine Tissue Extraction. *J Minim Invasive Gynecol.* 2014;21(4):517–30.

[5] Driessen SRC, Arkenbout EA, Thurkow AL, Jansen FW. Electromechanical morcellators in minimally invasive gynecologic surgery: An update. *J Minim Invasive Gynecol.* 2014;21(3):377–83.

[6] Kho KA, Brown DN. Surgical treatment of uterine fibroids within a containment system and without power morcellation. *Clin Obstet Gynecol.* 2016;59(1):85–92.

[7] Bolland MJ, Grey A, Reid IR. Vitamin D supplements do not reduce mortality risk. *BMJ.* 2014; 21(3):377-83.

[8] Alessandri F, Lijoi D, Mistrangelo E, Ferrero S, Ragni N. Randomized study of laparoscopic versus minilaparotomic myomectomy for uterine myomas. *J Minim Invasive Gynecol.* 2006;13(2):92–7.

[9] Damasco MR, Chan PWK, Slonim M, Ang WEC, Healey MG. Incidence of Malignancy and Myoma Variants at Surgery for Presumed Benign Symptomatic Myomas. *J Minim Invasive Gynecol.* 2017;24(4):659–64.

[10] FDA, U.S. Food and Drug Administration. *Laparoscopic Uterine Power Morcellation in Hysterectomy and Myomectomy: FDA Safety Communication.* http://www.fda.gov/MedicalDevices/Safety. 2014. p. Available at: http://www.fda.gov/MedicalDevices/S.

[11] Barron KI, Richard T, Robinson PS, Lamvu G. Association of the U.S. Food and Drug Administration Morcellation Warning with Rates of Minimally Invasive Hysterectomy and Myomectomy. *Obstetrics and Gynecology.* 2015;126(6):1174-80.

[12] Kapp DS, Shin JY, Chan JK. Prognostic factors and survival in 1396 patients with uterine leiomyosarcomas: Emphasis on impact of lymphadenectomy and oophorectomy. *Cancer*. 2008;112(4):820–30.

[13] Toubia T, Moulder JK, Schiff LD, Clarke-Pearson D, O'Connor SM, Siedhoff MT. Peritoneal Washings After Power Morcellation in Laparoscopic Myomectomy: A Pilot Study. *J Minim Invasive Gynecol.* 2016; 22(6S):S62-S63.

[14] Nugent W, Engelke G, Reicke S, Söder R, Hennefründ J, Hasskamp T, et al. Laparoscopic Supracervical Hysterectomy or Myomectomy With Power Morcellation: Risk of Uterine Leiomyosarcomas. A Retrospective Trial Including 35.161 Women in Germany. *J Minim Invasive Gynecol.* 2015;22(6):S2–3.

[15] Thomassin-Naggara I, Dechoux S, Bonneau C, Morel A, Rouzier R, Carette MF, et al. How to differentiate benign from malignant myometrial tumours using MR imaging. *Eur Radiol.* 2013;23(8):2306–14.

[16] Halaska MJ, Haidopoulos D, Guyon F, Morice P, Zapardiel I, Kesic V, et al. European Society of Gynecological Oncology Statement on Fibroid and Uterine Morcellation. *Int J Gynecol Cancer.* 2017;27(1):189–92.

[17] Donnez O, Squifflet J, Leconte I, Jadoul P, Donnez J. Posthysterectomy pelvic adenomyotic masses observed in 8 cases out of a series of 1405 laparoscopic subtotal hysterectomies. *J Minim Invasive Gynecol.* 2007;14(2):156–60.

[18] Leal MA, Piñera A, De Santiago J, Zapardiel I. Novel Technique for Contained Power Morcellation through Umbilicus with Insufflated Bag. *Gynecol Obstet Invest.* 2017;82(2):205–7.

[19] Kanade TT, McKenna JB, Choi S, Tsai BP, Rosen DM, Cario GM, et al. Sydney Contained in Bag Morcellation for Laparoscopic Myomectomy. *J Minim Invasive Gynecol.* 2014;21(6):981.

[20] Cholkeri-Singh A, Miller CE. Power Morcellation in a Specimen Bag. *J Minim Invasive Gynecol.* 2015;22(2):160.

[21] Donnez O, Jadoul P, Squifflet J, Donnez J. Iatrogenic peritoneal adenomyoma after laparoscopic subtotal hysterectomy and uterine morcellation. *Fertil Steril.* 2006;86(5):1511–2.

[22] Donnez O, Donnez J. A series of 400 laparoscopic hysterectomies for benign disease: A single centre, single surgeon prospective study of complications confirming previous retrospective study. *BJOG An Int J Obstet Gynaecol.* 2010;117(6):752–5.

[23] Barra F, Evangelisti G, Ferro Desideri L, Di Domenico S, Ferraioli D, Vellone VG, De Cian F, Ferrero S. Investigational PI3K/AKT/mTOR inhibitors in development for endometrial cancer. *Expert Opin Investig Drugs.* 2019;28(2):131-142.

[24] Barra F, Evangelisti G, Damiano G, Mammoliti S, Ferrero, S. New perspectives with targeted drugs. Ferrero S, editor. *Endometrial cancer: risk factors, management and prognosis.* New York (NY): Nova Science Publisher. 2018;301-314.

[25] Barra F, Lorusso D, Leone Roberti Maggiore U, Ditto A, Bogani G, Raspagliesi F,

Ferrero S. Investigational drugs for the treatment of cervical cancer. *Expert Opin Investig Drugs.* 2017;26(4):389-402.

[26] Tantari M, Barra F, Di Domenico S, Ferraioli D, Vellone VG, De Cian F, Ferrero S. Current state of the art and emerging pharmacotherapy for uterine leiomyosarcomas. *Expert Opin Pharmacother.* 2019:6:1-11.

In: Uterine Fibroids
Editors: S. Ferrero and F. Barra
ISBN: 978-1-53615-046-9

Chapter 15

ROBOTIC-ASSISTED MYOMECTOMY

Giulio Evangelisti, MD, Fabio Barra, MD and Simone Ferrero*, MD, PhD

Obstetrics and Gynecology, Department of Neurosciences, Rehabilitation, Ophthalmology, Genetics, Maternal and Child Health (DiNOGMI), University of Genoa, Italy
Academic Unit of Obstetrics and Gynecology, IRCCS Ospedale San Martino, Genoa, Italy

ABSTRACT

In the early 2000s, the Food and Drug Administration (FDA) approved robotic-assisted laparoscopic surgery as treatment for gynecological diseases. For treating uterine fibroids, myomectomy can be successfully performed by abdominal, laparoscopic or robotic surgery on the basis of several factors including patient age, status, desire to preserve fertility and myomas features (in particular, number, size or location). Although mini-invasive surgery has demonstrated several advantages, a high number of myomectomies is still performed via traditional abdominal route. Since 2004, surgeons have started to employ mini-invasive robotic technology for performing myomectomy. Anyway, to date, there is a lack of knowledge about surgical or fertility rate after myomectomy performed with robotic surgery, not being available randomized controlled studies on this setting in the literature. In addition, different types of robotic surgery have been developed; these procedures have weak or strength points that should be evaluated in each single patient before being planned and performed. However, all of them require further validation about safety, feasibility and effectiveness before being adopted routinely in the clinical practice. This chapter aims to review the main steps of the robotic surgery development for myomectomy.

* Corresponding Author's Email: simoneferrero@me.com.

Keywords: mini-invasive surgery, myomectomy, robotic-surgical outcomes, robotic-assisted laparoscopic myomectomy, robotic single site surgery, reduced port robotic surgery

INTRODUCTION

In the complex management of uterine fibroids, myomectomy is the preferred surgical modality for patients with symptomatic myomas who desire to preserve their future fertility [1–3].

Healthy status of the single patient, localization, size and number of myomas as well as level of surgeon experience play a crucial role in determining if myomectomy should be performed by open surgery, laparoscopic surgery or by the recently introduced robot-assisted surgery. Moreover, several preoperative medical options are available for the treatment of myomas, with the aim of shrinking myomas size and ameliorating the anemia due to eventual uterine bleeding.

The better surgical methods for performing myomectomy is still an important matter of debate. Currently, the majority of myomectomies are performed via laparotomic route although the advantages of the laparoscopic approach are today well known [4, 5]. In fact, the persistence of the open abdominal approach in the surgical practice is related to ensure a high strength of the scar after the reparation of uterine myometrium.

In order to reduce the rate of sequelae after surgery, including pelvic adhesions or the need to use cesarean sections, in the last years laparoscopic myomectomy emerged as a better surgical method of treatment.

Many studies demonstrated relevant advantages like shorter hospitalization, lesser pain, decreased blood loss and fewer surgical complications, when laparoscopic surgery was compared to the abdominal approach [4,6–8]. However, laparoscopic myomectomy presents some technical challenges. Firstly, the operator performing this approach is faced with the lack of tactile feel; in addition, limitations in moves caused by the use of fixed port can lead to an inappropriate closure of the myometrial wall [7,9,10]. Moreover, a mini-invasive access results also in a more complex extraction of the myomas through the port. These challenges are related to prolonged operative time, major risk of postoperative bleeding, conversion to open procedure, uterine rupture in further pregnancy and risk of recurrence [11–13].

Because of these limitations, laparoscopic myomectomy is not potentially useful in all the patients with myomas.

In early 2000s, robotic surgical techniques have been developed as alternative way to overcome limits and difficulties of both laparoscopic and open surgery. Several studies confirmed that surgical outcomes between traditional laparoscopic and robot-assisted myomectomies are comparable [10,14–16].

The only commercially available robotic surgical system is the Da Vinci Surgical System® (Intuitive Surgical Inc., Sunnyvale, CA, USA). In 2005, it has been approved by the Food and Drug Administration (FDA) for performing gynecological surgical procedures.

This system uses a 3-dimensional camera that requires a 12 mm port (rather than 5- or 10-mm port of the conventional laparoscopy) and 8 mm robotic trocars (rather than conventional 5 mm). Unlike conventional laparoscopy, the ports are more spaced and the camera is usually placed upper the umbilicus in order to increase the range of instruments motions [17]. The first robotic-assisted laparoscopic myomectomy (RALM) was performed by Adavicula et al. [18] in 2004.

To date, no guidelines are still available to better contextualize the role of RALM. In general, there is consensus that the introduction of robotic surgery has expanded the indications for minimally invasive myomectomy to more complex cases previously performed by laparotomy [16].

Some studies have reported surgeon preference for RALM in the case of ≥10 myomas, diameter ≤7 cm or patient' obesity. However, skilled surgeons currently tend to perform laparoscopic myomectomy also in these specific cases without reporting any complications [19,20].

Overall, RALM presents some advantages like improved access to myomas in difficult locations and a more precise and adequate layered closure of the myoma bed [18]. However, apart the higher cost of this technology, limitations of RALM include reduced range of movements that results in difficult removal of very large myomas, inability to apply an adequate hemostatic pressure as well as lack of tactile feedback.

Nowadays, no randomized trials comparing robotic to either laparoscopic or abdominal myomectomy are available in literature. A recent meta-analysis compared 2027 patients who underwent myomectomy performed by laparoscopic (8 studies) or laparotomic (9 studies) approach with those who received RALM. No significant differences were found among robotic or laparoscopic approach regarding to surgical time, estimated blood loss, blood transfusion, length of hospital stay, complications as well as postoperative fertility. Anyway, when comparing minimally invasive techniques with the abdominal approach some advantages were found with regard to blood loss, need for blood transfusion, rate of postoperative complications and duration of hospital recovery [21].

The role of RALM was also assessed for fertility-related outcomes. Anyway, only few studies are currently available on this topic.

The literature reports 50-60% of pregnancy rates after laparoscopic myomectomy [22–24]. Two retrospective studies demonstrated comparable pregnancy rates when intramural myomas are removed using robotic surgery (68-75%) [12,25]. Another retrospective study by Pitter et al. [26] examined pregnancy outcomes in 107 women who tried to conceive after RALM; 127 pregnancies resulted in 92 deliveries, less than 5% of patients delivered vaginally; one uterine rupture was reported. Moreover, preterm delivery prior to 35 weeks of gestational age occurred in 17.4% of patients. Higher preterm delivery rates were significantly associated with a greater number of myomas removed [26]. Overall, these small studies, despite of being non-randomized, support the feasibility of RALM in terms of pregnancy rate and surgical outcomes, but further trials are needed to evaluate the safety and effectiveness of this procedure.

Recently, single-incision laparoscopic surgery (SILS) has been introduced as a more mini-invasive laparoscopic option that requires only an umbilical access. This approach allows to achieve some additional relevant advantages like fewer scars, less pain and risk of surgical site infection after surgery as well as a better cosmetic result [27–29]. However, SILS may be difficult to be performed due to the limited range of movements and conflict between instruments. This is the main cause of its limited spreading [30–32].

With the advent of robotic surgery, interest in single-incision approach has been reborn. In fact, one of the greatest challenges of this surgery is the suture of the myometrial layer. It has been suggested that the robotic single-site (RSS) system may be particularly suitable for performing the complex suture of the uterine incision after myomectomy.

The first attempt to perform myomectomy using RSS has been reported by Lewis et al. [33] in 2015 who proposed a step-by-step guide for this procedure [34].

Several studies have shown RSS as a feasible and safe procedure even in case of large, multiple or intramural myomas [34,35]. Anyway, no studies comparing RSS myomectomy to conventional laparoscopic or multiport robotic myomectomy have been published yet.

Besides, RSS approach presents limitations, including reduced extracorporeal triangulation and a limited repertoire of non-articulating instruments and electrosurgical options compared with multiport robotic surgery [28,30].

In 2017, Kim et al. [36] described a newer approach, called reduced port robotic surgery (RPRS). This technique requires only two scars: one at umbilical level for multiport instruments (Octo-Port plus) and one on the right side of the patient to be used as conventional robotic port. In their prospective study, the authors reported a success rate of 89.5% for myomectomy with no cases of conversion to open laparotomy, proving that RPRS port can be performed with comparable operative outcomes to robotic single-site surgery, overcoming also its main limitations [36]. In addition, RPRS for myomectomy seems technically feasible and safe, having short-term perioperative outcomes similar to those of multiport RALM [37]. Anyway, large-cohort and randomized prospective studies with long-term follow-up are necessary to validate the best indications and safety profile of RPRS myomectomy.

REFERENCES

[1] Koo YJ, Lee JK, Lee YK, Kwak DW, Lee IH, Lim KT, et al. Pregnancy Outcomes and Risk Factors for Uterine Rupture After Laparoscopic Myomectomy: A Single-

Center Experience and Literature Review. *J Minim Invasive Gynecol.* 2015;22(6):1022–8.

[2] Begum N, Anwary SA, Alfazzaman M, Sultana P, Banu J, Deeba F, et al. Pregnancy outcome following myomectomy. *Mymensingh Med J.* 2015; 24(1):84-8.

[3] Ferrero S, Abbamonte LH, Giordano M, Parisi M, Ragni N, Remorgida V. Uterine myomas, dyspareunia, and sexual function. *Fertility and Sterility*. 2006;86(5):1504-10.

[4] Bhave Chittawar P, Franik S, Pouwer AW, Farquhar C. Minimally invasive surgical techniques versus open myomectomy for uterine fibroids. *Cochrane Database of Systematic Reviews.* 2014.

[5] Alessandri F, Lijoi D, Mistrangelo E, Ferrero S, Ragni N. Randomized study of laparoscopic versus minilaparotomic myomectomy for uterine myomas. *J Minim Invasive Gynecol.* 2006;13(2):92–7.

[6] Liu G, Zolis L, Kung R, Melchior M, Singh S, Francis Cook E. The Laparoscopic Myomectomy: A Survey of Canadian Gynaecologists. *J Obstet Gynaecol Canada.* 2010;32(2):139–48.

[7] Morita M. Laparoscopic myomectomy for symptomatic uterine myomas. Vol. 55, *Journal of the Medical Society of Toho University.* 2008. p. 218–22.

[8] Leone Roberti Maggiore U, Scala C, Venturini PL, Ferrero S. Preoperative treatment with letrozole in patients undergoing laparoscopic myomectomy of large uterine myomas: A prospective non-randomized study. *Eur J Obstet Gynecol Reprod Biol.* 2014;181:157–62.

[9] Alessandri F, Remorgida V, Venturini PL, Ferrero S. Unidirectional barbed suture versus continuous suture with intracorporeal knots in laparoscopic myomectomy: A randomized study. *J Minim Invasive Gynecol.* 2010;17(6):725–9.

[10] Cooper AR, Powell MA, Jimenez PT, Johnson MD, Rabinov A, Graseck AS. Comparison of robotic and laparoscopic myomectomy. *Am J Obstet Gynecol.* 2009;201(6):625–7.

[11] Takeuchi H, Kuwatsuru R. The indications, surgical techniques, and limitations of laparoscopic myomectomy. *JSLS.* 2003;7(2): 89–95.

[12] Tusheva OA, Gyang A, Patel SD. Reproductive outcomes following robotic-assisted laparoscopic myomectomy (RALM). *J Robot Surg.* 2013;7(1):65–9.

[13] Saccardi C, Gizzo S, Noventa M, Ancona E, Borghero A, Litta PS. Limits and complications of laparoscopic myomectomy: which are the best predictors? A large cohort single-center experience. *Arch Gynecol Obstet.* 2014;290(5):951–6.

[14] Nezhat C, Lavie O, Hsu S, Watson J, Barnett O, Lemyre M. Robotic-assisted laparoscopic myomectomy compared with standard laparoscopic myomectomy-a retrospective matched control study. *Fertil Steril.* 2009;91(2):556–9.

[15] Gobern JM, Rosemeyer CJ, Barter JF, Steren AJ. Comparison of Robotic, Laparoscopic, and Abdominal Myomectomy in a Community Hospital. *JSLS J Soc Laparoendosc Surg.* 2013;17(1):116–20.

[16] Barakat EE, Bedaiwy MA, Zimberg S, Nutter B, Nosseir M, Falcone T. Robotic-assisted, laparoscopic, and abdominal myomectomy: a comparison of surgical outcomes. *Obstet Gynecol.* 2011;117(2):256–66.

[17] Gingold JA, Gueye NA, Falcone T. Minimally Invasive Approaches to Myoma Management. Vol. 25, *Journal of Minimally Invasive Gynecology.* 2018. p. 237–50.

[18] Advincula AP, Song A, Burke W, Reynolds RK. Preliminary experience with robot-assisted laparoscopic myomectomy. *J Am Assoc Gynecol Laparosc.* 2004; 11(4):511–8.

[19] Kim H, Shim S, Hwang Y, Kim M, Hwang H, Chung Y, et al. Is robot-assisted laparoscopic myomectomy limited in multiple myomas?: a feasibility for ten or more myomas. *Obstet Gynecol Sci.* 2018;61(1):135.

[20] Vargas M V., Moawad GN, Sievers C, Opoku-Anane J, Marfori CQ, Tyan P, et al. Feasibility, Safety, and Prediction of Complications for Minimally Invasive Myomectomy in Women With Large and Numerous Myomata. *J Minim Invasive Gynecol.* 2017;24(2):315–22.

[21] Iavazzo C, Mamais I, Gkegkes ID. Robotic assisted vs laparoscopic and/or open myomectomy: systematic review and meta-analysis of the clinical evidence. *Archives of Gynecology and Obstetrics.* 2016;294(1):5-17.

[22] Goldberg J, Pereira L. Pregnancy outcomes following treatment for fibroids: Uterine fibroid embolization versus laparoscopic myomectomy. *Curr Opin Obstet Gynecol.* 2006;18(4):402–6.

[23] Seracchioli R, Rossi S, Govoni F, Rossi E, Venturoli S, Bulletti C, et al. Fertility and obstetric outcome after laparoscopic myomectomy of large myomata: A randomized comparison with abdominal myomectomy. *Hum Reprod.* 2000;15(12):2663–8.

[24] Kučera E, Dvorská M, Křepelka P, Heřman H. Pregnancy after laparoscopic myomectomy - Long-term follow up. *Ces Gynekol.* 2006;71(5):389–93.

[25] LÖnnerfors C, Persson J. Pregnancy following robot-assisted laparoscopic myomectomy in women with deep intramural myomas. *Acta Obstet Gynecol Scand.* 2011;90(9):972–7.

[26] Pitter MC, Gargiulo AR, Bonaventura LM, Stefano Lehman J, Srouji SS. Pregnancy outcomes following robot-assisted myomectomy. *Hum Reprod.* 2013;28(1):99–108.

[27] Gargiulo AR, Choussein S, Srouji SS, Cedo LE, Escobar PF. Coaxial robot-assisted laparoendoscopic single-site myomectomy. *J Robot Surg.* 2017;11(1):27–35.

[28] Scheib SA, Fader AN. Gynecologic robotic laparoendoscopic single-site surgery: Prospective analysis of feasibility, safety, and technique. *Am J Obstet Gynecol.* 2015;212(2):179.e1-179.e8.

[29] Escobar PF, Fader AN, Paraiso MF, Kaouk JH, Falcone T. Robotic-Assisted Laparoendoscopic Single-Site Surgery in Gynecology: Initial Report and Technique. *J Minim Invasive Gynecol.* 2009;16(5):589–91.

[30] Eisenberg D, Vidovszky TJ, Lau J, Guiroy B, Rivas H. Comparison of robotic and laparoendoscopic single-site surgery systems in a suturing and knot tying task. *Surg Endosc.* 2013;27(9):3182–6.

[31] Nam EJ, Kim SW, Lee M, Yim GW, Paek JH, Lee SH, et al. Robotic single-port transumbilical total hysterectomy: A pilot study. Vol. 22, *Journal of Gynecologic Oncology*. 2011. p. 120–6.

[32] Escobar PF, Knight J, Rao S, Weinberg L. da Vinci® single-site platform: Anthropometrical, docking and suturing considerations for hysterectomy in the cadaver model. *Int J Med Robot Comput Assist Surg.* 2012;8(2):191–5.

[33] Lewis EI, Srouji SS, Gargiulo AR. Robotic single-site myomectomy: Initial report and technique. *Fertil Steril.* 2015;103(5):1370–1377.

[34] Gargiulo AR, Lewis EI, Kaser DJ, Srouji SS. Robotic single-site myomectomy: a step-by-step tutorial. *Fertil Steril.* 2015;104(5):e13.

[35] Choi EJ, Rho AM, Lee SR, Jeong K, Moon HS. Robotic Single-Site Myomectomy: Clinical Analysis of 61 Consecutive Cases. *J Minim Invasive Gynecol.* 2017;24(4):632–9.

[36] Kim JJ, Choi C, Nam SH, Kim WY. Feasibility of Reduced-Port Robotic Surgery for Myomectomy with the da Vinci Surgical System. *J Minim Invasive Gynecol.* 2017;24(6):926–31.

[37] Nam SH, Paek J, Choi C, Nam SH, Kim WY. A comparison between reduced-port robotic surgery and multiport robot-assisted laparoscopy for myomectomy. *Eur J Obstet Gynecol Reprod Biol.* 2017;213:53–7.

About the Editors

Simone Ferrero, MD, PhD

Simone Ferrero obtained his specialization in Gynecology and Obstetrics at the University of Genoa (Genoa, Italy) and the title of Doctor of Philosophy (PhD) at the Queen Mary Hospital (London, UK). He currently is Associate Professor of Gynecology & Obstetrics at the University of Genoa, working at IRCCS San Martino Policlinic Hospital (Genoa, Italy). Simone Ferrero is author of over 280 publications in scientific journals indexed in PubMed with impact factor. He has already been editor of a book entitled "Endometrial Cancer: Risk Factors, Management and prognosis" published by Nova Publisher.

Simone Ferrero is currently recognized as the 6th world expert in the field of endometriosis by Expertscape and is member of several editorial boards of gynecological international journals.

Fabio Barra, MD

Fabio Barra got the degree in Medicine and Surgery at the University of Genoa (Genoa, Italy). Currently, he is resident in Gynecology and Obstetrics at the IRCCS San Martino Policlinic Hospital (Genoa, Italy). He is author of over 30 publications in scientific journal indexed in PubMed with impact factor and chapters of international book.

INDEX

B

C

D

E

F

G

H

I

L

M

N

O

S

Related Nova Publications

Ovulation: Detection, Signs/Symptoms and Outcomes

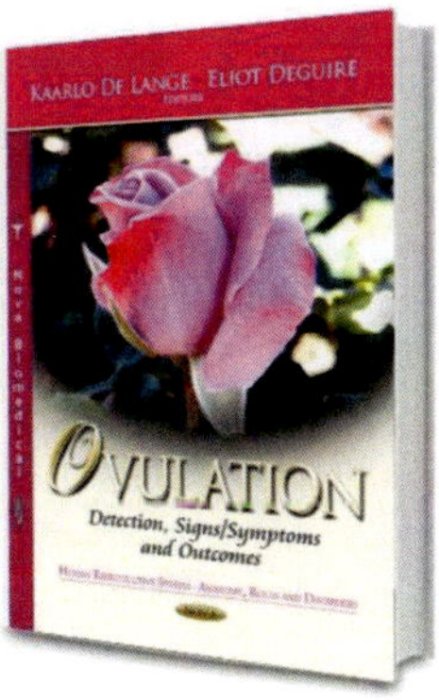

Editors: Kaarlo De Lange and Eliot Deguire

Series: Human Reproductive System - Anatomy, Roles and Disorders

Book Description: In this book, the authors present current research in the study of ovulation detection, its signs, symptoms and outcomes. Topics discussed in this compilation include the importance of up and down regulation of receptors for FSH, progesterone and GnRH in the ovary, and endometrium and lymphocytes in correcting various ovulatory disorders and achieving live deliveries.

Hardcover ISBN: 978-1-62618-472-5
Retail Price: $130

Menstrual Cycle: Signs and Symptoms, Psychological/Behavioral Changes and Abnormalities

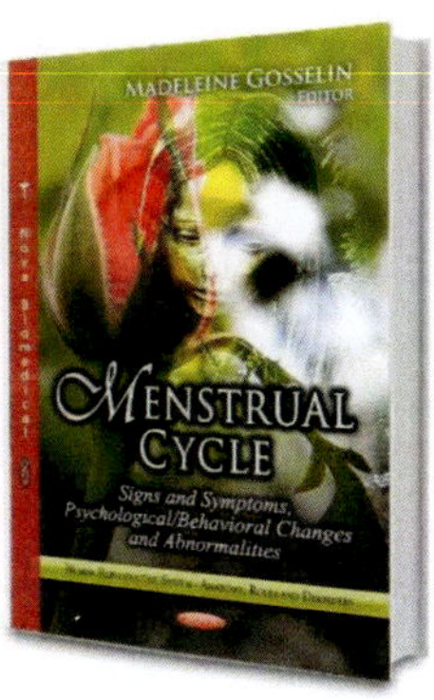

Editor: Madeleine Gosselin

Series: Human Reproductive System - Anatomy, Roles and Disorders

Book Description: The menstrual cycle is the scientific term for the physiological changes that occur in fertile women and other female primates for the purposes of sexual reproduction. In this book, the authors discuss the signs and symptoms, psychological/behavioral changes and abnormalities of the menstrual cycle.

Hardcover ISBN: 978-1-62417-945-7
Retail Price: $130

Related Nova Publications

Estradiol: Synthesis, Functions and Effectiveness

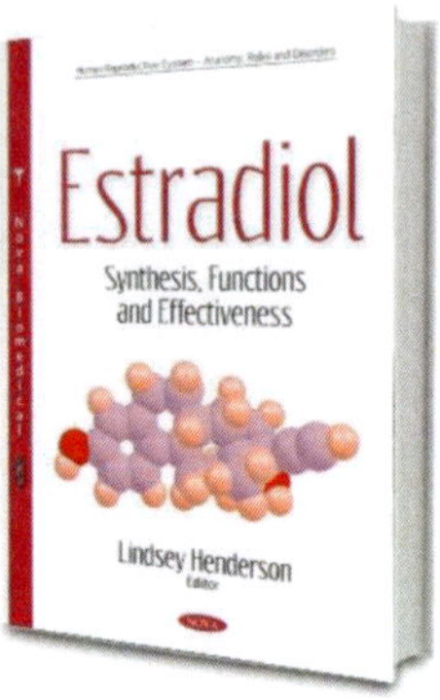

Editor: Lindsey Henderson

Series: Human Reproductive System – Anatomy, Roles and Disorders

Book Description: Estrogens comprise a group of structurally related and hormonally active molecules derived from cholesterol. 17¦Â-estradiol (E2) is the most potent member of this group. In Chapter One, the authors summarize various aspects of estradiol signaling, with special emphasis in the fast action of the hormone.

Softcover ISBN: 978-1-53612-298-5
Retail Price: $82

Endometriosis: A Multidisciplinary Approach

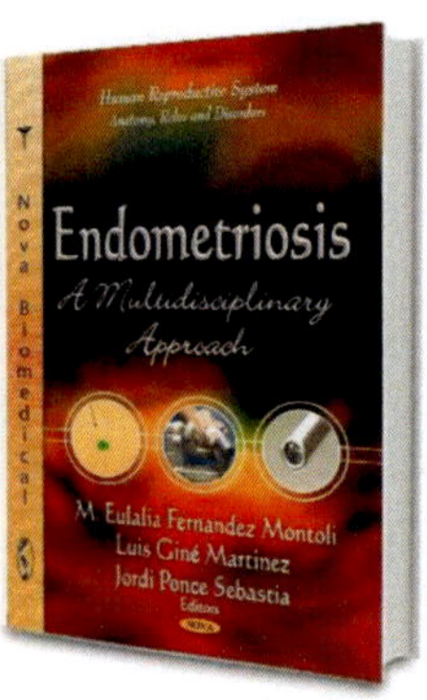

Editors: M. Eulalia Fernandez Montoli, Luis Giné Martinez and

Series: Human Reproductive System - Anatomy, Roles and Disorders

Book Description: The book reviews the diagnosis and surgical management of deep infiltrating endometriosis, endometrioma, urological endometriosis, and other localizations of the disease, as thoracic endometriosis. New approaches to manage endometrioma (sclerosis of endometriomas) are described.

Hardcover ISBN: 978-1-62618-611-8
Retail Price: $205

To see complete list of Nova publications, please visit our website at www.novapublishers.com